Essentials of Obstetrics and Gynaecology

SECOND EDITION

BARRY O'REILLY
MD FRCOG FRANZCOG

Consultant Obstetrician and Gynaecologist, Cork University Maternity Hospital, Cork, Ireland

CECILIA BOTTOMLEY
MA MB BCHIR MRCOG

Specialist Registrar in Obstetrics and Gynaecology, Guy's and St Thomas' Hospital Trust, London, UK

JANICE RYMER
MD MRCOG FRANZCOG ILTM

Senior Lecturer and Honorary Consultant in Obstetrics and Gynaecology, Guy's, Kings' and St Thomas' Hospital Trust, London, UK

SAUNDERS

ELSEVIER

EDINBURGH   LONDON   NEW YORK   OXFORD
PHILADELPHIA   ST LOUIS   SYDNEY   TORONTO   2012

SAUNDERS
ELSEVIER

© 2012, Elsevier Ltd. All rights reserved.

No part of this publication may be reproduced or transmitted in any form or by any means, electronic or mechanical, including photocopying, recording, or any information storage and retrieval system, without permission in writing from the publisher. Details on how to seek permission, further information about the Publisher's permissions policies and our arrangements with organizations such as the Copyright Clearance Centre and the Copyright Licensing Agency, can be found at our website: www.elsevier.com/permissions.

This book and the individual contributions contained in it are protected under copyright by the Publisher (other than as may be noted herein).

First edition 2005
Second edition 2012
  Reprinted 2013

ISBN 978 0 7020 4361 1

British Library Cataloguing in Publication Data
A catalogue record for this book is available from the British Library

Library of Congress Cataloging in Publication Data
A catalogue record for this book is available from the Library of Congress

ELSEVIER your source for books,
journals and multimedia
in the health sciences

www.elsevierhealth.com

Working together to grow
libraries in developing countries

www.elsevier.com | www.bookaid.org | www.sabre.org

ELSEVIER   BOOK AID International   Sabre Foundation

The Publisher's policy is to use **paper manufactured from sustainable forests**

Printed in China

Series preface

Medical students and doctors in training are expected to travel to different hospitals and community health centres as part of their education. Many books are too large to carry around, but the information they contain is often vital for the basic understanding of disease processes.

The *Pocket Essentials* series is designed to provide portable, pocket-sized companions to larger texts, such as our own *Kumar & Clark's Clinical Medicine*. They are most useful for clinical practice, whether in hospital or the community, and for exam revision.

All the books in the series have the same helpful features:

- succinct text
- simple line drawings
- emergency and other boxes
- tables that summarize causes and clinical features of disease
- exam questions and answers.

They contain core material for quick revision, easy reference and practical management. The format makes them easy to read, providing an indispensable 'pocket essential'.

Parveen Kumar and Michael Clark
Series Editors

Preface

This is the second edition of the very successful *Essentials of Obstetrics and Gynaecology*.

This book continues to fill the gap for a compact textbook that gives a concise yet comprehensive account of all topics covered by undergraduate and postgraduate curricula. It has a strong emphasis on obstetric and gynaecological management, in particular through the use of management flow charts and in the emergency and procedures section.

This book has three strengths – it is a pocket book and therefore easy to carry around with you at all times, it is a part of a well-recognized series, and it is written by three authors who have been actively practising obstetrics and gynaecology at consultant level for many years, and are actively involved in undergraduate and postgraduate education.

The information is easy to access, easy to read, evidence-based and very up to date.

The information available on the web and the Cochrane database, as well as college guidelines, have been the lynchpin of our information but we have collated it to provide a comprehensive cover of obstetrics and gynaecology, concentrating on the core curriculum.

In addition we have included sample examination questions, which inevitably assist learning. In this latest edition we have modified the question section to the newer exam format of 'single best answer' and 'extended matching' questions, which will be invaluable to all those taking examinations in obstetrics and gynaecology.

We would like to thank Mike Clark and Parveen Kumar for their support in the preparation of this latest in the *Pocket Essentials* series.

Barry O'Reilly
Janice Rymer
Cecilia Bottomley

Contents

Contents

Section 4 – Emergencies and practical procedures

History-taking and examination in obstetrics and gynaecology

Gynaecology history-taking 1

CHAPTER CONTENTS

The importance of taking an accurate and detailed history cannot be overemphasized, particularly in gynaecology where the symptoms are often embarrassing and patients may not wish to discuss them unless specifically asked. The very nature of the specialty requires the history-taker to be respectful, sensitive and on the alert for both verbal and non-verbal cues. It is essential that during the consultation one tries to put the patient at ease so that she feels as comfortable as she can discussing her symptoms.

THE CONSULTATION

The consultation should commence with a professional introduction assuming one has looked at the referral letter or the notes beforehand so that the woman can be addressed appropriately. As with all histories, it is easiest to start with the presenting complaint. When did the problem first begin, how long has it been present and how frequently does it occur? How much does it affect her quality of life? If the problem is pain, then one must elicit what exacerbates the pain and what alleviates it. The site and nature of the pain must be determined. As with all history-taking it is important to ask open questions rather than direct questions initially. Enquire whether she has ever consulted anyone else about this problem, and if so, what was the management?

PRESENTING COMPLAINT

Abnormal bleeding

If the problem is abnormal bleeding, a more detailed menstrual history should be taken. When did menarche occur? How often does she menstruate and how long does it last?

Is it regular or irregular, heavy, or painful? If the bleeding is heavy, it is important to enquire as to the number of tampons/pads used and whether extra protection is also needed. Is there any premenstrual pain or inter-menstrual or postcoital bleeding? If she is of reproductive age, then enquire as to her last menstrual period.

Enquire whether the woman is sexually active and if so, whether there are any problems with intercourse. What type of contraception is she currently using and what has she used in the past?

Does she suffer with a vaginal discharge and has she ever had pelvic inflammatory disease?

With regard to cervical smear history, one needs to know the date of the last smear and whether or not it was abnormal, and whether or not she has ever had an abnormal smear in the past, and if so, what was the treatment?

Urinary symptoms

With regards to urinary symptoms one needs to enquire about frequency, dysuria, nocturia, urgency or incontinence. If she does suffer from urinary incontinence, then one needs to assess how often it is occurring and whether it is affecting her quality of life; are there any aggravating factors, for example smoking, coughing, constipation? She should be asked specifically whether she has ever had a dragging sensation in the pelvis or felt a lump coming through the vagina.

It is important to ascertain whether or not she has a normal bowel habit and whether she has any pain or bleeding with defecation.

PAST HISTORY

With regard to past history one should ascertain whether the woman has had any previous gynaecological problems and whether she has had any gynaecological surgery in the past (Fig. 1.1).

It is best to enquire with a general statement about the obstetric history, for example: 'Have you ever been pregnant?' If the answer is no, then one proceeds, but if the answer is yes, then it is best to record the pregnancies in chronological order, noting the year, gestation and outcome. If there were

---

Name

DOB

Age   Parity   Last menstrual period –/–/–

Cycle   Contraception   Last cervical smear –/–/–

Presenting problem

Previous obstetric and gynaecological history

Previous medical history

Functional enquiry

Social history/family history   Drugs

Allergies

Figure 1.1 History sheet.

deliveries, then enquire about the length of pregnancy and whether there were any problems, the duration of labour and second stage and the mode of delivery. Check that there were no complications during the pregnancy or labour. If there were miscarriages or terminations, enquire about the gestation and the method of termination or, in the case of a miscarriage, whether an evacuation was performed.

Past medical history

As with any history, one asks if she has or has had any medical problems or if she has ever been admitted to hospital.

Past surgical history

Any previous operations, apart from gynaecological operations, should be enquired about. Were there any postoperative complications?

Systems review

Symptoms relating to respiratory, cardiovascular, abdominal and neuro-logical systems should be ascertained.

Drug history

Is she currently taking any medications? Does she take any recreational drugs? Is she taking any prepregnancy vitamins? It is important to ascertain whether she is allergic to any drugs.

Family history

It is best to start with an open-ended question, such as: 'Are there any significant diseases in your family?' and then particularly enquire about a family history of breast, ovarian or cervical carcinoma, diabetes, heart disease, thromboembolic disease and hypertension.

Personal and social history

One should enquire as to occupation, whether she is currently smoking and whether she has smoked in the past, as well as weekly intake of alcohol. Is she in a stable relationship and, if not, does she live in a supportive environment?

Having taken a thorough history it is worth enquiring whether the patient feels that there is anything else that she should tell you. She should be asked what she thinks might be causing the problem and what she might be expecting from the consultation in terms of investigations or treatments.

PRESENTING A HISTORY

In presenting a gynaecological history one should start with name, age, presenting complaint, duration of presenting complaint and other significant features. For example, Mrs Fairhall is a 35-year-old nullipa-rous woman, presenting with a 6-month history of irregular heavy bleeding. Then go through the presenting complaint in detail, other relevant gynaecology or obstetric past history and then the other histories. Then summarize at the end, which usually means repeating the original sentence that you started with.

Gynaecological examination 2

As with the examination of any organ system, a gynaecological examination starts with a general examination. One should assess from the end of the bed whether the patient appears healthy or not, obese, average or thin, anxious or at ease. One should specifically examine for anaemia, jaundice or lymphadenopathy. If the patient is a young fit woman, then further general examination is unnecessary; however, if the patient is elderly or unwell then a more detailed examination is required. The practice of routine breast examination is controversial, but if it is performed one should initially observe for tethering or peau d'orange. All four breast quadrants are palpated, followed by the axilla on each side with the patient's arm resting on the examiner's arm so that there is no tension in the axilla.

ABDOMINAL EXAMINATION

This commences with inspection, and exposure must be from the symphysis pubis to the xyphisternum, taking care to respect the patient's dignity with regard to the genital and breast region, with appropriate drapes. It is important to ensure that the patient is lying comfortably and that she has emptied her bladder. On inspection one looks for asymmetry in the abdomen and scars, particularly above the symphysis pubis and in the umbilicus. The distribution of body hair should be noted and any striae or hernias.

Before moving on to palpation one should enquire whether there are any areas of tenderness. One then gently palpates around the abdomen looking for areas of tenderness or masses. If any masses are found, then they should be percussed, remembering that fluid-filled and solid cavities are dull, and free fluid in the abdomen will be percussed as shifting dullness on the change of position.

Auscultation is used to ascertain the nature of bowel sounds if the woman has presented with an acute problem.

PELVIC EXAMINATION

Pelvic examination may be both uncomfortable and embarrassing for the patient and one must be sensitive to ensure that the environment is as friendly as possible. It is important to ensure privacy and explain to the patient exactly what she needs to remove and what you plan to do. A chaperone is recommended in all situations and is mandatory when the examiner is male. If a Cusco's speculum is being used, the speculum should be warmed and lubricating jelly placed on the blades (a very small amount if a cervical smear needs to be taken). The examination may be uncomfortable, but it should not be painful in the absence of pathology.

The vulva and perineum should be inspected and one should observe any areas of discoloration, lumps or areas where the skin may have broken down. One should look for any evidence of prolapse. The Cusco's speculum allows inspection of the cervix so that a cervical smear or endo-cervical swabs may be easily taken. It may be difficult to observe the cervical walls with a traditional Cusco's speculum, but the plastic variety is now available where one can observe the entire vaginal wall. The patient lies in the supine position with the heels together and knees apart. The speculum is inserted with the blades closed and parallel to the labia and the opening mechanism towards the patient's right. The speculum is gently inserted and when it is halfway into the vagina it is rotated 90° (so the locking mechanism is anterior) and inserted as far as it will go. The blades are then opened slowly under direct vision and if there has been correct placement the cervix should come into view. The cervix should be closely observed to detect any abnormalities and then a cervical smear can be taken, plus or minus endocervical swabs depending upon the clinical presentation. A cervical smear is taken by inserting the spatula or brush into the endocervical canal and rotating it 360° in one direction and 360° in the other direction. The speculum is then withdrawn, watching carefully so that the blades do not clamp down on to the cervix. The vaginal walls are observed as the Cusco's speculum is withdrawn.

A Sims' speculum is used to assess women with uterovaginal pro-lapse or when the cervix is difficult to find. The patient should be placed in the Sims' position or the left lateral position. The patient's buttocks should be separated, with assistance if necessary, or by asking the woman to raise the upper leg, and the patient should be asked to cough in order to observe for obvious prolapse or stress incontinence. The blade of the Sims' speculum should then be inserted along the posterior vaginal wall and retracted posteriorly to display the anterior vaginal wall. The patient should be asked to cough again, to assess any degree of prolapse of the anterior vaginal wall and to note any stress incontinence. The anterior vag-inal wall is then supported with a sponge forceps and the patient is asked to cough again, while continuing to support the anterior vaginal wall with the sponge forceps. One can then observe for cervical descent. To assess cervical descent fully a sponge forceps can be placed on the anterior lip of the cervix and traction can be applied, but this can be uncomfortable for the patient and should only be done as a preoperative assessment to deter-mine the route of hysterectomy. The patient is asked to bear down again and the speculum is then slowly removed while the anterior vaginal wall is supported. The top of the vaginal vault and the posterior vaginal wall can thus be visualized sequentially to detect the presence of an enterocele or rectocele, respectively.

Both the Cusco's and the Sims' speculum examination should be followed by a bimanual examination. The patient lies in a similar position as for the Cusco's speculum examination and the left hand parts the labia as two fingers are inserted into the vagina and then placed behind the cervix. The left hand is then placed on the abdomen above the symphysis pubis and pushes down onto the pelvis so that the organs are palpated between the left hand and the two fingers within the vagina. The uterus, which is situated centrally, should be assessed for size, consistency, mobility, regu-larity, anteversion, retroversion and tenderness. The adnexae are palpated on each side, particularly looking for tenderness and any suggestion of a mass. In very thin women normal-size ovaries may be felt (Fig. 2.1).

The area behind the cervix is palpated for any areas of tenderness or masses.

The pelvic examination occasionally needs to be concluded with a rectal examination if indicated.

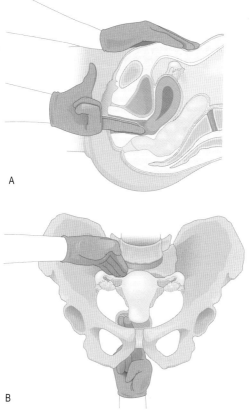

A

B

Figure 2.1 (A) Bimanual examination of the pelvis. (B) Examination of the lateral fornix.

PRESENTING AN EXAMINATION

To present the examination findings one should say: Ms Fairhall is a (describe general appearance) and abdominal examination was…and speculum examination revealed a normal/abnormal cervix and bimanual examination revealed a normal-sized anteverted uterus and the adnexae were unremarkable.

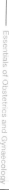

Obstetric history-taking 3

CHAPTER CONTENTS

Following an introduction to the obstetric patient, establish her name, age, parity and gestation.

PARITY

This is defined as the number of times a woman has delivered a potentially viable baby (viability in the UK is taken after 24 completed weeks of a pregnancy).

GRAVIDITY

This is defined as the total number of pregnancies achieved.

Confusion may arise with the use of 'gravidity' and so the term 'parity' is better to describe the obstetric status of the patient.

GESTATION

This is the number of weeks of pregnancy.

Gestation of the pregnancy must be calculated both from ultrasound scan estimation (most accurate up to 20 weeks' gestation) and from last menstrual period (LMP) dates using Naegele's rule or by an obstetric wheel. Ultrasound calculation of gestation is done by measuring the crown–rump length (CRL) in the first gestation and by measuring the biparietal diameter (BPD) and/or femur length (FL) in the second trimester.

NAEGELE'S RULE

The estimated date of delivery (EDD) is calculated by subtracting 3 months from the date of LMP, adding 7 days and 1 year. This calculation may not be accurate in women with irregular cycles or in those who had been using the oral contraceptive pill.

PRESENTING COMPLAINT

Establish the presenting complaint or reason for referral or admission of the patient in a short but concise manner. Common causes for admission include abdominal pain, hypertension, bleeding or ruptured membranes. Obstetric patients are often very well informed and can give a precise and detailed account of their admission and so it is always wise to ask them what their doctor has planned. At this stage enquire whether the pregnancy has been uncomplicated to date or outline previous admissions to hospital. Ask what tests have been performed, including ultrasound scans, blood tests and any screening investigations, including prenatal diagnostic tests. Also enquire whether the patient had taken preconception folic acid.

PAST HISTORY

Past obstetrical history

This includes details on all previous pregnancies. Specifically enquire about terminations of pregnancy or miscarriages. For each pregnancy enquire about date, any antenatal, intrapartum or postpartum problems, gestation at delivery, mode of delivery, birth weight and sex of the baby and any neonatal problems. If the patient has had any operative deliveries in the past, it is useful to establish the circumstances fully, including number of hours in labour, the use of oxytocin, fetal distress, cervical dilatation and perineal trauma and reason for that mode of delivery.

Past gynaecological history

This will include last cervical smear, previous contraception, any fertility investigations and any previous gynaecological surgery. It is important to include relevant points; for example, previous recurrent pregnancy loss, previous fibroid surgery or pelvic floor surgery, all of which would influence the management of this pregnancy.

Past medical history

This will include any previous surgery or medical conditions that may have required investigation. If the patient has any medical history, one must establish the severity of the problem; for example, the mild asthmatic requiring infrequent inhaler use, or the asthmatic on multiple medications requiring frequent hospital admissions. A drug history must be taken, including regular medication, recreational drug usage and allergies, specifically to penicillin.

Family history

Ask about family history of any genetic diseases, twins, hypertension or diabetes.

Personal and social history

A good social history will give valuable insight into the domestic circumstances of the patient, including smoking, alcohol intake, employment, relationships, support structure and accommodation.

At the end of the meeting always ask the patient if she feels there is something else important that you may have missed, and enquire what has been done for her during this admission and what her doctor's plans are for the management of the remainder of her pregnancy.

PRESENTING A HISTORY

If this history is to be presented to colleagues, then it is useful to construct a short, concise summary of the case.

Obstetric examination   4

CHAPTER CONTENTS

GENERAL EXAMINATION

Take note of the patient's general appearance: does she look healthy and well? Note her general demeanour and nutritional state. Take note of the patient's weight, height (or body mass index) and temperature. At the first visit a full medical examination should be conducted, including the neck (for goitre or lymphadenopathy), cardiovascular and respiratory systems, breasts, abdomen and periphery. The blood pressure is taken and urinalysis is performed at this and every subsequent visit. If the blood pressure is raised or there is proteinuria, then one must inspect for peripheral oedema and assess for hyperreflexia and clonus.

Oedema is defined as an increase in interstitial fluid and is a normal feature of pregnancy; however, it can be a manifestation of pre-eclampsia or renal disease. Peripheral oedema can be found around the eyes, sacrum or pretibial area.

Clonus is involuntary muscle spasm caused by cerebral irritation and can be assessed by rapidly dorsiflexing the ankle joint, holding it there and then observing for beats of clonus.

ABDOMINAL EXAMINATION

The patient is asked to lie as flat as is comfortable and to expose her abdomen from just below the breasts to the symphysis pubis. A sheet should be available to maintain modesty.

Inspection

During inspection of the abdomen make note of scars from previous surgery (especially laparoscopic and suprapubically), striae gravidarum and linea nigra. In later pregnancy one may note fetal movements.

Palpation

The uterus can be felt abdominally after about 12 weeks' gestation; by 20 weeks' gestation it is generally at the level of the umbilicus and by term it is at the xyphisternum. During palpation the questions that need to be answered are:

● Is the fetus appropriately grown for gestation? The symphyseal–fundal height of the uterus (in centimetres) should correspond with the gestation +1–2 weeks.

- Does the liquor volume feel normal? This could be considered in a larger-for-dates tense uterus in which the fetus is difficult to palpate (polyhydramnios) or, conversely, in a smaller-for-dates uterus in which very little fluid is palpated around the fetus (oligohydramnios).
- Is this a singleton or multiple pregnancy, i.e. greater than two fetal poles can be palpated?
- Is the lie of the fetus (the relation of the fetal spine to the longitudinal axis of the uterus) longitudinal or oblique or transverse?
- Is the presentation cephalic or breech? If cephalic, is it engaged or how palpable is it above the pelvis?

To measure the symphyseal–fundal height, feel for the fundus of the uterus with the tips of the fingers or ulnar surface of the hand and measure the distance to the symphysis pubis with a tape measure, turning it over so that the centimetre markings cannot be seen, to avoid bias (Fig. 4.1). The manoeuvres for palpation of the uterus include: lateral uterine grip with the hands, assessing the lie of the fetus by palpating the sides of the uterus (Fig. 4.2); fundal grip with the hands, assessing the fetus at the uterine fundus; the deep pelvic grip with both hands pointed towards the pelvis to assess for presentation and engagement, ensuring that one is not causing discomfort by observing the mother's face during palpation. An alternative to the latter is Pawlik's grip, which is the grasping of the presenting fetal part between the index finger and thumb, taking care to avoid patient discomfort. Engagement of the fetal head is said to occur when the largest diameter has passed into the pelvis.

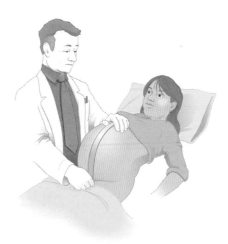

Figure 4.1 Measuring the height of the fundus. (Redrawn with permission from Hanretty K P 2003 Obstetrics Illustrated, 6th edn. Edinburgh: Churchill Livingstone, p. 76.)

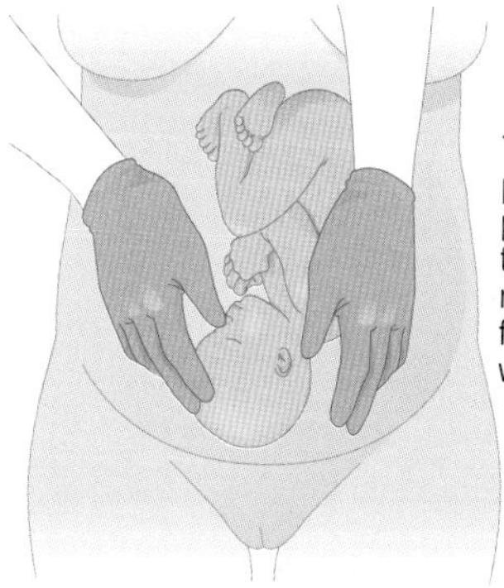

The examiner faces the patient's feet and gently pushes two fingers towards the pelvis. This is the best method of palpating the fetal head and determining whether it is fixed or mobile.

Figure 4.2 Abdominal palpation. (Redrawn with permission from Hanretty K P 2003 Obstetrics Illustrated, 6th edn. Edinburgh: Churchill Livingstone, p. 75.)

For a subjective description of this, the fetal head is divided into fifths palpable abdominally. The head is engaged if less than two-fifths of it can be palpated abdominally (Fig. 4.3).

Auscultation

The final part of the abdominal examination is auscultation of the fetal heart. To locate the best position to auscultate, palpate for the fetal shoulder and place the Pinard stethoscope or Sonicaid just behind this.

Just like in the obstetric history, a short summary of the clinical examination should be prepared, mentioning relevant negative findings also if necessary, e.g. in a case of pre-eclampsia it is important to mention the absence of hyperreflexia or clonus if these are not present.

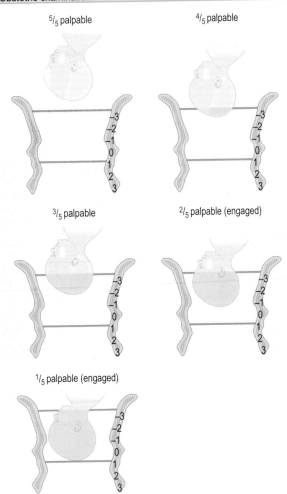

Figure 4.3 Palpation for engagement of fetal head with corresponding station of head on vaginal examination. (Reproduced with permission from Rymer J, Davis G, Rodin A et al. 2003 Preparation and Revision for the DRCOG, 3rd edn. Edinburgh: Churchill Livingstone, p. 210.)

Gynaecology

The menstrual cycle, menstrual disorders, infertility and the menopause

5

CHAPTER CONTENTS

THE MENSTRUAL CYCLE

The menstrual cycle is the pattern of hormonal changes, ovulation, endometrial changes and menstruation that are governed by the hypothalamus, anterior pituitary gland and ovaries. This interaction between the brain and the reproductive organs is known as the hypothalamo–pituitary–ovarian axis.

Hypothalamus and pituitary

Gonadotrophin-releasing hormone (GnRH) is released in a pulsatile fashion from the hypothalamus. The anterior pituitary releases the gonadotrophins, luteinizing hormone (LH) and follicular stimulating hormone (FSH) in a pulsatile manner in response to stimulation by GnRH. This is modulated by oestrogen and progesterone feedback to both the anterior pituitary and hypothalamus. Circulating oestrogen generally acts as negative feedback on the pituitary. However, when oestrogen production from the dominant follicle of the ovary peaks, an LH surge is stimulated.

Ovary

Follicular phase

At the start of each menstrual cycle 10–20 primordial follicles are developing. FSH causes growth of one or more dominant follicles, while the rest of the follicles regress. Oestrogen is released from the theca interna cells within the dominant (graafian) follicle.

Ovulation

The midcycle LH surge causes meiosis of the ovum to be completed, stimulates ovulation 36 hours later and encourages development of the corpus luteum.

Luteal phase

Oestrogen and progesterone are produced by the corpus luteum, which disintegrates after 9–11 days, if pregnancy has not occurred.

Endometrium

Proliferative phase

During the first half of the cycle oestrogen causes growth of glands and arterioles, with thickening of the endometrium.

Secretory phase

Oestrogen and progesterone produced by the corpus luteum during the second half of the cycle induce the endometrium to become vascular and the glands to become tortuous and coiled. The stroma becomes oedematous and the stromal cells become decidualized (change from fibroblast-like to large polyhedron-shaped) in preparation for a fertilized ovum.

Menstruation

Menstruation occurs when the spiral arteries constrict and the endometrium becomes necrotic and sloughs off in response to the cessation of progesterone support as the corpus luteum collapses.

The menstrual cycle showing all these changes is best illustrated diagrammatically, as shown in Figure 5.1.

The average cycle length (from the first day of one period until the first day of the next) is 28 days. The normal range is 21–35 days. Day 1 is defined as the first day of the period. The time from ovulation to menstruation is always 12–16 days, whereas the time from menstruation to the next ovulation may vary widely.

The normal length of bleeding is 3–5 days. Bleeding for less time is not pathological. Bleeding for more time may be normal or may be associated with anaemia and an underlying cause such as fibroids should be excluded. Bleeding is usually heaviest on days 2–3. The average blood loss per menstrual period is 30 ml.

The average age for menarche (the first menstrual period) is 13 years (range 11–15 years).

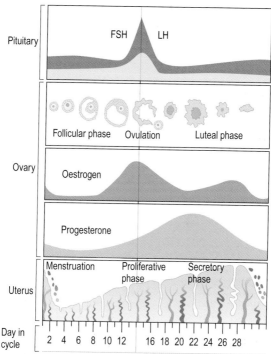

Figure 5.1 Pituitary, ovarian and endometrial changes during the menstrual cycle. FSH, follicle-stimulating hormone; LH, luteinizing hormone.

The average age of the menopause (the last menstrual period) is 51 years. Menstrual cycles shortly after the menarche and close to the menopause are commonly anovulatory and this commonly causes irregular periods in these women.

MENSTRUAL DISORDERS

Menorrhagia

Menorrhagia is heavy cyclical menstrual bleeding over several consecutive cycles. Historically, the definition of menorrhagia has been the loss of more than 80 ml of blood per menstrual period. In practice, actual loss is rarely calculated and menorrhagia is said to occur if the woman finds the heaviness of the bleeding a problem.

Dysfunctional uterine bleeding is excessively heavy, prolonged or frequent uterine bleeding that is not due to pregnancy or recognizable pelvic or systemic disease.

Prevalence

One-third of women describe heavy periods.

Age

Menorrhagia can occur at any age, but is particularly common just prior to the menopause. One in 20 women aged 30–49 years consult their general practitioner each year with heavy periods. Until recent advancements in medical treatment and ablation techniques, menorrhagia was the indication for 50% of all hysterectomies.

Aetiology

Pathological causes for menorrhagia are:

- Uterine fibroids (submucosal)
- Anovulatory bleeds, e.g. menarche, perimenopausal and with polycystic ovarian syndrome (PCOS)
- Endometrial pathology, e.g. endometrial polyps or hyperplasia
- Coagulation disorders, e.g. von Willebrand's disease or anticoagulant treatment
- Iatrogenic, e.g. intrauterine contraceptive device (IUCD)
- Endocrine, e.g. hypothyroidism.

In 40–60% of women no cause is found and the condition is termed dysfunctional uterine bleeding.

Presentation

Women may complain of heavy periods or be referred after a diagnosis of iron-deficiency anaemia.

History

In addition to a full gynaecological and obstetric history, it is important to elucidate how bad the bleeding is, what effect it has on daily life, whether there are symptoms of anaemia and whether there are features suggestive of pathology. Specific questions to ask are:

- What is the cycle length, including the longest and shortest cycles?
- For how many days does the bleeding last?
- For how many days is bleeding heavy?
- How much sanitary protection is needed – how often does the woman need to change her sanitary towel or tampon? Does she ever need to wear both together or 'double up' towels?
- Does she experience flooding (sudden loss of blood, which exceeds the absorbency of the protection, causing embarrassing blood leak through to clothes or bed linen)?
- Does she pass clots of blood? If so, what size?
- Does she need to take time off work during her period?
- How else does her bleeding affect her life (social life, sex life)?
- What contraception is being used?
- Are there any anaemia symptoms (tiredness, shortness of breath, palpitations)?
- Is there pain associated with the period?

Features suspicious of a pathological cause are:

- Intermenstrual or postcoital bleeding
- Dyspareunia
- Pelvic pain
- Premenstrual pain.

Examination

Signs of anaemia (pale conjunctivae, tachycardia, breathlessness) may be present. Fibroids may be palpable as an abdominal mass. Tenderness, uterine size and any adnexal masses should be assessed bimanually.

Investigations

Full blood count should be performed and, if anaemic, a blood film and serum ferritin and B_{12} should be checked. Thyroid function should only be tested if there are clinical signs of hypothyroidism. Coagulation tests are useful for women on warfarin or with other features of a coagulopathy (e.g. easy bruising).

Transvaginal pelvic ultrasound should be arranged for fibroids and endometrial thickness (ideally on day 5).

Endometrial biopsy or hysteroscopy is indicated only for irregular bleeding or that which is not helped by first- and second-line treatment.

The alkaline haematinic method for measuring actual blood loss is time-consuming and unpopular with women. It is generally reserved for research situations.

Management

Anaemia should be treated with ferrous sulphate 200 mg three times daily. If a cause for the menorrhagia is found, then this should be treated. This may involve myomectomy for fibroids, resection of endometrial polyps, removal of IUCD or correction of international normalized ratio on warfarinized patients.

First-line treatments

The choice of first-line treatment depends on the contraception need, any associated symptoms (e.g. dysmenorrhoea) and the woman's preference.

The most effective treatment in randomized controlled trials is tranexamic acid 1 g three times daily from the first day of bleeding until the bleeding is tailing off.

The following three alternative treatments have equal efficacy:

- Mefenamic acid – mefenamic acid 500 mg is taken three times daily from the first day of bleeding until the bleeding is tailing off. This, or another non-steroidal anti-inflammatory agent, is particularly helpful if there is associated dysmenorrhoea.
- Combined oral contraceptive pill (COCP) – this may be suitable where contraception is also required or the cycle is irregular.
- Progestogens – continuous progestogens usually cause amenorrhoea and may be helpful in women who are severely anaemic and who can tolerate the side effects. Depot medroxyprogesterone acetate is an effective long-term treatment, or oral norethisterone three times daily may be used in the short term.

The levonorgestrel-releasing intrauterine system (LNG-IUS) is extremely effective at reducing menorrhagia. However, irregular bleeding in the first 3 months is a significant side effect in some women and is the commonest reason for the device to be removed.

Second-line treatments

- **Levonorgestrel-releasing intrauterine system:** The LNG-IUS should always be considered after failure of other medical treatments and prior to any surgical procedure, as it can be inserted easily as an outpatient and does not have the operative risks associated with endometrial ablation or hysterectomy.
- **Endometrial ablation techniques:** Various techniques are effective at treating menorrhagia by destroying the endometrium down to the basal layer, with the aim of preventing endometrial regeneration. The advantages over hysterectomy are shorter operating time, return home on the same day, shorter time off work and lower morbidity. However,

endometrial ablation techniques have a lower cure rate and some women require a repeat ablation procedure or hysterectomy at a later stage.

Endometrial ablation is not suitable for women who may wish to become pregnant, and all women should be advised to continue to use contraception after the procedure.

- Hysteroscopic endometrial ablation techniques:
  - *Transcervical resection of the endometrium* - Transcervical resection of the endometrium (TCRE) is a hysteroscopic technique involving the use of an electrodiathermy loop to resect the endometrium, in strips, to a depth of 3 mm (with a further 2 mm thermal damage). The endometrium is prepared with preoperative GnRH analogues to thin the endometrium, which further reduces operative time, reduces fluid absorption and improves outcome. The procedure is carried out as a day case under general anaesthesia. Most women return to work within 2 weeks. They should be advised to expect bleeding and discharge for up to 2 weeks and some pain. They should also be advised to return immediately if they experience severe pain, pyrexia, heavy bleeding or shortness of breath.

    TCRE is contraindicated with suspicion of malignancy, uterine size greater than 12 weeks or in the presence of active infection.
- Complications of transcervical resection of the endometrium:
  - *Uterine perforation* - The risk of perforation (1% risk) may be reduced by use of the rollerball, rather than the loop, at the cornu and fundus where the myometrium is thinner.
  - *Fluid overload* - Glycine is absorbed into the myometrial vessels during the TCRE procedure. This causes hyponatraemia and fluid overload (6% risk), which can lead to pulmonary oedema. Prevention involves limiting the amount of fluid absorbed (calculated by subtracting the volume out from the volume in) to 1000 ml. Treatment of fluid overload is mostly supportive, with monitoring of fluid balance, haemoglobin, haematocrit and electrolytes.
  - *Bleeding* - Heavy bleeding is rare, but may be controlled with a 14-gauge Foley catheter with 30 ml balloon inflated above the cervix. This allows tamponade and can be removed after 12 hours. Hysterectomy for bleeding is very rarely indicated.
  - *Infection* - Women should all be given antibiotic prophylaxis with azithromycin (1 g) orally as a single dose.
- Late complications: Pregnancies can occur after ablation techniques due to regrowth of endometrial tissue, so effective contraception should be used. Haematometra, from cervical fibrosis, is rare and should be drained. Endometrial cancer may occur in islands of residual endometrium, with the risk of delayed diagnosis if the malignant area is 'walled off' by fibrotic tissue.
- Outcome of transcervical resection of the endometrium: At 1 year up to 66–87% of women are satisfied with TCRE, with 42% reporting amenorrhoea, 33% light periods and 16% no improvement. However, 10–38% have repeat surgery within 5 years and some eventually go on to have a hysterectomy. Endometrial ablation is more effective in older women. It may help with associated dysmenorrhoea and premenstrual symptoms, but is less likely to help if there is premenstrual pain. Success and complication rates both relate to the operator's experience.

- *Rollerball endometrial ablation* - Rollerball endometrial ablation uses an electrosurgical rollerball to destroy the endometrium. It is less effective than resection and is generally only used for the cornu and fundal areas, where there is less risk of uterine perforation than with the resection loop.

- *Endometrial laser ablation* - The neodymium:yttrium-aluminium-garnet (Nd:YAG) laser effectively destroys the endometrium. Results and complications are equivalent to TCRE. Fluid overload may still occur, but as saline is used rather than glycine, hyponatraemia is not a problem.

- Non-hysteroscopic endometrial ablation techniques: Non-hysteroscopic endometrial ablation procedures, as described below, are known as the 'second-generation' ablation techniques and are performed 'blind'. As such, endometrial polyps and small fibroids may be missed at the time of the procedure. However, the advantages of second-generation techniques are that they are generally simpler and quicker to perform, require less operator training and can often be carried out under local anaesthetic in the outpatient or day-surgery setting. Fluid overload does not occur and complications such as uterine perforation are very rare.

  There is no significant difference in efficacy between the hysteroscopic and non-hysteroscopic techniques for patient satisfaction and reduction in heavy bleeding. Thirty to 60% of women become amenorrhoeic after the procedure.

  Long-term safety and efficacy evidence is still awaited for these procedures.

- *Thermal balloon ablation* - Thermal balloon ablation involves the insertion of a soft flexible balloon into the uterine cavity through the cervix. The balloon is then inflated with a pressurized solution so that it fits the shape of the cavity. The solution is heated to 87 °C for 8 minutes to destroy the endometrium.

- *Microwave endometrial ablation* - Microwave endometrial ablation is performed by inserting a microwave probe into the uterine cavity and heating it to 75–80 °C for 3 minutes while the probe is moved from side to side to ablate the endometrium.

- *Photodynamic therapy, cryotherapy, radiofrequency ablation and free fluid endometrial ablation* - These are other less common second-generation endometrial ablation techniques.

Third-line treatment

Hysterectomy as a treatment for menorrhagia has a 100% cure rate and greater than 90% satisfaction rate. It also has the advantage of removing the need for contraception and eliminating the risk of endometrial and cervical cancer (in total hysterectomy). However, 3% of women experience life-threatening complications from hysterectomy. There are also common emotional side effects relating to loss of fertility, and physical side effects in terms of time to full recovery. The economic cost to the National Health Service and the woman are higher for hysterectomy than for medical treatment or ablation techniques.

If hysterectomy is performed for heavy bleeding with a normal-sized uterus, then vaginal hysterectomy, or laparoscopically assisted hysterectomy is preferable as these procedures have lower complication rates and faster recovery times than abdominal hysterectomy.

Dysmenorrhoea

Definition

Dysmenorrhoea is cyclical pelvic pain occurring just before or during the menstrual period. Dysmenorrhoea may be primary (onset soon after the menarche and no identifiable cause) or secondary (later onset and usually associated with pathology such as endometriosis).

Prevalence

Between 50 and 97% of women experience some degree of pain with their periods and 10% have severe symptoms.

Aetiology

Causes of secondary dysmenorrhoea include endometriosis, adenomyosis, pelvic inflammatory disease and submucosal pedunculated fibroids. The pain may also be secondary to heavy blood flow or a symptom of premenstrual syndrome. Iatrogenic causes are the IUCD and cervical stenosis after large loop excision of transformation zone or TCRE.

Clinical features

Dysmenorrhoea generally starts 1–2 days prior to the period and is often relieved within the first day of bleeding. It always stops before the end of the period. The pain may radiate down the thighs or to the back.

Important questions in the history are:
- What is the nature of the pain?
- When does the pain start in relation to the period?
- When does the pain stop?
- Does the pain radiate?
- What medication does the woman take to relieve the pain?
- Does she have any non-menstrual pain or dyspareunia?
- How does the pain impact on her life – does she take time off work, does it limit her social life?

Examination

Abdominal tenderness or masses may be palpable. Bimanual examination detects uterine size, orientation, cervical excitation and adnexal tenderness or masses. In the presence of endometriosis, palpation of the uterosacral ligaments and pouch of Douglas may reveal a mass, nodules or tenderness. Adenomyosis may cause a mildly enlarged and soft uterus.

Investigations

Swabs should be taken for infection. Ultrasound scan will usually be normal, but can exclude a pelvic mass. Laparoscopy is indicated if simple analgesia is not effective, to look for evidence of endometriosis, pelvic inflammatory disease or adhesions.

Management

Identifiable causes should be treated. This may include antibiotics for pelvic inflammatory disease or ablation of endometriosis.

Anti-inflammatory analgesia, such as mefenamic acid, reduces the pain in up to 70% of women and also reduces blood loss to an extent. Paracetamol and dihydrocodeine are alternatives. The COCP is also effective at reducing dysmenorrhoea in up to 80% of women.

Locally applied heat (hot-water bottle), transcutaneous electrical nerve stimulations and acupuncture have all been shown to have some effect. In intractable cases, there is some evidence for laparoscopic uterosacral nerve ablation, but this evidence is controversial.

Amenorrhoea and oligomenorrhoea

Definitions

- Amenorrhoea is the absence of menstruation.
- Primary amenorrhoea is the failure to establish menstruation.
- Secondary amenorrhoea is the absence of periods for 6 months or more after previously regular menstruation.
- Oligomenorrhoea is fewer than four periods occurring within a 12-month interval.

Incidence

Primary amenorrhoea is experienced by 0.3% of girls and 3% of women have secondary amenorrhoea.

Primary amenorrhoea

- Aetiology: The two commonest causes of primary amenorrhoea are Turner's syndrome and constitutional delay (Fig. 5.2). Other causes include pregnancy, hypothalamic causes (stress, excessive exercise, anorexia), androgen insensitivity syndrome, hypothyroidism, primary ovarian failure and anatomical causes (uterine malformation, imperforate hymen and vaginal septum). Drugs that cause amenorrhoea are chemotherapeutic agents (damage to ovaries) or others such as phenothiazines, which are dopamine antagonists.

- Clinical features: A family history of female relatives with late onset of periods is suggestive of constitutional delay. Autoimmune disease or androgen insensitivity syndrome may also be suggested in the family history. Excessive exercise and any change in weight should be elicited. Chronic illnesses or medications should be asked about. An imperforate hymen or vaginal septum may present with a history of amenorrhoea and cyclical abdominal pain.

- Examination: The important examination feature is the presence or absence of secondary sex characteristics such as breast development, pubic and axillary hair. Absence of such features by 14 years suggests ovarian dysgenesis (e.g. Turner's), a hypothalamic cause or hypothyroidism.

  The weight and height should be checked for calculation of body mass index.

  Other features to note are signs of Turner's syndrome (such as webbed neck and short stature), hypothyroidism or abnormal visual fields from a possible prolactinoma. Acne or hirsutism suggests androgen excess and clitoromegaly may suggest virilization or may represent ambiguous genitalia of congenital adrenal hyperplasia or an androgen-secreting tumour.

- Investigations: Investigations should be initiated in a girl who has no periods by the age of 16 years if secondary sexual characteristics are present and at 14 if there is no secondary sex development.

  A pregnancy test should be performed if there is a possibility of pregnancy. Thyroid function and prolactin levels should be checked. Serum gonadotrophin levels are high with low oestrogen in ovarian causes, such as Turner's syndrome, previous chemotherapy or premature ovarian failure. Low gonadotrophins are found in hypothalamic causes such as weight-related and exercise-induced amenorrhoea. In PCOS, the testosterone and LH levels are high, with normal FSH.

  Karyotype confirms the presence of Turner's syndrome or other rare abnormalities, such as fragile X syndrome, and aids the diagnosis of androgen insensitivity.

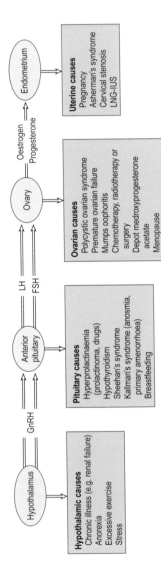

Figure 5.2 Causes of amenorrhoea in relation to the hypothalamopituitary–ovarian–endometrial axis. GnRH, gonadotrophin-releasing hormone; LH, luteinizing hormone; FSH, follicle-stimulating hormone; LNG-IUS, levonorgestrel-releasing intrauterine system.

Ultrasound scan should be arranged to confirm the presence of a uterus and exclude haematometra or haematocolpos.

In constitutional delay, the commonest cause of primary amenorrhoea, the examination and gonadotrophin results are normal.

- **Management:** Girls with constitutional delay will menstruate spontaneously and reassurance should be given.

Other causes of primary amenorrhoea should be treated where possible; for example, thyroxine for hypothyroidism, bromocriptine or surgery for prolactinoma, hymenal division for haematocolpos. Exercise should be limited in those with exercise-induced amenorrhoea and weight gain encouraged if the body mass index is less than 19.

In causes such as Turner's syndrome, androgen insensitivity and premature ovarian failure, extensive counselling is required for both the girl and her parents. Support groups exist for all these disorders and cover issues of self-image, sexuality and fertility. Osteoporosis should be prevented by long-term hormone replacement, usually in the form of the COCP.

Secondary amenorrhoea

The causes of amenorrhoea are illustrated in relation to the hypothalamo-pituitary–ovarian–endometrial axis in Figure 5.2.

After physiological causes, such as pregnancy, breastfeeding and contraceptives, the commonest causes are polycystic ovaries, hyperprolactinaemia and premature ovarian failure.

- **History:**

The questions to ask include:

- Is there a possibility of pregnancy?
- What contraception is used – could it be causing amenorrhoea?
- Is there a history of previous pregnancy complications, such as post-partum haemorrhage, evacuation of retained products of conception or termination of pregnancy?
- What was the nature of the periods when present – regularity, length, heaviness of flow?
- Is exercise excessive? Has there been recent weight loss?
- Is there a history of chronic illness, radiotherapy or chemotherapy?
- Does the woman experience headaches or visual symptoms?
- Are there associated endocrine symptoms such as obesity, hirsutism, acne or symptoms of hypothyroidism?
- Are there associated menopausal symptoms such as hot flushes, night sweats or vaginal dryness?
- What medications are being taken?
- **Examination:** Examination should be directed by the history, looking for signs of PCOS (obesity, hirsutism and acne) or endocrine disease such as hypothyroidism. If a prolactinoma is suspected then the visual fields should be checked.

All women should have body mass index calculated. A bimanual examination may be indicated, for example to check for uterine size in suspected haematometra.

- **Investigations:** A pregnancy test is usually indicated in secondary amenorrhoea. A hormone profile should then generally indicate the diagnosis.

In PCOS, a raised LH and moderately high testosterone are found in the majority of women. A very high testosterone level indicates further investigation for a possible androgen-secreting tumour, for example from the ovary or adrenal gland.

Premature ovarian failure is associated with raised FSH (>10 IU/l) and LH and with low oestradiol.

Hypothyroidism is associated with low thyroxine and raised thyroid-stimulating hormone.

Serum prolactin should always be checked, but caution is needed in interpreting the result as a prolactin level up to 1000 mU/ml may be due to stress, breast examination, PCOS or the venepuncture itself. True hyper-prolactinaemia is usually caused by a microprolactinoma or occasionally a macroadenoma. Computed tomography or magnetic resonance imaging of the pituitary fossa and formal visual field testing should be arranged in cases of suspected prolactinoma.

Pelvic ultrasound is helpful where haematometra is suspected.

If premature ovarian failure is confirmed by gonadotrophin levels, then karyotype and autoimmune tests should be arranged for genetic causes and associated autoimmune disease, respectively.

If Asherman's syndrome is suspected from previous uterine evacuation, then a hysteroscopy is indicated.

Management

Management of secondary amenorrhoea depends on the cause of the problem. As with primary ovarian failure, counselling is an essential part of the management of women in whom the amenorrhoea is permanent, in view of the anxiety caused about fertility, sexuality and long-term health issues such as osteoporosis.

Polycystic ovaries

Treatment with a COCP will restore periods and should be used if the woman has had fewer than four periods per year. Co-cyprindiol (ethinyloestradiol with cyproterone acetate) has been used in the past, as cyproterone acetate acts as an antiandrogen, thus also improving hirsutism and acne. However, the incidence of thrombosis exceeds that with low-dose oestrogen preparations and, therefore, co-cyprindiol should only be used after appropriate counselling.

If obesity is a problem in these women, then weight loss usually restores periods and fertility. If the woman is trying to conceive, then ovulation may be induced with clomifene.

Premature ovarian failure (spontaneous or iatrogenic)

Hormone replacement therapy (HRT) for osteoporosis prevention is necessary and counselling support should be offered. Fertility is only a possibility by ovum donation and in vitro fertilization (IVF).

Anorexia- or exercise-related amenorrhoea

Clear advice about lifestyle and diet is essential to restore periods. Most women recommence menstruating once exercise is reduced or the body mass index is above 19. If a woman continues to be amenorrhoeic, then some form of hormone replacement with COCP or HRT is needed to prevent osteoporosis.

Prolactinoma

Prolactinoma is generally managed by endocrinologists with bromocriptine or cabergoline. Surgery is only indicated for macroadenomas or cases resistant to medication.

Hypothyroidism

Hypothyroidism should be treated with thyroxine replacement.

Asherman's syndrome

Adhesions can be broken down hysteroscopically and a combination of an IUCD with a 3-month course of systemic oestrogen is necessary to prevent reformation. However, although periods may return, pregnancy is unlikely.

Contraceptive-related amenorrhoea

Amenorrhoea related to depot medroxyprogesterone acetate may continue for 12–18 months after the last injection. The management is, therefore, expectant. However, ovulation is likely to occur before a period and effective contraception should still be advised. Women who are amenorrhoeic with the progesterone-only pill, LNG-IUS or implant should be reassured that this is normal and that the contraceptive method does not need to be changed. There is no evidence for 'postpill amenorrhoea' occurring after discontinuation of the COCP.

INTERMENSTRUAL AND POSTCOITAL BLEEDING

Intermenstrual bleeding (vaginal bleeding not due to a regular menstrual period) and postcoital bleeding (bleeding after sexual intercourse) are almost always pathological.

Aetiology of intermenstrual and postcoital bleeding

Hormonal and contraception-related causes

Long-acting progestogens, the LNG-IUS and progesterone-only pill can all cause irregular bleeding, as can poor compliance with the COCP.

Uterine causes

The most important cause of intermenstrual bleeding and postcoital bleeding, especially in older women, is endometrial carcinoma. Other uterine causes are endometrial hyperplasia, endometrial polyps and pedunculated submucosal fibroids. Retained products of conception are an uncommon cause.

Cervical causes

Cervical carcinoma can present with intermenstrual or postcoital bleeding. More commonly, cervical ectropion, infection (*Trichomonas*, gonorrhoea) or endocervical polyps may be the cause of the irregular bleeding.

Vaginal causes

Candida, carcinoma and hypo-oestrogenic atrophy are vaginal causes of intermenstrual and postcoital bleeding.

Non-gynaecological causes

Rectal bleeding (e.g. from haemorrhoids) and urethral bleeding (e.g. from a caruncle) can be mistaken for vaginal bleeding.

Clinical features

The history should include the amount and timing of the bleeding, contraceptive use and any previous infections. The cervical smear history is important. Some risk factors may suggest a more likely cause. For example, obesity, diabetes and nulliparity are associated with endometrial hyperplasia and malignancy.

Examination

Careful examination of the anus, external genitalia and urethral orifice may reveal the site of bleeding. Speculum examination may show an ectropion, inflamed cervix or features suggestive of malignancy. Endocervical polyps may be visualized. Bimanual examination may show an enlarged uterus suggestive of fibroids or malignancy.

Investigations

Triple swabs should be taken for infection (high vaginal swab for *Candida* and *Trichomonas*, endocervical for gonorrhoea, endocervical for *Chlamydia*).

Cervical smear should be taken if it has not been performed within the last 3 years.

Colposcopy and cervical biopsy should be performed if there is suspicion of cervical malignancy.

Transvaginal ultrasound scan, preferably around day 5, may suggest endometrial thickening or a polyp.

Hysteroscopy should be arranged in women where no other cause has been found for the irregular bleeding and a biopsy should be taken.

Management

The management of intermenstrual and postcoital bleeding depends on the cause.

Sexually transmitted infections or *Candida* should be treated. Visible endocervical polyps should be removed in the outpatient clinic by grasping with polyp forceps and twisting repeatedly until the polyp is avulsed. Larger endocervical or intrauterine polyps or fibroids should be resected hysteroscopically. All specimens should be sent for histological analysis to confirm they are benign.

Continuous progestogens can be used for the treatment of endometrial hyperplasia. Oncological assessment is necessary if uterine, cervical or vaginal malignancy is diagnosed.

Cervical ectropion usually resolves by stopping the COCP, or it may be cauterized in the colposcopy unit, only after a normal smear.

For women taking a COCP in whom a cervical ectropion is not present, it is important to check that compliance is good and that there are no other factors influencing the effect, such as enzyme-inducing drugs or diarrhoea and vomiting. Otherwise, a biphasic or triphasic preparation can be considered, or a preparation containing a different progestogen or a lower oestrogen.

PREMENSTRUAL SYNDROME

One in three women experience some degree of premenstrual symptoms. In 3–5% these symptoms are severe, and when mood and behaviour symptoms dominate, the term 'premenstrual dysphoric disorder (PMDD)' is used.

Pathophysiology

Premenstrual syndrome and PMDD are poorly understood, but increased sensitivity to progesterone is thought to cause a fall in the concentration of neurotransmitters, including serotonin, hence the benefit of serotonin-specific reuptake inhibitors in treatment.

Clinical features

The symptoms of premenstrual syndrome always start after ovulation, worsen as menstruation approaches and resolve within the first few days of bleeding. Symptoms may be physical, emotional or behavioural.

Physical symptoms include breast swelling and discomfort, abdominal bloating, oedema, weight gain, headaches or deterioration in asthma, migraine or epilepsy. Emotional and behavioural symptoms include aggression, anger, irritability, tearfulness, low mood, anxiety, altered eating habits and disturbed sleep.

In severe cases, women may become violent or suicidal. Relationship difficulties and occupational problems are commonly reported.

Diagnosis

The diagnosis is made clinically with a symptom diary kept over a few months. The symptoms must be seen to occur in most months, develop in the luteal phase and resolve soon after the onset of menstruation. There must be at least 1 week without symptoms and if any symptoms persist throughout the menstrual cycle then an alternative diagnosis, such as anxiety or depression, is likely.

Treatment

Ovulation inhibition

Preventing ovulation with the COCP is effective for many women. Oestrogen may also be administered in other forms, for example as patches, as long as the endometrium is protected. The LNG-IUS is a useful method of protection for the endometrium as it acts locally on the endometrium with minimal systemic progestogen absorption.

Serotonin-specific reuptake inhibitors

There is good evidence that serotonin-specific reuptake inhibitors, particularly fluoxetine and sertraline, improve physical, emotional and behavioural symptoms of premenstrual syndrome and PMDD. Long-term treatment is generally needed, as symptoms tend to relapse after stopping.

Alternative treatments

Evening primrose oil has some benefit for reducing breast tenderness and pain. There is no evidence of benefit from vitamin B_6 (pyridoxine), though it may be an effective placebo treatment.

Progesterone treatment has no role in the treatment of premenstrual syndrome or PMDD.

POLYCYSTIC OVARIAN SYNDROME

Definition

The classic definition of PCOS (Stein–Leventhal syndrome) is a triad of obesity, oligomenorrhoea and infertility. 'Polycystic ovaries' is the term used to describe a typical appearance of ovaries on ultrasound scan.

PCOS is now known to involve a disturbance of metabolic function. There are no specific diagnostic criteria, but the diagnosis is made on a combination of any of the following features:

- Clinical features
  - oligomenorrhoea or amenorrhoea
  - subfertility
  - acne and greasy skin
  - hirsutism
  - obesity
  - male-pattern baldness.
- Biochemical features
  - raised testosterone or androstenedione
  - raised LH and increased LH:FSH ratio

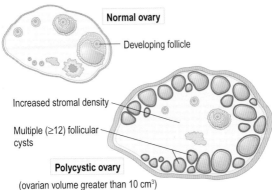

Figure 5.3 Schematic representation of normal and polycystic ovary.

- decreased sex hormone-binding globulin
- impaired glucose tolerance.
- Ultrasound features: three features are found, as illustrated in Figure 5.3
  - increased stromal density (echolucency similar to or greater than myometrium)
  - enlarged ovaries (typically 2–4 times normal volume)
  - multiple (>10) follicular cysts (each >8 mm) typically peripherally arranged around the ovary, like a 'string of pearls'.

Incidence

The typical appearance of polycystic ovaries is found in 20% of women on pelvic scan. Of these, 50% have other features suggestive of PCOS.

Aetiology

The aetiology of PCOS is poorly understood, but there is a genetic correlation.

Pathophysiology

Infrequent periods result from anovulation in most cycles. Greasy skin, acne and hirsutism arise from the androgen excess. The underlying metabolic disorder is insulin resistance (hyperinsulinaemia in the presence of normoglycaemia) and this accounts for the common symptom of obesity.

Presentation

Women may present with a history of subfertility or irregular periods. Others present with hirsutism, skin problems or obesity. Polycystic ovaries are also a common incidental finding on ultrasound scans for other indications.

Clinical features

The spectrum of clinical features is described above. The presentation of PCOS varies enormously between different women. For example, many women have normal body mass index despite the typical features of oligomenorrhoea, ultrasound features and abnormal androgen concentrations. Other women may have regular periods with obesity and abnormal lipids.

In PCOS, irregular periods are often very heavy or prolonged as they result from endometrial shedding after prolonged oestrogen priming without a progesterone-induced withdrawal bleed.

Examination

A general examination may reveal hirsutism, greasy skin, acne and obesity. Abdominal and pelvic examinations are usually unremarkable and the ovaries are not usually palpable.

Investigations

A hormone profile should be taken around day 5. The investigations usually show:

- LH greater than 10 IU/l
- Raised LH:FSH ratio
- Testosterone greater than 2.5 nmol/l
- Decreased sex hormone-binding globulin.

Serum FSH, thyroid function tests and prolactin levels are usually normal in women with PCOS.

Other causes of hyperandrogenism should be screened for if there are other virilizing features (such as clitoromegaly, voice changes or altered body habitus) or if the serum testosterone concentration is greater than 4.8 nmol/l. Such causes include adrenal or ovarian tumours, Cushing's syndrome and atypical congenital adrenal hyperplasia.

Transvaginal ultrasound scan usually confirms the typical features of polycystic ovaries, but the diagnosis of PCOS is not dependent on this.

Management

Women with PCOS need a careful explanation of the diagnosis and its implications. Further management should be determined by the symptoms and in women with no symptoms reassurance alone is needed.

The COCP is the most effective method used to regulate periods. Oligomenorrhoeic or amenorrhoeic women with PCOS may be at risk of endometrial hyperplasia or malignancy from persistent oestrogen stimulation. In these women regular menstruation should be induced by the COCP or by a 14-day course of progesterone.

Hirsutism may be treated by local treatments, such as waxing, electrolysis and bleaching, though these are expensive and need repeating regularly. Oral and topical antibiotics may help with acne.

The COCP is also effective in women with hirsutism and acne, especially where contraception or regulation of periods is also desirable. A COCP containing cyproterone acetate, an antiandrogen with progestogenic effects (co-cyprindiol), helps to improve acne by 3 months and hirsutism by 6–9 months, as well as regulate menstruation. Extra cyproterone acetate, up to 100 mg daily, may be added if the COCP alone is not effective, but evidence for this is unclear. Co-cyprindiol has a higher associated risk of thrombosis than other low-dose pills and this should be explained to the woman. Spironolactone is an unlicensed treatment that may be of benefit in hirsutism by acting as an androgen receptor antagonist.

Weight loss may be difficult in women with PCOS, but is important for reducing long-term cardiovascular risks, self-image, menstruation and fertility. Referral to a dietician and exercise advice are helpful.

Ovarian stimulation with clomifene citrate or laparoscopic ovarian drilling is effective for PCOS-related subfertility. However, simple weight loss alone also has a dramatic effect on restoring ovulation.

Evidence suggests that metformin regulates ovulation, improves fertility and improves the lipid profile in women with PCOS. The presumed mechanism is that, by reducing insulin resistance, it breaks the chain of events that leads to the symptoms and signs of the disease. However, it is not licensed for these indications and no evidence is yet available to indicate whether it has a long-term benefit in preventing the metabolic consequences of PCOS. It is generally reserved for women who are significantly overweight and who have not been successful in reducing weight by diet control and exercise.

Contraception in polycystic ovarian syndrome

Women with PCOS may ovulate in some cycles, but not in others, so effective contraception should be used if pregnancy is not desirable.

Prognosis

The risk of type 2 diabetes developing in women with PCOS is significantly increased. Yearly screening for glycosuria and raised random blood glucose should be considered, though there is no evidence for the effectiveness of this yet.

Other cardiovascular disease risk factors are also more common in women with PCOS, such as hypertriglyceridaemia, reduced high-density lipoprotein cholesterol and obesity. Cerebrovascular accident (CVA) is more common, but mortality from cardiac disease has not been shown to be increased in these women.

Endometrial carcinoma is more common in women with PCOS. However, this may relate to obesity and the evidence is not clear that inducing a regular withdrawal bleed in these women reduces the malignancy risk.

Women with PCOS have a higher chance of miscarriage, but no effective treatment has been shown to reduce this.

Women with PCOS have an increased chance of developing gestational diabetes if they become pregnant. Screening with random blood glucose or glucose tolerance test should be considered for all PCOS women in pregnancy.

INFERTILITY

Definitions

- Subfertility – failure to conceive after 1 year of regular unprotected sexual intercourse.
- Infertility – no chance of spontaneous conception, for example because of bilateral salpingectomy or azoospermia.
- Primary subfertility – the woman has never been pregnant.
- Secondary subfertility – the woman has had at least one pregnancy before.

Incidence

Thirty per cent of all women will become pregnant after 1 month of regular unprotected intercourse. The number of women becoming pregnant in each consecutive month then reduces so that only 10% of couples will not achieve pregnancy after 1 year (5% after 2 years).

Fifteen per cent of couples are referred for investigation or treatment for subfertility, usually after 1 year of trying, though many of these still conceive spontaneously while waiting for investigation or treatment. Some couples will be referred earlier if they are known to have fertility problems. Examples include women with previous salpingectomies or men with cystic fibrosis.

Age

Female fertility declines naturally with age, such that the chance of pregnancy at 35–39 years of age is half that at 19–26 years of age. Recently, male fertility has also been shown to decline with age, to a lesser extent.

Aetiology

Fifteen per cent of couples have more than one cause for their infertility. The causes of infertility are shown in Table 5.1.

History

A full medical history should be taken from both partners. Important questions for the woman are:
- Has the woman been pregnant before and what were the outcomes of the pregnancies? Has she had an ectopic pregnancy or evacuation of the uterus or other previous pregnancy complications?

Table 5.1. Causes of infertility

Male factor (30–50%):
Erectile problems (e.g. psychological or neurological disease)
Ejaculatory dysfunction (e.g. retrograde ejaculation after prostatic surgery)
Sperm dysfunction (motility, normality, survival)
Testicular failure (e.g. cryptorchidism, mumps orchitis, torsion, chemo- or radiotherapy, Klinefelter's, hypogonadotrophic hypogonadism)
Genital tract obstruction (e.g. vasectomy, incidental ligation of vas deferens at hernia surgery, infection with gonorrhoea, *Chlamydia* or tuberculosis)
Congenital absence of the vas (e.g. cystic fibrosis)

Ovulatory problems (30%):
Polycystic ovary syndrome (70% of anovulatory infertility)
Hypogonadotrophic anovulation (e.g. excess exercise, anorexia, Sheehan's, Kallman's syndrome)
Hyperprolactinaemia (e.g. prolactinoma, drugs)
Genetic causes (e.g. Turner's syndrome, androgen insensitivity)
Premature ovarian failure

Tubal problems (20%):
Infection (e.g. *Chlamydia*, gonorrhoea, pelvic inflammatory disease, tuberculosis)
Adhesions (e.g. surgery or endometriosis, but not unruptured appendicitis)
Previous ectopic pregnancy

Other causes:
Endometriosis (5%)
Fibroids (up to 10%)
Uterine anomalies (1%)
Unexplained infertility (25%)

- Has she had any previous abdominal operations?
- Is there a history of sexually transmitted infection or pelvic inflammatory disease?
- Have there been any other medical problems, such as previous radiotherapy, chemotherapy or thyroid disease?
- Does the woman take any medication that might affect her fertility?
- What is the menstrual cycle length and regularity?
- Does she experience dysmenorrhoea, dyspareunia or menorrhagia?
- What is the frequency of sexual intercourse?
- How much alcohol does she drink?
- Does she smoke, and if so, how many cigarettes per day?

The partner should also be asked specifically:

- Have any previous partners become pregnant by him?
- Has he had any previous operations, such as inguinal hernia repair or orchidopexy?
- Have there been any recent or previous serious illnesses?
- Is there a history of chemotherapy or radiotherapy?
- Has he had mumps?
- Has he ever been diagnosed with a sexually transmitted infection?
- Does he experience any erectile or ejaculatory difficulty?
- Does he take any medications which might affect spermatogenesis, such as cimetidine, antihypertensives or anabolic steroids?
- Does he smoke and, if so, how many cigarettes per day?
- How much alcohol does he drink?
- Does his occupation involve possible exposure to chemicals or an adverse testicular environment (e.g. long-distance lorry driver)?

Examination

A general gynaecological examination should be performed for all women, though commonly no abnormality is found. Body mass index should be calculated.

The man may be examined for the presence of both testes in the scrotum and the vas deferens should be palpated bilaterally. However, this is usually helpful only if semen analysis has shown oligozoospermia or azoospermia. If azoospermia is present, there may also be signs of hypoandrogenism (e.g. lack of body hair).

Investigations

Female investigations

- Hormone profile: The following tests should be requested on all women complaining of subfertility:
- LH (day 2–5 of the menstrual cycle) – LH greater than 10 IU/l and a raised LH:FSH ratio suggests PCOS.
- FSH (day 2–5 of the menstrual cycle) – FSH greater than 10 IU/l suggests a poor prognosis as it is associated with poor ovarian reserve (ovarian failure) and a likely poor outcome from assisted conception, unless donor eggs are used.
- Progesterone (day 21 for a 28-day cycle, otherwise about 8 days before expected menstruation) – progesterone greater than 30 nmol/l suggests that ovulation has occurred.
- Testosterone – testosterone concentration 2.5–5 nmol/l is consistent with PCOS. If testosterone is greater than 5 nmol/l, then further investigation is needed for other causes of androgen excess.

- Prolactin – prolactin >1000 mU/ml suggests hyperprolactinaemia and if repeat test confirms this, then investigations for prolactinoma should be initiated. Prolactin levels less than 1000 mU/ml may be due to stress, exercise or venepuncture.
- Blood tests: Full blood count should be checked to confirm that the woman is not anaemic.

  Thyroid function tests are only indicated where there are other signs or symptoms of thyroid disease.

  Rubella immunity should be confirmed in order that immunization can take place, if indicated, before pregnancy.
- Transvaginal ultrasound scan: Ultrasound scan should identify fibroids or polyps. Other anatomical uterine anomalies, such as a uterine septum, may also be seen.
- Further investigations:
  - *Tests for tubal patency* - All tests of tubal patency should be performed in the first 10 days of the menstrual cycle to avoid disruption to a potential early pregnancy. Various tests are employed, as described below, depending on the skills of the clinicians and the likely diagnosis from the history. As all tests involve some degree of instrumentation of the uterus, prophylactic antibiotics should be given.
  - *Hysterosalpingogram* - Hysterosalpingogram involves contrast medium injected into the cervix and real-time X-ray to visualize its progress through the uterus and tubes. It demonstrates the shape of the uterine cavity as well as tubal patency and morphology.
  - *Hystercontrastsalpingography* - Hystercontrastsalpingography involves saline injection through the cervix and visualization with transvaginal ultrasound. It shows polyps and fibroids more clearly than hysterosalpingogram as well as demonstrating tubal patency.
  - *Laparoscopy and dye* - Laparoscopy is performed, under general anaesthetic, and methylene blue dye is injected through the cervix into the uterus. If the tubes are patent, the dye can be visualized as it fills the tubes and spills from the fimbrial ends into the peritoneal cavity. Any tubal blockage identified can be assessed for suitability for tubal microsurgery. The procedure also has the advantage of demonstrating and allowing immediate treatment of any endometriosis.
  - *Postcoital test* - The postcoital test provides little useful information.

Male investigations

- Semen analysis: A semen sample must be given by masturbation without lubrication into a sterile pot and transported to the laboratory within 1 hour for analysis. If the man cannot masturbate then a coital specimen in a non-spermicidal condom may be sufficient. The man should not have ejaculated for at least 3 days prior to providing the specimen.

  The normal values for semen analysis are given in Table 5.2.

Table 5.2. Normal values for semen analysis	
Volume	2–5 ml
Count	>20 million per ml
Motile forms	>50% progressively mobile and >25% rapidly progressive
Normal forms	>15% normal shape

- Semen deficiency definitions:
- Teratozoospermia is an abnormally high number of abnormal forms.
- Asthenozoospermia is reduced sperm motility.
- Oligozoospermia is a reduced sperm count.
- Azoospermia is the absence of sperm in the ejaculate.

    Abnormal sperm counts often consist of a reduced number of poorly motile sperm with excessive abnormal forms, rather than a single problem. If the result is abnormal, the sample should be repeated after 6 weeks. If there is a history of a recent serious illness then it may take 3–4 months for return of normal spermatogenesis and a normal semen analysis result.

- Further investigations: Testicular biopsy will confirm whether azoospermia has an obstructive cause (mature sperm seen) or is due to testicular failure (Sertoli cell-only syndrome or maturation arrest).

    LH and FSH can help diagnose hypogonadotrophic causes. Karyotype will identify Klinefelter's (XXY) and Y chromosome microdeletions. Cystic fibrosis testing should be arranged in cases of obstructive azoospermia.

Management

The chance of successful spontaneous or assisted pregnancy relates to age, previous pregnancy, duration of subfertility, body mass and the cause of the problem.

Couples often feel they have failed in not achieving a pregnancy and need careful counselling for subfertility. Realistic pregnancy rates should be given with emphasis on the stress placed on couples and the treatment failure in many cases. Options, including donor insemination for sperm problems, ovum donation, adoption or accepting childlessness, are all difficult issues for couples to consider.

Sperm dysfunction

Any abnormal specimen should be repeated after 6 weeks to exclude illness as a cause. In the meantime, advice should include avoiding alcohol, nicotine, very hot baths or tight underpants, all of which are known to inhibit sperm quality. If the sperm quality does not improve, then referral can be made to an andrologist for further investigation. Testosterone injections stimulate spermatogenesis in hypogonadotrophic hypogonadism. Sperm may be retrieved from the testis in obstructive cases. This sperm may then be used for intracytoplasmic sperm injection (ICSI). ICSI is also very effective, even for poor sperm quality or oligozoospermia.

Reversal of vasectomy depends on the time since the operation, with almost no pregnancies if the procedure was more than 10 years earlier. However, early reversal results in sperm in the ejaculate in up to 90% of samples and pregnancy in up to 50% of couples after 2 years.

Tubal infertility

Some women will become pregnant spontaneously despite apparently non-patent tubes. However, most women with tubal infertility will need IVF to bypass the damaged tubes.

Surgical options are available for a few specific tubal problems. For example, open or laparoscopic salpingotomy or reanastomosis may be possible after previous sterilization and proximal tubal obstruction is sometimes helped by hysteroscopic cannulation of the tube. Severely damaged tubes and hydrosalpinges should be removed by bilateral salpingectomy to reduce the complications of IVF.

Anovulatory infertility

Where possible, the cause of anovulation should be treated. Prolactinomas are treated with 1.25 mg bromocriptine at night, gradually increased to 7.5 mg daily in divided doses, though much higher doses can be required. The serum prolactin level should be maintained below 1000 mU/ml for ovulation to return in 70–80% of women. Bromocriptine should then be discontinued once pregnancy is confirmed.

Cabergoline is an alternative treatment for hyperprolactinaemia, but should be discontinued at least 1 month prior to pregnancy due to theoretical risks of teratogenicity.

Other medication should be reviewed where this may be the cause of anovulation.

Women should be encouraged to maintain their body mass index at between 20 and 30 to maximize the chance of conception. Most underweight women will ovulate once their body mass index exceeds 20, but those who do not may need further GnRH pulsatile stimulation.

Polycystic ovarian syndrome

Weight loss is the simplest treatment for anovulatory women with PCOS and they should all have clear advice about improved diet and exercise.

Ovarian stimulation with clomifene results in a 40–60% conception rate after 6 months, though twins occur in 10% and triplets in 1%. Hyperstimulation also occurs in 1% of women taking clomifene. The clomifene dose is 50 mg daily from day 2 to 6 of the cycle. Day 21 progesterone is checked in the first cycle to confirm that ovulation has occurred. If ovulation has not occurred, then the dose is increased to 100 mg daily. The maximum course is 6 months due to fears of ovarian carcinoma from repeated stimulation. Those women who do not respond to clomifene may need FSH injections to stimulate ovulation.

Metformin also improves ovulation (20% pregnancy after 6 months), with no reported teratogenic effects. However, it is not licensed for this use.

Ovarian drilling (laparoscopic diathermy to make several holes in the ovaries) is another effective method of inducing ovulation in women with PCOS and does not result in hyperstimulation or increased risk of multiple pregnancy. There are, however, associated operative complications.

Endometriosis

Infertility with endometriosis does not necessarily relate to tubal obstruction, as many women will have normal tubal patency, but possibly impaired tubal function, limited fimbrial mobility or adhesions. Surgical treatment to ablate the endometriosis has been shown to improve fertility in moderate to severe endometriosis. Endometriomas should be drained or excised as they may inhibit follicular development and also increase the chance of infection at egg retrieval in IVF.

Women with minimal disease do not benefit from surgery and should be treated initially with intrauterine insemination (IUI).

IVF is the most effective treatment where the above measures have not been successful.

Fibroids

Submucosal fibroids may interfere with implantation and IVF cycles are 50% less successful in the presence of fibroids. Intracavity fibroids should, therefore, be removed hysteroscopically after shrinking with

GnRH analogues. Laparoscopic or open myomectomy is performed for intramural fibroids where no other cause for the infertility has been identified.

Social factors

Alcohol, caffeine and smoking may reduce fertility in women and should be discouraged.

Unexplained infertility

Women with unexplained infertility should be offered superovulation and IUI. IVF is then indicated for those who have not responded to IUI. Women over 38 years may be offered IVF as a first-line treatment.

Assisted conception techniques

Assisted conception techniques aim to:
- Pharmacologically stimulate ovaries to produce several eggs.
- Prepare the semen by washing, and in ICSI selecting a highly motile normal form.
- Optimize fertilization by approximating the sperm and egg closely (IUI) or facilitating fertilization in vitro (IVF or ICSI).

Ovulation induction

Oral drugs such as clomifene and tamoxifen or parenteral drugs such as FSH can stimulate ovulation.

FSH can be 'natural', from the urine of postmenopausal women, or more commonly recombinant. The side effects are increased multiple pregnancy rates and ovarian hyperstimulation. Down-regulation of the pituitary–gonadal axis with GnRH analogues or antagonists prior to FSH stimulation reduces the chance of these side effects, but carries menopausal-type side effects itself.

The follicles are monitored during stimulation and eggs collected or ovulation triggered when the leading follicle reaches 18 mm. Ovulation is triggered by human chorionic gonadotrophin (hCG), which mimics the normal LH surge.

Intrauterine insemination

IUI involves placing a small volume of prepared motile sperm high in the uterine cavity on the day of ovulation. It bypasses cervical mucus, introduces sperm at the right time in the cycle and places them close to the fallopian tubes. It may be used in natural cycles or be combined with controlled ovarian stimulation (with gonadotrophins or clomifene). The success is 10–17% pregnancy per cycle and it is cheaper and much less invasive than IVF. If used as a first-line treatment, IUI probably prevents 20% of couples from having to move on to IVF.

Indications for IUI are mild sperm defects, unexplained infertility, failure to conceive with ovulation induction alone, ejaculatory failure or retrograde ejaculation.

In vitro fertilization

IVF involves ovulation induction with FSH, usually after GnRH down-regulation, to produce several eggs. Once the dominant follicle reaches 18 mm in diameter, maturation of the eggs is stimulated by injection of hCG 38–48 hours later; the eggs are then collected by ultrasound-guided aspiration, usually under sedation. Sperm is collected by masturbation and washed. Each egg is then cultured with a small sample of the washed sperm.

On the second or third day, at the four- to eight-cell stage, one to three embryos are transferred back into the uterus, via a transcervical cannula.

The pregnancy is supported with hCG injections or progesterone pessaries, tablets or injections as there is no corpus luteum to produce natural progesterone.

A pregnancy test is taken after 2 weeks and, if positive, an ultrasound scan is performed to confirm the presence of an intrauterine sac. Vaginal bleeding in the meantime usually implies failed implantation. Indications for IVF are severe tubal damage, endometriosis, bilateral salpingo-oophorectomy, unexplained infertility and mild male factor infertility.

Success rates are variable, up to 25–30% live birth rate per cycle, depending on the age of the mother, whether donated eggs are used and the number of embryos transferred. The overall national average success rate, however, is about 17%.

- Complications of in vitro fertilization:
  - *Ovarian hyperstimulation* - Ovarian hyperstimulation may occur with FSH or clomifene stimulation. It is more common when GnRH analogues have been used prior to stimulation, in women with PCOS and in successful implantations. The pathophysiology involves massively enlarged ovaries, extravasation of fluid causing ascites and haemoconcentration causing thrombosis.

  Clinical features are:

- Mild ovarian hyperstimulation syndrome (OHSS) – abdominal discomfort
- Moderate OHSS – abdominal distension and pain, nausea, vomiting, constipation or diarrhoea, dark urine and oedema
- Severe OHSS – pulmonary oedema or thrombosis.

Management for mild OHSS is to increase the oral fluid intake and review regularly. For moderate OHSS, admission is indicated for daily weight and girth measurement, fluid balance monitoring, thromboprophylaxis and monitoring of liver function, albumin, electrolytes and haematocrit. Severe OHSS may need intravenous fluids and drainage of ascites or pleural effusions.

  - *Multiple pregnancies* - Multiple pregnancies are common after assisted conception. The risks of multiple pregnancies include maternal obstetric complications (e.g. pre-eclampsia), extreme prematurity, cerebral palsy and increased perinatal mortality. Strategies to prevent this include implantation of a maximum of two embryos, with cryopreservation of extra embryos for use in future cycles.
  - *Ectopic pregnancy* - Ectopic pregnancy occurs in about 4% of assisted conception pregnancies. Heterotopic pregnancies (simultaneous intrauterine and ectopic pregnancies) are also much more common and diagnosis (with a combination of clinical symptoms, biochemical markers and ultrasound) is difficult.

Intracytoplasmic sperm injection

ICSI is the injection of a single sperm into an oocyte. Similar egg retrieval methods are used as for IVF. The sperm may be from a semen sample or may be retrieved from the epididymis or testis in obstructive azoospermia. Indications for ICSI include severe oligozoospermia, severe sperm morphological abnormalities, poor motility and obstructive azoospermia.

The success rates are up to 20–30% live births per cycle where oligozoospermia is the only cause and the woman is under 35 years.

There is some evidence that sex chromosome anomalies, congenital abnormalities and developmental delay may be more common with ICSI.

Gamete intrafallopian transfer

Gamete intrafallopian transfer involves retrieval of eggs as for IVF and injection of the sperm and eggs directly into the fallopian tube under laparoscopic guidance. It has largely been replaced by IVF and ICSI and is not commonly used.

Alternative infertility options

Donor insemination, embryo donation and egg donation are all possible ways of achieving pregnancy in cases of failure of other methods. Surrogacy, where another woman carries the pregnancy in her uterus, using the partner's sperm and either her own or the infertile woman's egg, is also possible, but has no legal backing in the UK.

Acceptance of childlessness and adoption should also be discussed from an early stage.

Human Fertilisation and Embryology Authority

The Human Fertilisation and Embryology Authority (HFEA) regulates all assisted conception units in the UK. It licenses units involved in ICSI, IVF, preimplantation genetic diagnosis, embryo, egg or sperm donation and surrogacy, as well as storage of embryos and sperm (occasionally eggs) and research involving human embryos.

The HFEA also sets standards for assisted conception, which include consideration of the welfare of the potential child, information to be given to couples, counselling to be given, confidentiality issues and consent issues.

OVARIAN FAILURE

Ovarian function declines gradually from birth and the climax of this is the menopause, which normally occurs in the fifth or sixth decade. Some women experience earlier ovarian failure, which may be spontaneous or secondary to medical or surgical treatment.

Definitions

Menopause

Menopause is the permanent cessation of periods resulting from the loss of ovarian follicular activity.

The menopause can only be diagnosed retrospectively, 1 year after the last menstrual period.

The climacteric (menopause transition)

The climacteric is the time prior to the menopause, when menopausal symptoms are present and periods are usually irregular.

The average duration of such symptoms before cessation of periods is 4 years.

Premature ovarian failure

Premature ovarian failure is the cessation of periods due to ovarian failure under 40 years.

Age

The average age of the menopause is 51 years. Smoking reduces the age of menopause by 2 years. There is a genetic tendency, with daughters experiencing the menopause at about the same age as their mothers.

Pathophysiology

Women have a finite number of oocytes within the ovary, which undergo atresia with time. In the climacteric, failing ovarian follicular activity causes lower circulating oestrogen levels and thus higher levels of LH and FSH from the pituitary. Although ovarian oestrogenic hormone production falls, androstenedione continues to be produced by the ovarian stroma, which is converted peripherally to oestrogen, so measured oestradiol levels may remain high.

Bleeding is often irregular and prolonged as oestrogen induces endometrial proliferation, but anovulation means no progesterone to induce a regular bleed.

Clinical features of menopause

Symptoms, which commonly start about 4 years before the last period, are experienced by 75–80% of women. Irregular periods are one of the commonest features, with only 10% of women having a sudden cessation of periods. Other features of oestrogen deficiency are hot flushes (a feeling of heat, flushing and perspiration of the head, neck and chest), palpitations, night sweats, headaches, tiredness, sleep disturbance, depressed mood, irritability, loss of concentration, vaginal dryness, decreased libido and urinary tract infections. Thin skin, brittle nails and hair loss are also reported.

Psychosexual changes also occur relating to self-image, libido, loss of fertility and the 'empty nest'. However, these symptoms have complex aetiology and may relate to ageing and relationship changes rather than low oestrogen levels.

Signs

Vaginal and labial atrophy may be recognizable on examination. However, other features such as thin skin and brittle nails may simply reflect the ageing process.

Investigations

Investigations are only indicated if there is diagnostic difficulty. FSH and LH are both raised. However, hormone levels fluctuate during the climacteric and women with very high gonadotrophin levels may still menstruate intermittently. Similarly, women with severe menopausal symptoms may have normal gonadotrophin levels at times.

Oestradiol measurement is not helpful.

Management

Hormone replacement therapy

Until recently, up to 60% of women had used HRT at some stage between the ages of 51 and 57. The current indications for treatment are symptom control and osteoporosis risk.

Symptom control

Oestrogen-containing systemic HRT, in the form of tablets, patches, gels or implants, improves hot flushes, vaginal dryness and urinary symptoms. Cognitive function, tiredness and mood symptoms also improve with systemic oestrogen, but this may relate to better sleep once the sweats and flushes have been treated. Systemic HRT may regulate irregular perimenopausal bleeding if no other pathology is present.

Topical oestrogens, in the form of creams, pessaries or rings, are only effective at reducing vaginal atrophy and urinary symptoms.

Low libido is sometimes improved with HRT, but counselling or androgen supplementation may be indicated.

Osteoporosis prevention

Bone density declines with age and this is accelerated by the menopause. Systemic HRT reduces this bone loss for the duration of the therapy.

Types of hormone replacement therapy

Oestrogen (oestradiol, oestrone, oestriol or conjugated equine oestrogens) is the active hormone in all HRT, but if the uterus is present then some form of progestogen is needed to prevent endometrial hyperplasia or malignancy from the unopposed oestrogen.

- **Sequential hormone replacement therapy:** Sequential HRT consists of continuous oestrogen with an additional 12–14 days of progestogen every month to induce a withdrawal bleed. 'Long cycle' preparations use a progestogen to induce a bleed only every 3 months.
- **Continuous combined hormone replacement therapy:** Continuous combined HRT (CCT) consists of continuous oestrogen and low-dose progestogen. The advantage of this regime is the absence of periods – women usually experience irregular bleeding for the first few months and are then bleed-free. However, CCT is only suitable for women who have stopped menstruating for at least 1 year or who are over 55 years. This is because persistent irregular bleeding is likely if the woman still has significant endogenous hormone production.
- **Unopposed oestrogen:** Unopposed oestrogen preparations are only suitable in women without a uterus (generally after hysterectomy). They are not suitable for women who have had a resection of the endometrium for menorrhagia, as small islands of endometrial tissue may still be present.
- **Tibolone:** Tibolone is a synthetic steroid with oestrogen, progestogen and androgen activity. It is used, like CCT, as a bleed-free preparation. An advantage is the improvement in libido for some women from the androgenic component.

Modes of administration

- **Oral:** Daily HRT tablets are easy to take and there is a wide choice of preparations. However, some women may not remember to take them or may object to tablets and there is variable absorption between women.
- **Transdermal:** Patches are the commonest transdermal preparation, with twice-weekly or weekly application. Disadvantages include variable absorption, skin irritation, possible dislodgement and the need to remember to change the patch. Transdermal gels are also available.
- **Implants:** Oestradiol may be given as a subcutaneous implant under local anaesthetic every 6 months. The advantage is that there are no compliance issues and testosterone implants can be co-administered for libido problems. However, tachyphylaxis may occur, where the woman becomes less responsive to successive implants and experiences menopausal symptoms despite high blood levels of oestradiol. Other disadvantages are occasional infections at the wound site, difficulty with removal if side effects occur and the need to give a progestogen by a different route.
- **Topical:** Oestrogen cream, pessaries or rings are very effective for urogenital symptoms. If long courses are required in women with a uterus, then to protect the endometrium a progestogen should also be administered.

- **Combined approach:** Many different combinations of approaches may be used to administer HRT. For example, oestrogen patches may be used with 14 days of progesterone tablets each month, or oestrogen tablets may be used in a woman with the LNG-IUS, though it is not licensed for this use.

Side effects of hormone replacement therapy

- **Vaginal bleeding:** Unwanted withdrawal bleeds may occur with sequential HRT and irregular bleeding can occur with CCT. This may be managed by altering the oestrogen or progestogen dose, changing to tibolone or considering an LNG-IUS.
- **Oestrogenic effects:** Breast tenderness, nausea and leg cramps may occur with systemic oestrogen. Such symptoms often settle after a few months.
- **Progestogenic effects:** Fluid retention, breast tenderness, headache, acne and greasy skin may occur. These may be intermittent with sequential regimes. Three-monthly sequential preparations, CCT or the LNG-IUS may improve the symptoms.
- **Weight gain:** Weight gain is reported by some women taking HRT, but probably relates to age and lack of exercise rather than to HRT.
- **Contraindications to hormone replacement therapy:** HRT is contraindicated in women with a history of endometrial cancer, undiagnosed vaginal bleeding, thromboembolic disease or thrombophilia and porphyria.

  Relative contraindications are breast cancer, obesity, cardiovascular disease, diabetes, migraine and a family history of deep-vein thrombosis.

  Malignant melanoma contains oestrogen receptors, but there is no current evidence to support avoidance of HRT in these women.
- **Risks of hormone replacement therapy:**
  - *Breast cancer* - There is an overall 26% increase in breast cancer in HRT users. This means an extra eight cases per 10 000 women (38 versus 30 cases). This should be seen in the context of a 1 in 9 background risk of breast cancer by the age of 74.

    The risk increases by 2.3% for each year of HRT use (Table 5.3) and declines to a normal risk 5 years after stopping. The risk is higher for oestrogen and progestogen preparations than for oestrogen alone. The risk of breast cancer with tibolone is somewhere between that of oestrogen alone and that of combined preparations.

    There is no evidence for an increased risk of recurrence if HRT is given after breast cancer and it is occasionally prescribed by specialists, depending on the need in terms of vasomotor or osteoporosis problems and the type of tumour.

Table 5.3. Breast cancer cases per year of hormone replacement therapy (HRT) use

No HRT	45 cases per 1000 women
5-year HRT	47 cases per 1000 women
10-year HRT	51 cases per 1000 women
15-year HRT	57 cases per 1000 women

(Reproduced from Collaborative Group on Hormonal Factors in Breast Cancer. Breast cancer and hormone replacement therapy: collaborative reanalysis of data from 51 epidemiological studies of 52705 women with breast cancer and 108411 women without breast cancer. Lancet 1997; 350: 1047–1059, with permission.)

- *Thrombosis* - The relative risk for venous thromboembolism (VTE) for women on HRT is 2.1–2.7. This means an extra eight cases per 10 000 women per year. The risk of VTE with HRT is probably highest in the first year of use.
- *Endometrial cancer* - The risk of endometrial cancer is increased with unopposed oestrogens and to a lesser extent by sequential regimes. CCT is thought to have a lower risk than oestrogen alone or sequential regimes.
- *Cardiovascular disease* - Cardiovascular morbidity and mortality increase after the menopause and oestrogens appear to reduce this risk in epidemiological studies. However, a recent prospective randomized trial of daily equine oestrogens and medroxyprogesterone acetate showed an increase in cardiovascular events (41% increase in coronary heart disease and CVA, that is, seven extra cases of coronary heart disease and eight extra cases of CVA per 10 000 users). Therefore, HRT should not be prescribed for the prevention of cardiovascular disease or for women with a high risk of cardiovascular disease.

  HRT has no effect on blood pressure in randomized controlled trials.

- Benefits of hormone replacement therapy: Symptom control has been discussed above.
  - *Osteoporosis* - HRT reduces the rate of bone loss in postmenopausal women. Approximately five fewer hip fractures occur per 10 000 women per year. This effect lasts for the duration of therapy and the bone loss restarts once therapy is stopped.
  - *Bowel cancer* - There are six fewer cases of colorectal cancer per 10 000 women per year when HRT is taken.
  - *Alzheimer's disease and rheumatoid arthritis* - HRT is associated with a possible reduction in the incidence of Alzheimer's disease and rheumatoid arthritis.
- Counselling about hormone replacement therapy: All women considering HRT need careful counselling about the risks, benefits and uncertainties. Indications for use are hypo-oestrogenic symptoms and osteoporosis prevention. Many women feel their quality of life is improved overall by HRT, such that the risks are justified. Women with cardiovascular disease, deep-vein thrombosis and breast cancer risks should usually be discouraged from taking HRT.

  Women with premature menopause should be encouraged to take HRT until the age of 50. These women are a different group from those experiencing a normal menopause as their risks from oestrogen deficiency, particularly of osteoporosis, outweigh their risks from HRT. They should be advised that evidence surrounding the risks from HRT applies to older women with much higher background rates of disease and it is generally believed that the risks are lower in younger women undergoing premature menopause.
- Alternatives to hormone replacement therapy: There is no clear evidence for a beneficial effect of evening primrose oil, vitamin E or ginseng for the relief of menopausal symptoms. However, there is evidence of a possible benefit from phyto-oestrogens, plant-derived chemicals with a similar structure to oestrogen. Isoflavones, found in soy products, are one example of a phyto-oestrogen.
  - *Selective oestrogen receptor modulators* - Raloxifene is a selective oestrogen receptor modulator (SERM), which reduces osteoporotic fractures (relative risk 0.5–0.7) and has no adverse effect on the

endometrium. However, it does not help with vasomotor symptoms and has a similar VTE risk to HRT. Tamoxifen is another SERM, but is not used for HRT due to the increased incidence of vaginal bleeding and endometrial cancer.

- *Clonidine* - Clonidine is an alpha-receptor blocker which may be useful for short-term relief of vasomotor symptoms.

Osteoporosis

Osteoporosis is a disease characterized by low bone mass and microarchitectural deterioration of bone tissue. It is a clinically silent disease unless fractures occur as a result of bone fragility. Bone loss accelerates after menopause and one in three women develop fractures over the age of 50. Fractures occur most commonly in the vertebral bodies, hip and wrist.

Risk factors

Particular risk factors for osteoporosis are premature menopause, prolonged amenorrhoea, Cushing's syndrome, thyrotoxicosis, anorexia, family history of osteoporosis, alcohol, long-term heparin and systemic disease (e.g. renal failure).

Dual X-ray absorptiometry is used for diagnosis of osteoporosis and monitoring treatment. Bone mineral density (BMD) is expressed as a standard deviation (SD) score in relation to the reference range and correlates well with fracture risk. Dual X-ray absorptiometry results are expressed as T-scores and Z-scores, for the vertebral body and hip:

- The T-score relates BMD to the young adult range.
- The Z-score relates BMD to sex and age matched controls.
- Osteopenia is defined as BMD 1–2.5 SD below the young adult mean and osteoporosis is defined as BMD 2.5 or more SD below the young adult mean.

Management

All women at risk of osteoporosis and fractures should be offered lifestyle and dietary advice to maximize bone density. Women with established osteoporosis should be treated with HRT or bisphosphonates, after discussion of the risks associated with each. Bone density should be reviewed every 6–12 months to ensure that improvement is occurring.

Lifestyle and diet

The risk of fracture is reduced by weight-bearing exercise (running, climbing stairs). Chronic excessive alcohol is associated with fractures and the normal weekly recommended limits for women should not be exceeded. The evidence does not clearly support a link between smoking and osteoporosis.

Calcium (in dairy products, green leafy vegetables and fish) should be encouraged and supplements of 700 mg/day for osteoporosis prophylaxis or 1000–1500 mg for treatment can be given to those with poor diets. In combination, vitamin D and calcium reduce the risk of fractures by 26% in institutionalized elderly people.

Hormone replacement therapy

HRT has been discussed above and reduces bone loss at the spine by 50% and at the hip by 30%, with a relative risk of 0.66 for fractures when compared with placebo.

Bisphosphonates

Bisphosphonates such as alendronate, risedronate and etidronate decrease bone resorption by inhibiting osteoclasts. They are used for both the prevention and treatment of osteoporosis, with a significant reduction (about 50%) in fracture risk. However, they are difficult to administer, needing to be taken with water, followed by remaining upright for 30 minutes. They also have risks of gastrointestinal side effects such as indigestion, abdominal pain, diarrhoea and peptic ulcers. The once-weekly preparations are preferred.

Calcium supplements and vitamin D should be co-administered with bisphosphonates if dietary intake is insufficient.

Contraception and the menopause

Although fertility declines with age, pregnancy in older women carries significant emotional and medical problems. Woman should be considered fertile for 2 years after the menopause if aged under 50 and 1 year if aged 50 or over, with contraception encouraged until this time. Common methods of contraception in older women are sterilization, IUCDs and the progesterone-only pill.

Premature ovarian failure

Incidence
One per cent of women experience ovarian failure before the age of 40.

Aetiology
Most premature ovarian failure is idiopathic. From 5% to 30% of these women have another affected relative and 10–30% have concurrent auto-immune disease such as hypothyroidism. Spontaneous return of ovarian function does occur in a few women, but it cannot be predicted.

Other causes for premature ovarian failure are genetic (Turner's syndrome, fragile X, Down's syndrome), surgical (bilateral oophorectomy for endometriosis, infection or ovarian cancer prophylaxis), radiotherapy-related or ischaemic (after uterine artery embolization). Chemotherapy for Hodgkin's disease or leukaemia causes ovarian failure in 50% of women.

Clinical features
Amenorrhoea may be present, or the woman may complain of irregular periods or menopausal symptoms such as hot flushes, night sweats or vaginal dryness.

Investigations
The diagnosis of premature ovarian failure is made with a raised FSH (> 30 IU/l) and high LH. The oestradiol may also be low (< 100 pmol/l). The sample should always be repeated at least once to confirm the diagnosis.

Chromosome analysis and autoimmune screen will help to identify any underlying cause of the ovarian failure or associated problems. Dual X-ray absorptiometry should be arranged for a baseline bone density measurement and to monitor treatment.

Ultrasound and ovarian biopsy are not helpful.

Management
The risk of osteoporosis is increased in women with premature ovarian failure. In addition, the psychological and fertility issues are very different from those in women experiencing a normal menopause.

Oestrogen replacement
Oestrogen replacement is given for symptom control, maintenance of bone density and to control periods. It may be given as the COCP or as HRT. Younger women may feel more 'normal' taking the COCP and

having regular bleeds. Older women may be happier with HRT and CCT is suitable for women who would rather avoid bleeding. Treatment until the age of 50 restores the normal background risk of osteoporosis in these women.

Fertility options

It is very rare for natural cycles to return, so assisted conception techniques are the only option for fertility. There is a low probability of success with ovulation stimulation because the ovaries are insensitive to FSH. However, the reported success rate for pregnancy using a donor egg with oestrogen and progesterone support is 30% per cycle.

Psychological issues

Counselling support should be offered to women diagnosed with premature ovarian failure and details given of a support group. Women may experience difficulty with issues of self-esteem, femininity and sexuality as well as fertility.

Summary

- Menorrhagia is one of the commonest presenting complaints to gynaecologists.
- Tranexamic acid is the most effective first-line treatment for menorrhagia.
- The LNG-IUS and endometrial ablation techniques are highly effective after failure of medical treatment for menorrhagia.
- Constitutional delay and Turner's syndrome are the usual causes of primary amenorrhoea.
- Intermenstrual and postcoital bleeding are almost always pathological and should be investigated.
- PCOS can present with a spectrum of clinical, biochemical or ultrasonographic manifestations.
- Subfertility is often multifactorial – male factor (30–50%), ovulatory (30%), tubal (20%) and unexplained (25%).
- Symptom control and osteoporosis prevention are important indications for HRT.
- All women considering HRT need individual assessment and careful counselling about the risks, benefits and uncertainties.
- Osteoporosis prevention is vital for women with premature ovarian failure.

PELVIC PAIN

Pelvic pain is a common reason for referral to a gynaecologist. The origin of the pain may be gynaecological, but non-gynaecological causes such as irritable bowel syndrome (IBS) and constipation can have similar clinical features, including exacerbations in the premenstrual period or during menses. Diagnosis depends on a detailed genitourinary and gastrointestinal as well as gynaecological history. Often no specific cause is identified.

Aetiology

Acute pelvic pain
- Pregnancy-related:
- Ectopic
- Threatened miscarriage
- Miscarriage
- Corpus luteum cyst.
- Non-pregnancy-related:
- Pelvic inflammatory disease (PID)
- Ovarian cyst torsion
- Ovarian cyst haemorrhage or rupture.
- Non-gynaecological:
- Appendicitis
- Appendix abscess
- Urinary tract infection
- Renal colic
- Gastroenteritis.

Chronic pelvic pain
- Gynaecological:
- Endometriosis
- Adhesions from former PID or surgery

- Chronic PID
- Ovarian cysts
- Fibroid degeneration
- Dysmenorrhoea
- Chronic pelvic pain syndrome.
- **Non-gynaecological:**
- Constipation
- IBS
- Urinary tract infection
- Renal calculus
- Functional pain.

Clinical features

Ectopic pregnancy is suggested by pain associated with dizziness, fainting, shoulder pain or collapse.

Ovarian cyst torsion presents with sudden onset of unilateral pain, which is colic-like or twisting and severe. Vomiting is usual and tachycardia, hypotension and pyrexia are found on examination. The pain may be intermittent if torsion is incomplete.

Ovarian cyst rupture presents with constant pain and signs of peritonism, but systemic features are less common.

A full gynaecological and obstetric history is important to make an accurate diagnosis. The diagnosis will often be made by paying particular attention to the nature, timing and associated features of the pain:

- What is the nature, site, type and onset of the pain? Is it constant or intermittent? Is it colic-like?
- What are the exacerbating and relieving factors?
- How does it relate to periods? A 3-month symptom diary is helpful in relating the pain to the hormonal cycle.
- How does the pain vary with defecation or micturition? Are there associated factors such as nausea, vomiting, bloating or malaise?
- A thorough urinary and bowel history is always necessary.
- Is there any significant previous surgical history?
- Is there dyspareunia?
- Is there a history of sexually transmitted infection?
- Is there a history of fertility problems?
- Have there been previous pregnancy complications, such as ectopic, evacuation of retained products of conception or termination of pregnancy?
- Is the woman currently in a relationship? Are there any relationship or sexual problems?
- Is there a history of sexual abuse in childhood or adult life?

Examination

Inspection of the abdomen will identify scars from previous surgery. Abdominal palpation may reveal tenderness, peritonism, masses, renal-angle tenderness or a loaded colon. Sims speculum may show abnormal bleeding or discharge. Bimanual examination features may include cervical motion tenderness ('cervical excitation'), adnexal tenderness, pelvic masses, uterine immobility or uterosacral nodules.

Investigations

All women with acute pelvic pain must have a pregnancy test. Other investigations should be performed according to the history and examination findings and generally include:

- Endocervical swabs and high vaginal swabs for *Chlamydia*, gonorrhoea and *Trichomonas*
- Midstream urine
- Pelvic ultrasound to exclude ovarian cysts, tubal masses or uterine pathology
- Renal tract ultrasound and/or intravenous urogram if a renal cause cannot be excluded.

Laparoscopy is the gold-standard investigation for gynaecological pathology and may reveal adhesions, endometriosis or evidence of PID (dilated, oedematous, tortuous or scarred tubes, with fine filmy adhesions). Fitz-Hugh–Curtis syndrome is the association of perihepatic adhesions (seen at laparoscopy) with previous *Chlamydia* or gonorrhoeal infection and supports the diagnosis of PID as the cause of the pain, even in the absence of obvious tubal damage.

Management

Acute pelvic pain

- **Pelvic pain in early pregnancy:** Women with a positive pregnancy test need urgent ultrasound and serial human chorionic gonadotrophin beta-subunit to exclude an ectopic pregnancy. If an intrauterine pregnancy is confirmed, then the commonest cause of pain is an enlarged or haemorrhagic corpus luteum. This should be identified on ultrasound scan and managed conservatively. Other ovarian cysts, urinary tract infection or appendicitis should also be considered and managed accordingly.
- **Acute pelvic inflammatory disease:** Suspected PID must be managed urgently, as described in Chapter 9. A low threshold for antibiotic treatment is important to minimize complications of tubo-ovarian abscess, chronic pain, subfertility or ectopic pregnancy.
- **Ovarian cyst accident:** Ovarian cyst haemorrhage or rupture is managed conservatively with admission and analgesia. Laparoscopy is indicated if the pain does not settle within 24–48 hours.

  Ovarian cyst torsion should not be missed, as failure to recognize the symptoms and signs may lead to irreversible ischaemia of the ovary. Urgent laparoscopy is indicated, after initial resuscitation, to confirm the diagnosis. Cystectomy may be possible, but signs of ischaemia or necrosis indicate oophorectomy by either laparoscopy or laparotomy.
- **Appendicitis:** Women with appendicitis generally complain of anorexia, malaise, nausea and abdominal pain, which originates centrally and moves to the right iliac fossa. A low-grade pyrexia, tachycardia and localized tenderness and peritonism are clinical signs. The white blood count is usually raised.

  Urgent referral to the general surgical team should be made, and the woman kept fasted, with intravenous fluids and analgesia given. Appendicectomy is performed laparoscopically or through an open procedure using a right iliac fossa incision. The appendix is normal in 10–20% of appendicectomy specimens.

- **Appendix mass and abscess:** An appendix mass forms when an inflamed appendix becomes walled off by omentum and small bowel. This presents with a longer history of several days localized pain and pyrexia. A mass is palpable in the right iliac fossa and the diagnosis is confirmed with ultrasound or computed tomography (CT) scan. Management is conservative with fluids, analgesia and antibiotics, with consideration of appendicectomy after 6–8 weeks.

  An appendix abscess is a collection of pus associated with appendicitis. Management depends on the clinical situation and may involve CT or ultrasound-guided drainage or an open procedure as well as fluids, analgesia and antibiotics.

Chronic pelvic pain

- **Pelvic inflammatory disease:** PID can present with chronic pelvic pain. This may be associated with a history of previous sexually transmitted infection, a change of partner, an abnormal discharge or irregular bleeding. Reinfection may be occurring where a woman who has been treated for PID continues to have unprotected intercourse with an untreated partner. Even where the diagnosis is not certain, a trial of antibiotic treatment can be helpful, with appropriate treatment for the partner and avoidance of unprotected intercourse until treatment for both partners has been completed.

- **Adhesions:** Adhesions may be present as a result of previous infection or surgery. The benefit of division of adhesions to relieve pelvic pain is not clear, but it is likely to be more helpful in women with severe adhesions and where division is performed laparoscopically. Adhesiolysis is associated with a high risk of visceral damage. The development of further adhesions is common after adhesiolysis, especially if an open (rather than laparoscopic) approach is used.

- **Ovarian cysts (see Chapter 7):** Ovarian cysts are managed according to the symptoms and investigation findings. Simple cysts should be managed conservatively and usually resolve spontaneously over 6–12 weeks. However, persistent pain is an indication for cystectomy. Endometriomas and dermoid cysts may be managed expectantly if small, but should be removed, preferably laparoscopically, if there is persistent pain or subfertility.

  Suspicious ultrasound features of ovarian cysts or raised cancer antigen 125 (CA 125) are also indications for surgical removal.

- **Fibroids (see Chapter 7):** Fibroids do not normally cause pain. However, they may be painful where the size of the fibroid causes a pressure effect, where the fibroid is degenerating or where an intracavity fibroid is being expelled from the uterus. Myomectomy should be performed for intracavity fibroids causing pain or for large fibroids causing a pressure effect. Fibroid degeneration is managed conservatively initially, with analgesia, fluids and antibiotics, but persistent or recurrent pain is an indication for surgery.

- **Chronic pelvic pain syndrome:** Chronic pelvic pain syndrome is long-term pelvic pain with no identifiable pathology at laparoscopy. The aetiology of chronic pelvic pain syndrome is poorly understood. Theories include undiagnosed IBS, congested dilated pelvic veins (pelvic congestion syndrome), disordered neurological signalling to the spinal cord (where normal sensation is perceived as painful) and functional pain.

Effective treatment options are laparoscopic uterosacral nerve ablation (effective in 30–90%), antidepressants and counselling.

- **Irritable bowel syndrome:** IBS affects up to 20% of people in the UK, with three times as many women affected as men. Diagnosis is clinical (after excluding other pathology) and symptoms include constipation, diarrhoea, pelvic pain, passage of mucus with the stool and bloating. The symptoms are often worse with eating, defecation, stress and in the premenstrual period. Treatment is with antispasmodic agents (e.g. mebeverine hydrochloride) for pain; antimotility agents (e.g. loperamide) for diarrhoea; and bulk-forming laxatives (e.g. ispaghula husk) for constipation, and increased dietary fibre may be of benefit.
- **Constipation:** Many women with pelvic pain are constipated and a detailed gastrointestinal history will elucidate this. On examination a palpable loaded colon may be present. Treatment is with laxatives and suppositories as well as dietary and fluid modification.
- **Urinary tract infection/interstitial cystitis/renal calculi:** Recurrent infections and irritative bladder symptoms are often associated with bladder pain. Thorough questioning about urinary symptoms is essential in a woman presenting with pelvic pain. Investigations should include urine microscopy and culture, and if necessary, cystoscopy and biopsy to exclude interstitial cystitis. Calculi may be identified in the ureters or bladder by ultrasound or intravenous urogram. Referral to the urologist should be made accordingly for treatment.
- **Functional pain:** All women undergoing investigation for pelvic pain should be informed that no specific cause might be found. This reassures most women and spontaneous resolution of symptoms is not uncommon. If pain persists, sensitive questioning around social and sexual circumstances may reveal an underlying problem, such as relationship difficulties, sexual abuse history or fears around sexuality or fertility.

ENDOMETRIOSIS

Definition

Endometriosis is the presence of functioning endometrial tissue outside the cavity of the uterus.

Incidence

Twenty-one per cent of women with infertility, 15% of women with chronic abdominal pain and 6% of women undergoing sterilization have endometriosis at laparoscopy.

Age

Endometriosis is most common in the 25–35-year age group, but can occur at any age from menarche until the menopause, or later if the woman is taking hormone replacement.

Aetiology

Various theories exist about the development of endometriosis:
- Retrograde menstruation
- Developmental (coelomic metaplasia)
- Immunological.

Retrograde menstruation is the passage of menstrual debris, containing endometrial cells, along the fallopian tubes to the peritoneal cavity. The cells are thought to adhere to the peritoneal surfaces and proliferate. This is the most likely aetiology. However, retrograde menstruation occurs in up to 90% of women and it is, therefore, likely that the development of endometriosis also depends on individual local peritoneal immunological factors.

Coelomic metaplasia is a more likely theory for endometriosis development at sites outside the pelvis.

There is also increasing evidence for a complex genetic predisposition to endometriosis.

Pathology

Endometriosis usually involves deposits of endometrial tissue anywhere in the pelvis, commonly the ovaries, uterosacral ligaments or ovarian fossae. Extrapelvic sites include operation scars, the vagina, the ureters, the bladder, the bowel, the umbilicus and, rarely, the lungs. Endometriomas (chocolate cysts) occur when the blood shed forms an encapsulated collection, usually on the ovary or in the pouch of Douglas. Adhesions are common from the monthly intraperitoneal bleeding.

History

The classic presentation is dyspareunia, dysmenorrhoea and subfertility. Non-menstrual pelvic pain may occur if adhesions or an endometrioma is present. Cyclical haematuria, rectal bleeding or haemoptysis can occur with endometriosis from other sites. The severity of disease at laparoscopy relates poorly to the symptoms reported and many women are asymptomatic.

Examination

Abdominal palpation

Tenderness is common. An endometrioma may be palpable as a mass if large. Vaginal endometriosis can be seen as blue nodules on speculum examination. Uterosacral nodules, endometriomas, adnexal tenderness or a fixed retroverted uterus may be palpated bimanually.

Investigations

Transvaginal ultrasound may suggest the presence of an endometrioma (ground-glass appearance) or a fixed retroverted uterus, and exclude other causes of a pelvic mass, but is not diagnostic for endometriosis.

Laparoscopy is needed to confirm the diagnosis, which is clinical, though biopsies may be indicated for unusual appearances.

Laparoscopic appearances include:

- Blue or black powder burn lesions
- Red, blue or white papular or flat lesions
- Peritoneal scarring and fenestrations ('peritoneal windows')
- Endometriomas
- Frozen pelvis (fixed, immobile uterus with dense adhesions to ovaries and tubes and obliterated pouch of Douglas).

The commonest sites of endometriosis are the ovaries, uterosacral ligaments and pouch of Douglas.

Endometriosis may be classified as stage I–IV by the revised American Fertility Society Score, according to the severity and extent of the disease at laparoscopy. More commonly, the laparoscopic findings are recorded diagrammatically and a judgement of mild, moderate or severe endometriosis assigned. Figure 6.1 illustrates some typical patterns of endometriosis found at laparoscopy.

Treatment

Treatment should be based on age, fertility wishes, location of disease, severity of symptoms and patient choice.

Medical

- **Analgesia:** Non-steroidal anti-inflammatory drugs may be effective for mild symptoms.
- **Hormonal medical treatment:** All hormonal treatments have an 80–90% rate of improvement of endometriosis symptoms. However, symptoms may recur within 12–24 months of stopping treatment. The recurrence rate after completion of medical treatment is up to 74% for severe disease.

   Hormonal medical treatment inhibits cyclical hormonal stimulation and causes atrophy of endometriotic tissue. Most treatments have significant side effects and long-term treatment is contraindicated for gonadotrophin-releasing hormone (GnRH) analogues and danazol or gestrinone.

   There is no difference in efficacy of treatments and a few women will not respond to any medical treatments. If an endometrioma is suspected, then medical treatment should not be first-line management.

   Fertility is not improved by hormonal treatments, all of which delay conception further.
- **Combined oral contraceptive pill:** The combined oral contraceptive pill suppresses ovulation and, therefore, inhibits cyclical stimulation of endometriosis, but is more effective if the monthly withdrawal bleed is omitted by taking three packs continuously (tri-cycling). It is reasonable to attempt a trial of therapy prior to laparoscopy for symptom control in a woman who is not attempting pregnancy and in whom a pelvic mass is not suspected.
- **Progestogens:** Continuous progestogens, such as medroxyprogesterone acetate, dydrogesterone and norethisterone, either oral or as depot form, are as effective as GnRH analogues and danazol for short-term pain relief. In the oral form they may be given continuously or cyclically (3-week course followed by a 1-week break). Medroxyprogesterone acetate can be given in the depot form, though this may delay ovulation for up to 18 months after stopping treatment, thus delaying fertility. Progestogens may be suitable for long-term management in women who are not planning to become pregnant.
- **Gonadotrophin-releasing hormone analogues:** GnRH analogues (leuprorelin, buserelin, nafarelin and goserelin) suppress gonadotrophin release from the anterior pituitary, thus interrupting the cyclical stimulation of endometriotic tissue. They are given subcutaneously or intranasally. Side effects include menopausal symptoms and loss of bone density (6% reduction over 6 months' treatment, which is reversed within 9 months of stopping treatment). Add-back hormone replacement therapy can be given to treat the menopausal symptoms and prevent the loss of bone density, without reducing efficacy.

Essentials of Obstetrics and Gynaecology

Mild

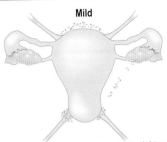

Superficial deposits on uterosacral ligaments, right ovary and uterovesical fold of peritoneum

Moderate

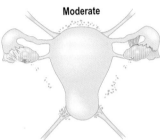

Superficial deposits on uterosacral ligaments and uterosacral fold of peritoneum. Deep deposits on left ovary with adhesions between fimbrial portion of tube and the ovary. Few adhesions between right ovary and tube

Severe

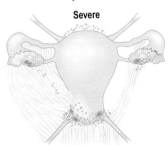

Dense adhesions and obliteration of the pouch of Douglas. Deep endometriosis on both ovaries. Dense adhesions in the left adnexa and moderate adhesions between right tube and pouch of Douglas. Endometrial deposits in uterovesical fold of peritoneum

Figure 6.1 Typical patterns of endometriosis found at laparoscopy.

Endometriomas may shrink by 20% with GnRH analogues, but surgical treatment should be first-line management of endometriomas if symptomatic or if fertility treatment is anticipated.

- **Antiandrogens:** Danazol and gestrinone are oral antiandrogens with antioestrogen and antiprogestogen properties. They inhibit endometriosis by inhibiting ovulation and directly suppressing the endometrial tissue. Side effects occur in 80% and include acne, hirsutism, weight gain and mood changes. Voice-lowering is a rare, but irreversible, side effect of treatment. They are not commonly used now as other treatments are equally effective, with better side effect profiles.

Surgical

- **Laparoscopic diathermy/laser ablation or excision:** The aim is to excise or ablate all visible endometriotic deposits and restore normal anatomy as far as possible. Care must be taken to avoid damage to other pelvic structures, particularly the ureters and rectum. From 60% to 70% of women experience cure or improvement in symptoms, more so if the disease was severe at the time of laparoscopy. Postoperative medical therapy may further improve the outcome for some women after laparoscopic treatment.

- **Surgical excision:** Endometrioma excision should be performed laparoscopically where possible. Cystectomy is the aim, but where this is not possible, the cyst is drained, fenestrated and the capsule ablated. Rarely, laparotomy is needed for cystectomy if adhesions are severe or the cyst is very large. Spillage of endometrioma contents is very irritable to the peritoneum and vigorous saline washout of the cavity should be performed if this occurs, with consideration of postoperative medical suppressive therapy.

- **Laparoscopic uterosacral nerve ablation:** Division of the uterosacral nerves by diathermy or laser is effective for 70–90% of women with chronic pelvic pain from endometriosis.

- **Total abdominal hysterectomy:** This is usually a last resort for patients with endometriosis. Bilateral salpingo-oophorectomy should also be performed to prevent the continued cyclical oestrogen and progestogen stimulation to any microscopic residual deposits of disease. Women under the age of 50 need hormone replacement therapy after bilateral salpingo-oophorectomy, and this should be a continuous combined preparation, as unopposed oestrogen may stimulate any residual endometriosis.

Support

Women with endometriosis should be given clear information about the disease and treatment options. Support groups are also helpful sources of information and psychological benefit.

Fertility

Endometriosis is associated with infertility, even where there is no demonstrable tubal blockage. Surgical treatment improves the fertility rate by 13% for mild to moderate disease, but not severe disease. Medical treatment does not improve the chance of pregnancy and prolongs the time to possible conception, as all medical hormonal treatments are contraceptive. In vitro fertilization is commonly indicated.

Prognosis

Endometriosis may recur after medical or surgical treatment and tends to regress spontaneously after the menopause.

ADENOMYOSIS

Adenomyosis is defined as the presence of functional endometrial tissue within the myometrium of the uterus. It may be focal or diffuse and occurs more commonly in the posterior uterine wall. It is found in 15–25% of hysterectomy specimens, whether pelvic pain had been a feature in the history or not.

It tends to occur in women over 35 years and it may be found in association with fibroids. Risk factors are parity, previous termination of pregnancy and previous caesarean section. Clinical features are predominantly severe dysmenorrhoea with a slightly bulky soft uterus.

The diagnosis can only be confirmed histologically after hysterectomy; however, the condition may be suspected on ultrasound or magnetic resonance imaging scan.

If adenomyosis is suspected, analgesia or medical suppression may be tried as for endometriosis. The only definitive surgical treatment is hysterectomy, though endometrial resection and shelling-out of diffuse areas of suspected disease have been attempted.

MINIMAL-ACCESS SURGERY

Minimal-access surgery (MAS) is the term used for surgical procedures where instruments are inserted through small access points and fibreoptic telescopes are used to facilitate diagnostic or therapeutic procedures without major incisions.

MAS aims to minimize the insult to the patient without compromising the safety or effectiveness of the treatment.

The advantages of MAS are reduced pain, reduced length of time in hospital, faster return to work, cost-effectiveness and a better cosmetic appearance.

The disadvantages are the specific surgical risks associated with minimal-access procedures, the training needed for the operator and the equipment investment needed.

Laparoscopy

Laparoscopy is the visualization of the abdominal viscera via a telescope inserted through a small incision in the anterior abdominal wall (usually just below the umbilicus), with carbon dioxide insufflation of the peritoneal cavity. The image is usually transmitted via a camera to a monitor. Other instruments may be inserted into the operative field through secondary entry sites in the abdominal wall. The procedure may be used for diagnostic purposes or for visualization during a therapeutic procedure. The procedure is performed under general anaesthetic, usually in a day-surgery unit.

The uses of laparoscopy in gynaecology are shown in Table 6.1.

Preoperative counselling

Preoperative counselling should cover the following points:

- Indication for the procedure – Is this the appropriate operation? Has the clinical situation changed since the outpatient consultation? If there was an ovarian cyst, has a repeat scan been performed to check it has not resolved?

Table 6.1. Uses of laparoscopy in gynaecology

Diagnostic uses of laparoscopy:
Pelvic pain (acute or chronic)
Subfertility (to assess for endometriosis and to look for spill of dye during a dye test)
Suspected ectopic pregnancy

Therapeutic uses of laparoscopy:
Sterilization
Adhesiolysis
Diathermy/laser/excision of endometriosis
Salpingectomy (ectopic pregnancy, hydrosalpinx)
Salpingotomy (ectopic pregnancy, hydrosalpinx)
Ovarian cystectomy
Oophorectomy
Myomectomy
Colposuspension
Laparoscopically assisted vaginal hysterectomy
Lymphadenectomy

- Last menstrual period: all premenopausal women should have a pregnancy test on the day of the procedure. If it is negative and they have had unprotected sex, they must be warned about the potential risk of instrumentation of the uterus to a very early pregnancy.
- Proposed procedure: women need an explanation of the proposed procedure, the reasons for it and the possible findings. It should be explained that images are printed out for the medical records and to help the patient understand the findings.
- Possible findings: it should be explained that laparoscopy is often normal in women with pelvic pain.
- Complications of the procedure and how they may be dealt with (laparotomy).
- Likely postoperative symptoms (e.g. pain, bleeding).
- Follow-up plans.

Technique

The essential steps involved with the basic laparoscopy procedure are the following:

- Ensure the woman has been fully counselled about the proposed procedure, reasons and risks for the operation, with informed consent given.
- Place patient level on the operating table with the legs at 45°; clean and drape the abdomen.
- Clean the external genitalia and vagina and catheterize.
- Examine bimanually to assess for uterine position, mobility, size and any pelvic masses.
- With a Sims speculum inserted along the posterior vaginal wall, insert an instrument (ideally, a Spackman-style) through the cervix into the uterine cavity for manipulation during the procedure and then remove the speculum.
- Check the instruments (light source, Veress needle, gas supply, trocar, laparoscope, any electrocautery equipment).
- Make a small vertical or horizontal infraumbilical incision (depending on the size of the trocar and laparoscope to be used, usually 5–10 mm) with a scalpel.

- Insert the Veress needle at 45° (towards the sacral promontory) and check the position by hearing a 'double click' as it passes through the rectus sheath and the peritoneum, saline test and by checking the gas flow and pressure once connected.
- Insufflate with carbon dioxide until the intra-abdominal pressure reaches 18 mmHg.
- Remove the Veress needle and insert the trocar through the same incision (the anterior abdominal wall can be lifted or pressure exerted superiorly to enhance tension).
- Remove the introducer from the trocar and insert the laparoscope. Once the correct position is confirmed then attach and switch on the gas, aiming for an operating pressure of 14–18 mmHg.
- Place the patient in the Trendelenburg position (head down).
- Under direct vision, insert secondary ports, commonly in the right or left iliac fossae, lateral to the inferior epigastric vessels or in the suprapubic region. These can be used for graspers, irrigation, scissors, diathermy or drains.

Closure of the wounds

- Secondary ports should be removed under direct vision to check for bleeding from the sites and for any entrapment of bowel or fat in the port site.
- Expel as much gas as possible through the trocar.
- Close the rectus sheath where the incisions are greater than 5 mm (except at the umbilicus).
- Close skin wounds with skin glue, absorbable sutures or Steri-strips.
- Remove the manipulator from the vagina.

Postoperative management

- Intraoperative and postoperative analgesia should be given as required.
- In recovery the woman is encouraged to eat and drink as soon as she feels ready.
- When the woman has had something to eat and drink, passed urine and is not in severe pain, she can usually be discharged within 2–4 hours.
- A 5-day course of paracetamol and non-steroidal anti-inflammatories (or dihydrocodeine) is usually sufficient for pain management and the patient should be advised about shoulder-tip pain, from peritoneal irritation by gas.

Complications

The overall complication rate is 6 per 1000 procedures. These include anaesthetic risks, infection (wound or urinary tract) and visceral (bowel or bladder) or vascular injury (port entry sites or major vessels). The risk of visceral or vascular injury is 0.6–1% for diagnostic procedures and 0.9–1.8% for therapeutic procedures.

Safety in laparoscopy

Important safety factors include the following:

- Checking the instruments.
- Good visualization. There may be a problem with the lens, light source or monitor. Alternatively, blood within the abdominal cavity may be absorbing light and decreasing view. The operating doctor or assistant should ensure that the area of interest and all instruments are at the centre of the view at all times.

- Alternative entry techniques. Where adhesions are suspected an open entry can be used (Hasson technique). Alternatively, Palmer's point can be used for entry, 2 cm below the left costal margin in the mid clavicular line, after excluding splenomegaly.

Contraindications

Absolute contraindications to laparoscopy are hypovolaemic shock, intestinal obstruction, a large abdominal mass and severe cardiac disease. Relative contraindications are peritonitis, obesity, previous major or multiple abdominal surgery, bleeding disorders and anaesthetic risks (e.g. heart disease or obstructive airways disease).

Electrosurgery in laparoscopy

Electrosurgery (diathermy, electrocautery) uses electrical energy to coagulate or cut tissues.

Risks from diathermy include capacitive coupling, direct coupling and thermal injury.

Risks are minimized by using equipment with an alarm system, ensuring correct positioning of the plate, using the lowest power setting needed for the surgery being performed, checking the insulation on the equipment before use and regular service checks.

- **Unipolar:** The electrical current returns to the ground electrode through the body and via the plate, usually positioned on the patient's thigh. A greater heat is produced around the operating area and the risk of visceral injury by thermal damage is, therefore, higher.
- **Bipolar:** The electrical current passes between the jaws of the forceps only. The surrounding thermal damage, for example causing bowel injury, is lower and the technique is safer. Bipolar diathermy should be used where possible.

Lasers in laparoscopy

Laser (light amplification by stimulated emission of radiation) uses a concentrated beam of light to cut or coagulate tissue. The advantages are that the laser is very precise and peripheral tissue damage is minimal. It is used most commonly during laparoscopy for adhesiolysis, ablation of endometriosis and uterosacral nerve ablation in women with pelvic pain. However, it can also be effective for salpingotomy in infertility management.

Different types of laser have different tissue penetration depths.

Hysteroscopy

Hysteroscopy is the use of a telescope through the cervix to visualize the uterine cavity. Diagnostic hysteroscopy is usually performed in the outpatient clinic, with or without local anaesthetic. Therapeutic procedures are generally performed under general anaesthetic in a day surgery unit.

Table 6.2 shows the diagnostic and therapeutic uses of hysteroscopy.

Preprocedure counselling

Preprocedure consultation should cover the following points:

- All premenopausal women must have a pregnancy test on the day of the procedure. If it is negative and they have had unprotected sex since the last menstrual period, they must be warned about the potential risk of instrumentation of the uterus to a very early pregnancy.
- Last menstrual period: menstruation at the time of hysteroscopy interferes with the operative view and theoretically increases the chance of

Table 6.2. Uses of hysteroscopy
Diagnostic uses of hysteroscopy:
Investigation of postmenopausal bleeding
Investigation of intermenstrual bleeding
Suspected polyp on ultrasound
Suspected uterine abnormality associated with infertility or miscarriage
Therapeutic uses of hysteroscopy:
Retrieval of an intrauterine contraceptive device
Resection of fibroid
Resection of a polyp
Resection of the endometrium
Resection of a septum (metroplasty)
Division of intrauterine adhesions (Asherman's syndrome)

retrograde flow of menstrual blood through the fallopian tubes, causing endometriosis. However, in some cases of intractable bleeding, not responsive to progestogen treatment, hysteroscopy may still be performed.

- The woman should have an explanation of the nature of the proposed procedure, the indication for it and the possible or expected findings.
- Explain that images will be printed or stored for the medical records and for the woman to see.
- Advise that the procedure takes only a few minutes, but that she may expect pain or discomfort during an outpatient hysteroscopy, similar to period pain, from dilatation of the cervical canal and spill of fluid into the peritoneal cavity through the fallopian tubes.
- Inform the woman of the rare complications of hysteroscopy.
- Explain that the woman should expect bleeding for up to 1 week after the procedure and may pass debris after a resection procedure.
- Simple analgesia may need to be taken for up to 24 hours.
- Explain that antibiotic prophylaxis is needed for women under 40 years.

Technique

The essential steps in the basic hysteroscopy procedure are:

- Place the patient in the Lloyd Davis position (and clean the vagina in an anaesthetized patient). Catheterization is not indicated.
- Insert a Cusco's speculum (and gently clean the vagina in a conscious patient).
- If indicated, inject the cervix with local anaesthetic with adrenaline (epinephrine) at the 12, 3, 6 and 9 o'clock positions.
- Grasp the anterior lip of the cervix using a vulsellum forceps or tenaculum.
- Depending on the diameter of the hysteroscope, dilate the cervix.
- Insert the hysteroscope with the gas or saline flowing and guide it along the cervical canal under direct vision.
- Inspect the uterine cavity, rotating the lens to visualize the tubal ostia (cornu) and anterior and posterior walls. Observe for polyps, submucous fibroids, adhesions or irregular lesions suggestive of malignancy.
- Visualize the cervical canal carefully as the hysteroscope is removed from the uterus.

Distension media

The uterine cavity is distended with saline or gas for diagnostic procedures and glycine for procedures where electrosurgery is anticipated.

Types of hysteroscope

Flexible hysteroscopes are generally of smaller diameter and more appropriate when dilatation of the cervix is difficult or if the cervix is atrophic or scarred. They are likely to cause less discomfort for the patient. However, the image may be less clear than with a rigid hysteroscope. Rigid hysteroscopes are always used for operative hysteroscopy.

Hysteroscopes vary from about 3 to 10 mm diameter. Smaller-diameter hysteroscopes are less painful to insert, but may give a more limited view and generally cannot be used in conjunction with instruments. The direction of view is usually 30° for diagnostic procedures and 12° for resection procedures.

All hysteroscopes have ports for fluid or gas input. Most also have outflow ports for effective irrigation of blood or debris from the field of view.

Operating hysteroscopes have channels for simple procedures such as inserting graspers for removal of a lost intrauterine contraceptive device. A resectoscope consists of a telescope, an attachment for electrosurgical instruments (e.g. resection loop, hook or rollerball) and inflow and outflow tracts for fluid distension and irrigation.

Antibiotic prophylaxis

All women of reproductive age should be screened for infections prior to a hysteroscopy. Any sexually transmitted infection should be treated prior to the procedure and consideration should be given to antibiotic prophylaxis for all premenopausal women.

A suggested prophylaxis regime is azithromycin (1 gram), given orally as a single dose.

Complications

- **Haemorrhage:** Haemorrhage may occur with resection procedures, especially transcervical resection of fibroids. This is usually controlled with electrocautery. In cases of intractable bleeding, a Foley catheter is inserted and the balloon inflated in the uterine cavity to create a tamponade effect. This is then removed after 12 hours.
- **Infection:** Endometritis and PID occur in less than 1% of women after hysteroscopy, but antibiotic prophylaxis should be used in all premenopausal women.
- **Cervical shock:** Instrumentation and dilatation of the cervix can induce a vagal response. This is associated, in the conscious patient, with dizziness and nausea and may result in loss of consciousness. The patient is bradycardic and hypotensive, but recovers when the instrument is removed. Treatment with atropine is rarely required.
- **False passage:** A false passage through the cervix may occur during difficult dilatation. It is diagnosed by visualization of a blind-ending canal when the hysteroscope is inserted. Occasionally, the false passage may go through to the peritoneal cavity and the features and management are as for perforation of the uterus.
- **Uterine perforation:** The instrument (dilator or hysteroscope) may pass through the uterus, most commonly into the pouch of Douglas. It is usually noticed by an abnormal feel and sudden loss of view as the distension fluid floods out into the peritoneal space. In most cases damage will be minimal if perforation is mechanical. However, if electrocautery

Essentials of Obstetrics and Gynaecology

is in use, then there is a more significant chance of damage to other structures. Laparoscopy must always be performed to check for uterine bleeding and bladder, bowel or vessel injury.

Occasionally, perforation is not noted at the time of the procedure and the woman may present with abdominal pain, pyrexia and systemic disturbance in the next few days. Ultrasound or CT scan may confirm the presence of free blood in the pouch of Douglas or haematoma around the uterus. Any suggestion of bowel injury necessitates urgent surgical review.

- **Fluid overload:** Operative hysteroscopy uses a non-electrolytic fluid (usually glycine) for distension and irrigation of the cavity. However, this fluid may be absorbed into the circulation through the open blood vessels within the myometrium, thus causing hyponatraemia. Prevention involves strict monitoring of fluid input and output with a continuous calculation of the presumed fluid absorbed. The procedure should be stopped once the fluid deficit exceeds 1000 ml. The management of fluid overload is mainly supportive with strict fluid balance recording, monitoring of electrolytes and treatment of any ensuing pulmonary oedema.

Contraindications

The absolute contraindications for hysteroscopy are acute endometritis, PID and pregnancy.

SUMMARY

- Pelvic pain is a common symptom, with both gynaecological and non-gynaecological causes. Genitourinary, gastrointestinal and gynaecological features are all important in the history.
- Pregnancy (and ectopic) must be excluded in all women with acute pelvic pain.
- Laparoscopy is the main diagnostic tool for women with pelvic pain.
- Endometriosis is a major cause of pelvic pain and infertility.
- The severity of symptoms of endometriosis correlates poorly with the extent of disease found at laparoscopy.
- All medical treatments for endometriosis have similar efficacy.
- Surgical treatment for endometriosis is more effective than medical treatment, especially in women wishing to become pregnant.
- All women undergoing hysteroscopy or laparoscopy should have a pregnancy test on the day of the procedure.

Problems of the female genital tract   7

CHAPTER CONTENTS

BENIGN CONDITIONS OF THE VULVA

Bartholin's cyst

Bartholin's glands are located on the posterolateral aspects of the introitus. Cysts can often be asymptomatic, but can become infected and result in pain, dyspareunia and often discomfort on sitting. If unresolved after a course of antibiotics, the infected cyst may need to be opened, drained and marsupialized under anaesthetic. Marsupialization involves a series of sutures between the cyst edge and vagina so that the cyst is left open to heal by secondary intention. Rarely, a recurrent cyst may need to be excised completely, although this is best done when the infection has resolved.

Vulvodynia

Definition

Vulvodynia is the term used to describe a specific type of vulval pain characterized by burning, stinging, irritation or rawness. However, the majority of women presenting with vulval symptoms will complain of pruritus.

Assessment

Management is aimed at identifying the cause and treating appropriately. A full history must include information about previous treatments, other skin or systemic disorders, hygiene measures, drugs taken and allergies known. Examination should include inspection of skin surfaces, the mouth, hands and nails, and palpation of the inguinal nodes. The vulva, including the mons pubis and the perianal skin, the vagina, urethral meatus and cervix should be inspected. Colposcopy of the vulva can define lesions that are not otherwise visible and a biopsy should be performed if epithelial abnormalities are suspected.

Causes of vulvodynia include vulvar dermatoses and vulvar vestibulitis.

Dermatoses

The dermatoses are classified as non-neoplastic epithelial disorders of the skin and mucosa, and they are outlined below.

Eczema

Allergic responses to substances such as perfume or washing powders can result in an acutely red, swollen, sharply demarcated area that is not only extremely itchy, but also may cause a burning raw sensation. Secondary infection leads to a wet, painful, often offensive-smelling lesion. Treatment is by removing the irritant or allergen and controlling the symptoms with soothing applications, bland emollients, local corticosteroid creams and appropriate therapy for secondary infection.

Lichen planus

This is usually idiopathic, but may be drug-related. Lesions occur in any keratinized skin and are flat, papular and purplish in colour. If the condition is erosive, the inner aspects of the vulva and vagina are affected: the vagina becomes friable with risk of adhesions and stenosis developing. Treatment is with potent steroids topically, or systemically with the addition of azathioprine.

Lichen sclerosus

The symptoms and signs are variable and may affect any age group and should always be considered in young women with dyspareunia. There is usually a long history of vulval irritation or pain and the affected area is usually thin and parchment-like. The affected areas may fuse together with associated genital atrophy. The treatment is with topical steroids or testosterone cream, often requiring maintenance therapy. If not resolving after first-line treatment, then a biopsy should be performed. There is a risk of progression to vulval carcinoma in 5–10% of cases and so patients should be followed up regularly with repeated biopsy of suspicious changes.

Vulvar vestibulitis

This is a very difficult condition to treat and is a diagnosis of exclusion. There are three cardinal criteria for this diagnosis: pain on entry or touch, vestibular erythema and tenderness to pressure.

Management of acute vulvar vestibulitis is medical, with the removal of any allergen or irritant, treatment of infection and local corticosteroid application. Treatment with a topical steroid preparation containing antifungal and antibacterial components (Trimovate) may relieve symptoms.

Vulvar intraepithelial neoplasia

Vulvar intraepithelial neoplasia (VIN) is a condition in which atypical or neoplastic cells are present within the boundaries of the surface epithelium of the vulva. Like its cervical counterpart (cervical intraepithelial neoplasia (CIN)), VIN has been divided into three categories depending on the extent of epithelial involvement and is also associated with CIN in around one-quarter of cases. VIN is uncommon, although it is believed that its incidence is increasing, particularly in young women. As well as the association with CIN there is also an association with human papillomavirus and lichen sclerosus. There are also strong associations between sexually transmitted diseases and VIN, in particular condyloma, herpes simplex, gonorrhoea, syphilis, trichomoniasis and *Gardnerella vaginalis*.

Clinical features
- Symptoms:
- Pruritus, present in 38–73% of cases
- Vulval pain/soreness
- Occasionally it can present with a vulval lump or lesions, often in the perianal region
- It can be asymptomatic, with many lesions detected at routine gynaecological examination.
- Physical signs: Clinical manifestations of VIN are highly variable, from papular (wart-like) or macular with irregular borders. Brown or black pigmentation of these lesions is common.

White lesions reflect hyperkeratosis and are commonly seen in the keratinized portion of the vulva.

Diagnosis

Diagnosis of VIN is made on microscopy and, therefore, a biopsy, which can be performed under local anaesthesia, is always required. Thorough assessment of the whole lower genital tract, including cervical cytology and colposcopy, is mandatory in patients with VIN.

Circumstances where excisional biopsies should be considered, rather than limited sampling, are:
- Elevated lesions, irregular surfaces
- Areas with distinct vascular patterns, e.g. mosaic, abnormal vessels
- Excessive hyperkeratosis in hair-bearing areas
- Pigmented lesions
- Elderly women with unifocal lesions.

Management

Management of VIN should be individualized, taking into consideration the presence or absence of symptoms and whether risk factors are present, i.e. postmenopausal presentation, immunosuppressed/immunodeficient patients, women with histologically progressive lesions on serial biopsy or excessively hyperkeratotic lesions.

If the risk of invasion is thought to be low and malignancy is excluded, then major vulval surgery can be avoided. Options include topical 5 fluorouracil, dinitrochlorobenzene, cryosurgery, carbon dioxide laser ablation, vulvectomy and wide local excision.

Small lesions can be dealt with in the outpatient clinic using local anaesthesia. Large areas of VIN require general anaesthesia for laser treatment.

CARCINOMA OF THE VULVA

This accounts for approximately 5% of genital tract cancers, with just over 1000 cases diagnosed in the UK each year. It is most common (over 80% of cases) after the menopause in the 60–70-year age group, although it can occur in younger women with a history of premalignant VIN.

The majority are squamous cell in origin, with the remainder including the rarer lesions of melanoma, basal cell carcinoma, sarcoma and adenocarcinomas of the Bartholin's gland.

Clinical features

Patients will usually experience symptoms of pruritus, bleeding or discharge or may present with a vulval mass. Examination will reveal an ulcer or mass, usually on the labia majora or clitoris, and often palpable inguinal lymph nodes.

FIGO staging

Staging is performed following surgical removal and histological assessment. Approximately one-half present with stage 1 disease and spread is via the lymphatic drainage of the vulva to the superficial and then deep inguinal nodes, and finally to the external iliac nodes. Pelvic lymph node spread is slow and will, therefore, indicate advanced disease with poor prognosis.

- Stage 0 – carcinoma in situ (preinvasive)
- Stage 1 – tumour confined to vulva or vulva and perineum <2cm in diameter with no nodal involvement
  - stage 1a – stromal invasion <1mm
  - stage 1b – stromal invasion >1mm with negative nodes
- Stage 2 – tumour >2cm in diameter with no nodal involvement
- Stage 3 – spread of tumour to urethra, vagina or anus or unilateral involvement of nodes. This stage has been subdivided into A, B or C according to number and nature of lymph node metastases. These changes reflect the fact that the number of nodes involved is a more significant prognostic factor than fully resected local disease
- Stage 4 – tumour within rectum, bladder, bone or distant metastases and bilateral nodal involvement.

Investigations

A biopsy is taken for histological diagnosis. Following diagnosis, the patient is prepared for surgery with routine bloods (including full blood count, urea and electrolytes, group and crossmatch) and chest X-ray and electrocardiograph. For tumours >2cm, computed tomography (CT) of chest, abdomen and pelvis can detect disease above the inguinal ligament.

Management

In stage 1a carcinoma, a wide local excision is appropriate with regular follow-up. In all other stages, a wide local excision and lymphadenectomy should be carried out. Sentinel lymph node mapping (the sentinel node receives the primary lymphatic drainage from the tumour) can be performed peroperatively as part of the staging procedure in order to reduce morbidity of radical lymphadenectomy. If the lesion is greater than 2 cm from the midline, then a unilateral inguinal lymphadenectomy is appropriate, but if <2 cm from the midline, a bilateral inguinal lymphadenectomy should be performed. This type of surgery can cause postoperative problems with wound breakdown, infection and lymphoedema.

Radiotherapy can be considered in cases of local recurrence or nodal disease but chemotherapy is rarely used, except in younger patients with positive nodes.

Prognosis

For stage 1 carcinoma the 5-year survival rate is 80%; it is 50% for stage 2, 30% for stage 3 and 10–15% for stage 4.

BENIGN CONDITIONS OF THE CERVIX

The outer surface of the cervix within the vagina is covered with stratified squamous epithelium, which becomes columnar within the cervical canal at the squamocolumnar junction. With the onset of puberty, the ovarian hormones cause eversion of the lower cervical canal so that this junction approaches the external cervical os. Squamous metaplasia occurs when the columnar epithelium at this junction is replaced by squamous epithelium.

Cervical ectropion

This is the florid appearance of the lower cervical canal that is often mistakenly described as an 'erosion' and is caused by the hormonal changes during puberty, pregnancy and by the oral contraceptive pill. It is usually asymptomatic, but may cause a persistent vaginal discharge or postcoital bleeding. In the presence of a normal smear test, this can be treated by diathermy or cryocautery in the office.

Cervical polyps

These are usually found protruding through the external cervical os and can either be asymptomatic or cause chronic discharge, postcoital or intermenstrual bleeding. In this situation they can simply be avulsed and the base cauterized with diathermy.

Cervical neoplasia

Role of human papillomavirus

Over 60 genotypes of human papillomavirus (HPV) have been identified; in particular, HPV 16, 18 and 33 have been shown to be associated with cervical neoplasia and with increasing grades of CIN.

Up to 10% of women will have HPV on cervical cytology at some stage and of these, 35–40% will have CIN. However, there is no increased risk of cancer in those patients with HPV without CIN. Most women will contract HPV at some point in their lives but will build up immunity and expel the virus before dysplasia can develop.

Cervical cytology
- Definitions:
- Inflammatory – this means that there are increased polymorphs and this may occur during the premenstrual or menstrual phases of the cycle.
- Mild squamous changes – mainly due to inflammation or an artefact of poor fixation, which will require a repeat smear in 6 months.

- Hyperkeratosis – may be due to HPV or uterovaginal prolapse, but CIN may be present in less than 5%.
- Dyskaryosis – this is the term used for cells that come from a dysplastic or neoplastic lesion.
- Transformation zone – this is the area between the original and existing squamocolumnar junction and is where the columnar epithelium undergoes metaplasia. This zone may extend up the cervical canal, especially in the postmenopausal patient.

Cervical screening

Screening for premalignant disease of the cervix is by cytology of cervical smears where cells are taken from the squamocolumnar junction using an Ayres spatula or cervical brush. This sample is spread on a glass slide and fixed with an alcohol spray. More recently liquid-based cytology has been introduced, with similar sampling of the cells with a brush instead of spatula. The slides are then screened for dyskaryosis. Cervical smears are best taken in midcycle and should be taken every 3–5 years from 20–25 to 60 years of age (depending on national protocols). If the woman has had a hysterectomy for benign disease, no further smears are necessary.

Cervical smears and cytology are 99.7% specific (false-positive rate of 0.3%), 80% sensitive (false-negative rate of 20%). Referral for colposcopy is advised if the cytology report shows moderate dyskaryosis or worse or if the woman has had two mildly dyskaryotic smears with 6 months.

Cervical intraepithelial neoplasia

CIN or cervical premalignant disease is classified from CIN 1 to CIN 3. Normally, cells differentiate and move to the surface, but abnormalities can occur, resulting in mitotic figures, nuclear pleomorphism and changes in nuclear to cytoplasmic ratio (dysplasia) or change to a different cell type (metaplasia).

CIN 1 is when two-thirds or more of the upper epithelium shows good differentiation, but the basal third of the epithelium demonstrates nuclear atypia. The majority of CIN 1 will resolve spontaneously. CIN 2 shows differentiation in the upper third of the epithelium, but with mitotic figures in the basal two-thirds. CIN 3 means that less than a third of the upper epithelium shows differentiation.

CIN 1 can progress to higher CIN lesions in approximately 20% of cases within 2–4 years. CIN 3 can progress to carcinoma in 20–30% of cases within 20 years.

Management

Colposcopy involves the microscopic examination of the transformation zone of the cervix to identify abnormal areas. This is not a diagnostic test, but simply a means of identifying an abnormal lesion on the cervix. To aid with identification, the cervix can be painted with various solutions. Acetoacetic acid will turn abnormal epithelium acetowhite since this epithelium contains more proteinaceous nuclei and less glycogenated cytoplasm. Aqueous iodine may also be used since it is taken up by normal epithelium, but not by columnar or abnormal squamous epithelium (Schiller's test). The identified area can then be biopsied or excised and the histology then will give the diagnosis.

Other CIN lesions include punctation (vessels running perpendicular to the surface), mosaic pattern (capillaries running parallel to the surface) and any other irregular vasculature.

Treatment

- Local ablative techniques:
  - laser vaporization
  - cold coagulation
  - diathermy
  - cryocautery (only for CIN 1).
- Excision techniques:
  - loop excision of the transformation zone, which can be performed in the clinic with local anaesthesia
  - 'cold knife' or laser cone biopsy, which is performed under general anaesthesia.

The excisional techniques are recommended to treat CIN 2 and 3 rather than ablative techniques. If smears are normal 12 months following treatment, then annual follow-up is recommended. Hysterectomy may be considered if there are any other gynaecological reasons and then the patient must be followed up annually with vaginal vault smears as there is an increased risk of vaginal intraepithelial neoplasia. If cervical abnormality occurs in pregnancy then a colposcopy can be performed, but the treatment of CIN is best left until postpartum. However, if invasion is suspected then resection must be performed.

Cervical intraepithelial glandular neoplasia

Adenocarcinoma coexists with CIN in 70% of cases.

CARCINOMA OF THE CERVIX

The development of cervical carcinoma occurs mainly in the squamous epithelium (within the transformation zone) or endocervix. Approximately 90% are squamous cell and the remainder are adenocarcinomas.

Cervical cancer is the second commonest malignancy in women worldwide after breast carcinoma, with approximately 470 000 cases occurring annually. The vast majority of women diagnosed with invasive carcinoma of the cervix have not had regular screening.

The mean age at diagnosis is 52 years, with two peaks at 35–39 and 60–64 years. It is associated with early onset of sexual activity, multiple partners and smoking.

The carcinoma can metastasize directly to the pelvic side wall, involving the ureters, bladder or rectum or via lymphatics to the pelvic nodes.

Presentation

Approximately 80% of affected patients are symptomatic. The most common presentation is with abnormal vaginal bleeding, e.g. postcoital, intermenstrual or postmenopausal or, alternatively, some may present with a chronic vaginal discharge that can be purulent, watery or mucoid and not necessarily malodorous. Pain is usually an indicator of advanced disease.

Examination should include general assessment for lymphadenopathy, speculum to assess the appearance of the cervix (bleeding, irregular or ulcerated), vaginal examination to assess for parametral extension and a rectal examination.

Investigations

These should include full blood count, urea and electrolytes (renal function), liver markers, chest X-ray, CT and occasionally renal ultrasound scan.

Formal surgical staging will include examination under anaesthesia, including pelvic and rectal examination, cervical biopsy and endocervical/uterine curettage, cystoscopy and occasionally proctoscopy.

International Federation of Gynecology and Obstetrics (FIGO) clinical staging for cervical carcinoma is as follows:

- Stage 1: carcinoma confined to the cervix
  - stage 1a: invasive carcinoma identified only microscopically
    - stage 1a1: invasion of stroma ≤3 mm and ≤7 mm diameter
    - stage 1a2: invasion of stroma >3 mm but <5 mm and <7 mm diameter
  - stage 1b: clinically obvious lesions confined to the cervix or preclinical lesions greater than stage 1a
    - stage inical lesions ≤4 cm
    - stage 1b2: clinical lesions >4 cm.
- Stage 2: carcinoma extending beyond the cervix but not to pelvic side walls. The carcinoma involves the vagina but not the lower third of vagina
  - stage 2a: no parametrial involvement
  - stage 2b: parametrial involvement
- Stage 3: carcinoma spread to pelvic side wall or lower third of vagina. Would include all cases of hydronephrosis or renal failure secondary to ureteric obstruction
- Stage 4: carcinoma extending beyond the true pelvis or involving the mucosa of bladder or rectum.

Management

Surgery

- Preoperative assessment:

This involves the following:

- Imaging – CT/magnetic resonance imaging (MRI)
- Routine bloods, including full blood count, urea and electrolytes, liver function test
- Group and crossmatch for 2 units of blood
- Bowel preparation
- Correction of medical problems
- Intraoperative antibiotic prophylaxis
- Anticoagulation prophylaxis.
- Technique:

Radical hysterectomy involves the following:

- Vertical midline or Cherney/Maylard incision. Minimal-access surgery is now an option, either laparoscopically or robot-assisted
- Assess for ascites, assess liver, spleen, undersurface of diaphragm, kidneys, ureters, omentum, appendix
- Removal of uterus, cervix, plus or minus ovaries and tubes, parametria, upper third of vagina and pelvic nodes.

    Locally radical fertility-sparing surgery (radical trachelectomy) should be considered in young women with early-stage cervical cancer.

- Complications:
- Haemorrhage, infection and thromboembolus
- Urinary tract infection – 10%
- Other infective morbidities, including pulmonary (secondary to atelectasis) infections, wound infection or pelvic haematoma – 10–20%
- Small-bowel obstruction – 1%
- Pelvic lymphocyst formation – 1–2%
- Fistula (ureteric or vesicovaginal).

Radiotherapy

Radiation treatment is used for stage 2b or greater, if the woman is unfit for surgery or as adjuvant therapy if the nodes are positive. The typical radiation dose is 60 Gray, or 30 Gray as a palliative dose, usually delivered in fractions over a 6-week period.

Complications of radiotherapy include proctitis, ileitis with diarrhoea and skin reactions. Other later complications may include bladder irritability and occasionally fistulae.

Chemoradiation is the incorporation of cisplatin-based chemotherapy with radiation therapy and has recently been recommended for patients with high-risk or advanced (stage 1b2 or greater) cervical carcinoma.

Early-stage cervical cancer
- Stage 1a1:
- lesions <1 mm: cone biopsy or simple hysterectomy
  - lesions <3 mm: simple hysterectomy
  - >3 mm: radical hysterectomy with adjuvant radiotherapy if nodes are positive
- Stage 1b:
  - radical hysterectomy or radiotherapy have identical survival rates
  - radiotherapy if unfit for surgery or adjuvant if nodes are positive
  - adjuvant chemoradiotherapy for stage 1b2 or greater
- Stage 2a:
  - treatment as for stage 1b
- Stage 2b:
  - radiotherapy.

Follow-up

Review patient for routine postoperative check at 6 weeks. Review 3-monthly for 2 years, 6-monthly until year 5, then annually until year 10. Assessment includes general examination, including breast (and nodes), abdominal examination, vault smear, vaginal and rectal examination. Other investigations, if appropriate, include chest X-ray or colposcopy/biopsy.

Prognosis

This depends on the stage of the disease and is usually expressed in terms of 5-year survival rates:
- Stage 1 – up to 90%
- Stage 2 – 55%
- Stage 3 – 30–55%
- Stage 4 – <10%.

Adenocarcinoma of the cervix

This occurs in approximately 30% of cervical cancers. It involves a greater tumour mass and, therefore, carries a worse prognosis than squamous cell carcinoma.

BENIGN TUMOURS OF THE UTERUS

Polyps

Endometrial polyps are very common and are usually multiple in premenopausal, but usually single in postmenopausal women. They are usually benign adenomatous lesions that are found in the body of the uterus and often occur as part of a hyperplastic endometrium, presenting with menstrual irregularity. Occasionally, they can protrude through the cervix to cause dysmenorrhoea or postcoital bleeding. Ideally, they should be removed with a hysteroscopic resectoscope and the excised tissue analysed histologically.

Uterine fibroids

Fibroids or leiomyomata are the commonest tumours of the female genital tract occurring in 20–30% of women over 30 years of age. They are particularly common in Afro-Caribbean and nulliparous women. Fibroids may be found in various sites; intramural are within the uterine wall; subserous are beneath the serosal surface of the uterus; and submucous are found beneath the mucosal surface of the uterus, often distorting it or increasing the surface area of the endometrium. Fibroids are usually multiple in number and can vary widely in size. They often undergo degenerative change as a result of poor vascularity, described as:

● Hyaline degeneration
● Cystic degeneration
● Calcification (in postmenopausal women)
● Necrosis and infection
● Red degeneration (during pregnancy).

Malignant change is rare (leiomyosarcoma), occurring in <0.5% of cases, but should be suspected in rapidly growing fibroids.

Presentation

The majority of fibroids are asymptomatic, but can cause symptoms depending on their size and position in the uterus.

Menorrhagia is the commonest symptom but symptoms can vary between menorrhagia, intermenstrual bleeding and abdominal swelling. If situated under the bladder, they can cause irritative bladder symptoms or incontinence. In pregnancy, fibroids may increase in size as they are hormone-dependent or degenerate (red degeneration), resulting in pain. They can also cause obstruction in labour, depending on their site.

Management

Fibroids are oestrogen-dependent and will, therefore, reduce in size after the menopause and so can be treated conservatively.

However, if symptomatic, fibroids can be treated either medically or surgically.

Medical

● Progesterone tablets
● Gonadotrophin-releasing hormone (GnRH) analogues – will cause rapid reduction in fibroid size, but will regrow when treatment is ceased. Side effects are unavoidable and include menopausal symptoms pelvic pain from fibroid necrosis and reduced bone density.

Surgery

Myomectomy can be performed through an abdominal incision, laparoscopically or hysteroscopically, depending on the site of the fibroid and skill of the operator. Pretreatment with GnRH analogues will shrink the fibroids and reduce blood loss during surgery. Myomectomy can be technically difficult and may result in excessive blood loss. It is, therefore, a procedure that is reserved for women who wish to preserve their fertility, but these patients should be carefully counselled regarding the risk of proceeding to hysterectomy in the case of excessive blood loss.

Adenomyosis

This is a benign condition of the uterus caused by invasion of endometrium and its underlying stroma into the myometrial layer of the uterus. It is often undiagnosed, but is found in at least 40% of hysterectomy specimens on histological examination. It is thought to be a variant of endometriosis and so it often presents in a similar way, with menstrual pain and also with menorrhagia.

Presentation

Adenomyosis may be asymptomatic, but characteristically will present as dysmenorrhoea and menorrhagia. On vaginal bimanual examination the uterus is often found to be enlarged and tender. Diagnosis, however, can usually only be made on histological examination of the removed uterus following hysterectomy.

Management

Management is aimed at control of dysmenorrhoea and menorrhagia. Non-steroidal anti-inflammatory medication or progestogens (either as an oral preparation or the intrauterine system) can be effective, but often hysterectomy may be necessary if the patient does not wish to preserve her fertility.

Congenital abnormalities of the uterus

The uterus is derived embryologically from fusion of the müllerian (paramesonephric) ducts. If these ducts fail to fuse during development varying degrees of uterine abnormality will result. Complete failure to fuse results in two separate uterine cavities and crevices often associated with a longitudinal vaginal septum (uterine didelphys). Partial failure to fuse will result in varying degrees of abnormality, including rudimentary horn (where one duct develops to a lesser extent than the other) or where a uterine septum is present to a varying degree (from an arcuate uterus to a bicornuate uterus to a subseptate uterus). These abnormalities are often discovered during investigation of pregnancy-related problems such as recurrent first- and second-trimester miscarriage, cervical incompetence or preterm labour.

ENDOMETRIAL CARCINOMA

Endometrial carcinoma is the most common gynaecological cancer in the developed world, particularly amongst postmenopausal women. The majority of tumours of the body of the uterus are adenocarcinomas of the endometrium, whereas malignant tumours of the myometrium, sarcomas, account for only 4%. Endometrial carcinoma usually presents with abnormal bleeding or discharge after 45 years of age or alternatively with postmenopausal bleeding. Most occur after the menopause, with only 5% of cases occurring in women under 40 years of age. These clinical situations should be investigated promptly with ultrasound, hysteroscopy and endometrial sampling.

There are two broad categories of endometrial cancer – type 1 (80% of cases) is slow-growing and oestrogen-dependent and is therefore associated with long-term unopposed oestrogen administration, oestrogen-secreting tumours of the ovary or adiposity (since adiposity increases oestrogen levels) and type 2 (20% of cases) is a more aggressive malignancy with a poorer prognosis than type 1. Other associations include nulliparity and late menopause.

FIGO staging of endometrial cancer (updated 2009)

- Stage 0 – carcinoma in situ
- Stage 1 – confined to the body of the uterus
  - stage 1a: tumour limited to the endometrium or <50% of myometrium
  - stage 1b: tumour invades >50% of endometrium
- Stage 2 – tumour invades cervical stroma but not beyond uterus
- Stage 3 – local and or regional spread of tumour
  - stage 3a: invasion of serosa, adnexae or peritoneum
  - stage 3b: vaginal or parametrial involvement
  - stage 3c: metastasis to pelvic and/or para-aortic nodes
- Stage 4 – tumour invades bladder mucosa and/or bowel mucosa and/or distant metastasis
  - stage 4a: invasion of bladder or bowel mucosa
  - stage 4b: distal metastases, including inguinal nodes.

Microscopic appearance

Most endometrial carcinomas are adenocarcinomas and are graded according to their differentiation. Grade 1 is well differentiated, grade 2 moderately differentiated and grade 3 is poorly differentiated. The pathology report should state the tumour type and the degree of differentiation.

Management

Approximately 90% of tumours will present at stage 1 or 2. When the diagnosis has been made, a total abdominal hysterectomy with bilateral salpingo-oophorectomy must be performed. Although it seems apparent that lymphadenectomy should be performed in order to stage the disease, the role of concurrent lymphadenectomy in the treatment of endometrial cancer remains controversial.

Radiotherapy has been shown to reduce the risk of vault recurrence in high-risk patients and should, therefore, be offered to patients with stage 2 or greater disease.

The role of chemotherapy is still debatable when balancing the morbidity associated with it with the short-term palliative benefits.

Prognosis

5-year survival
- Stage 1 – 85%
- Stage 2 – 75%
- Stage 3 – 45%
- Stage 4 – 25%.

Follow-up

It is essential that patients are routinely followed up with history and clinical examination but the routine use of vault smears is controversial. The role of hormone replacement treatment is also controversial, but combined oestrogen–progestogen therapy has been shown to have no effect on tumour recurrence and so should be considered, especially in young women.

OVARIAN CYSTS

Functional cysts of the ovaries are common and usually asymptomatic. Follicular cysts are usually found in women with anovulatory cycles or in women undergoing infertility treatment. They are usually <5 cm in diameter and can be diagnosed by ultrasound. They usually resolve and only rarely require surgery if the increased bulk of the ovary causes it to tort. Corpus luteal cysts are usually found in women with irregular cycles or with amenorrhoea followed by heavy vaginal bleeding. Functional cysts of the ovary usually resolve spontaneously. Occasionally, they can rupture, resulting in severe acute pelvic pain that again tends to resolve, but may require hospital admission for investigation. Persistent cysts can be removed laparoscopically and the combined oral contraceptive pill may be used to prevent recurrence by inhibiting ovulation.

Ovarian cysts in postmenopausal women

Ovarian cysts are less common after the menopause, but are increasingly picked up incidentally on routine screening or pelvic ultrasound for other reasons. Since diagnostic tests have become more accurate the need to resort to surgery has decreased. These tests include transvaginal ultrasound (or abdominal if the cyst is large) and cancer antigen 125 (CA 125), both of which can be useful in assessment, whereas the role of CT and MRI scanning is limited. The management of ovarian cysts in this age group can be influenced by these tests, which can classify the cyst according to its risk of malignancy.

Low risk

Ultrasound features include simple, unilateral, unilocular and a size <5 cm with a normal serum CA 125. These cysts can be managed conservatively, if the patient is asymptomatic, with 3–4-monthly follow-up, as more than 50% resolve. Otherwise these cysts can be removed laparoscopically, with the most appropriate surgery in this age group including a bilateral salpingo-oophorectomy.

High risk

Ultrasound features include complex (solid parts or papillary formation), bilateral, multilocular and size >5 cm with an elevated CA 125. These cysts need to be managed surgically in a specialist centre. The appropriate surgery is the same as for any ovarian malignancy – a total abdominal hysterectomy, bilateral salpingo-oophorectomy and full staging procedure (peritoneal washings, omentectomy and possibly para-aortic lymphadenectomy).

TUMOURS OF THE OVARY

Ovarian tumours can be primary or secondary. When considering primary neoplasms of the ovary, it is sensible to classify benign and malignant neoplasms together, as a benign cyst may undergo malignant change. There are three main groups of primary ovarian neoplasm: (1) epithelial tumours; (2) germ cell tumours; and (3) sex cord tumours.

Epithelial tumours

These are the most common ovarian tumours in postmenopausal women (85% of ovarian tumours) and may undergo malignant change. There are four types:

1. Serous cystadenoma or adenocarcinoma – this is the commonest form of ovarian carcinoma, accounting for 50% of ovarian malignancy, but both benign and malignant varieties exist.
2. Mucinous cystadenoma or adenocarcinoma – these are less commonly malignant, accounting for 10% of ovarian carcinomas. They are usually large ovarian cysts.

3. Endometrioid carcinoma – this malignant variety of ovarian carcinoma accounts for 25% of ovarian carcinomas and is associated with endometrial malignancy in 20% of cases.
4. Clear-cell carcinoma – this is a malignant tumour that accounts for 10% of ovarian carcinoma and carries a particularly poor prognosis.

Brenner's tumour is a rare form of ovarian neoplasm that is usually small and benign.

Germ cell tumours

Germ cell tumours arise from the undifferentiated germ cells of the ovary. There are two main varieties:

1. Teratoma (dermoid cyst) – this is a common benign cyst in young women that may contain tissue from all the cell lines derived from the primordial germ cells of the ovary, including hair and teeth. They are usually small, bilateral and asymptomatic, but can cause pain if the ovary torts or the cyst ruptures. They can, rarely, undergo malignant change to solid teratomas.
2. Dysgerminoma – this is a rare tumour of the ovary overall, but is the commonest type of ovarian malignancy in the younger age group.

Sex cord tumours

This type of ovarian tumour is derived from the ovarian stroma and there are three varieties:

1. Granulosa cell tumours – these are slow-growing malignant tumours of the ovary, which are usually malignant. They are rare and secrete oestrogen, and so may cause postmenopausal bleeding or endometrial hyperplasia or carcinoma in this group of women.
2. Thecomas – these are similar to the granulosa cell tumours, secreting oestrogen and, therefore, causing similar effects, but are rare and usually benign, e.g. Sertoli–Leydig tumours.
3. Fibromas – these are benign tumours that are uncommon and are often associated with ascites and pleural effusions as part of Meigs' syndrome.

Secondary ovarian malignancies are common, accounting for 10% of ovarian masses, since the ovary is a common area for metastatic spread from the breast, lung and gastrointestinal tract. The prognosis for secondary ovarian malignancy is poor.

OVARIAN CARCINOMA

This is the commonest gynaecological malignancy in the UK, where there are approximately 5000 cases per year. It characteristically presents late and is, therefore, the main cause of mortality from gynaecological cancer.

Aetiology

Benign ovarian cysts will frequently undergo malignant change and so all ovarian cysts need to be carefully managed. Risk factors include a history of early menarche, late menopause, nulliparity or infertility (i.e. increased number of ovulatory cycles), family history and other cancers that are linked include breast, endometrial or colonic cancer. Factors that reduce the number of ovulatory cycles are, therefore, protective, including the oral contraceptive pill, multiparity and breastfeeding. There is a familial predisposition in approximately 5% of cases, with mutations of the *BRCA1* and 2 genes being strongly implicated.

Microscopic appearance

The majority of ovarian carcinomas (85%) are epithelial, and germ cell tumours are more common in young women. Ovarian carcinoma will spread directly to the peritoneum and thereby to the peritoneal surfaces of the diaphragm, liver, bowel and omentum. In the later stages, metastatic spread occurs via the blood and lymphatic circulation. Ovarian carcinoma will vary from well to poorly differentiated with obvious prognostic implications.

Presentation

Ovarian carcinoma presents late (stage 3–4 disease) in over 70% of cases, as it is commonly asymptomatic in its early stages.

Typical non-specific symptoms or signs include weight loss, generalized abdominal pain or distension, back pain, urinary symptoms, constipation or deep venous thrombosis.

Examination may reveal an abdominal or pelvic mass, ascites or lymphadenopathy. It is therefore important to examine the abdomen, pelvis and rectum, as well as breasts and lymph nodes for evidence of metastases.

The clinical features consistent with malignancy include:
- Older age of patient: postmenopause
- Rapid growth of adnexal mass
- Bilateral adnexal masses
- Ascites.

Management

Ultrasound and tumour markers are useful in guiding the management of ovarian tumours. However, definitive staging is at the time of surgery.

Ultrasound
The features consistent with malignancy include:
- Solid appearance
- Thickened cyst wall
- Presence of septa within cyst
- Bleeding within cyst
- Bilateral cysts.

Tumour markers
CA 125 levels are raised in over 80% of epithelial ovarian malignancies and are useful in aiding diagnosis, monitoring treatment response during follow-up and in recurrence. Other tumour markers include alpha-fetoprotein and human chorionic gonadotrophin, which are characteristically raised in germ cell tumours amongst younger women.

Surgery
If malignancy is suspected, then laparotomy should be performed through a midline incision in order to stage the carcinoma accurately. This includes peritoneal washings, total abdominal hysterectomy, bilateral salpingo-oophorectomy and omentectomy. If extensive malignancy is present, then a debulking procedure is performed in which as much tumour as possible is removed. Surgery, is usually followed by chemotherapy in all patients except those with early stage 1a or borderline tumours. In young women with well-differentiated tumours who wish to preserve their fertility, a more conservative approach would involve a unilateral oophorectomy and partial omental biopsy.

Chemotherapy

This treatment is best performed under the supervision of a medical oncologist and usually involves a course of platinum-based compounds, e.g. carboplatin or cisplatin or alkylating agents such as cyclophosphamide in conjunction with taxol.

Regular follow-up is essential, with tracking of disease progression with CA 125 levels for epithelial tumours.

FIGO staging (and 5-year survival rate)

- Stage 1 – tumour confined to the ovaries (50–75%)
  - stage 1a: one ovary affected, capsule intact
  - stage 1b: both ovaries affected, capsule intact
  - stage 1c: either a or b, capsule ruptured or malignant cells in abdomen
- Stage 2 – pelvic extension beyond ovaries (40%)
  - stage 2a: spread to uterus or tubes
  - stage 2b: spread to other pelvic tissues
  - stage 2c: either of the above with ascites or positive peritoneal washings
- Stage 3 – extension beyond the pelvis, but within the abdomen, usually involving the omentum, small bowel and intestine (10–15%)
- Stage 4 – metastatic spread beyond the abdomen (5%).

GYNAECOLOGICAL CANCER IN PREGNANCY

Approximately 1 in 1000 pregnancies are complicated by gynaecological malignancy, of which cervical and ovarian carcinomas are the most common, and this figure is increasing as women delay childbirth into their later reproductive years.

Carcinoma of the cervix

Seventy per cent of cervical carcinoma in pregnancy is diagnosed at an early stage (2a or less). The antenatal clinic offers a good opportunity to follow up on cervical screening of pregnant women.

Management

1. Low-grade abnormality on smear – followed up with a further smear test in 12 months.
2. High-grade abnormality on smear – mandatory colposcopy, avoid biopsy if possible (but this will be unavoidable if invasive carcinoma is suspected), but repeat colposcopy at 24–28 weeks' gestation to exclude progression of disease. Follow up postpartum for biopsy if necessary.
3. Suspected microinvasion – may indicate need for cold-knife cone biopsy during pregnancy. This procedure carries a significant risk of morbidity for both mother and fetus.
4. Invasive carcinoma – adequate staging is essential. Management will depend on extent of stage, gestation at diagnosis and patient's wishes for continuing pregnancy. Generally, definitive treatment can be deferred if the carcinoma is diagnosed in the third trimester. If the carcinoma is at a stage that responds to surgery, most gynaecologists would advise elective caesarean section followed by a radical hysterectomy.

Carcinoma of the ovary

This is less common than cervical carcinoma in pregnancy. It also tends to be picked up at an earlier stage than in the non-pregnant setting, because of the routine use of ultrasound in pregnancy. Tumour markers are of limited value in pregnancy as their values tend to fluctuate and are generally elevated. Suspicious features on ultrasound include size >5 cm, persistence of cyst throughout pregnancy and bilateral or solid components within the cyst. Surgical intervention is usually delayed until 16–20 weeks' gestation and frozen-section analysis is useful to guide further management. Since the majority of ovarian carcinomas in pregnancy are germ cell in origin, often a unilateral salpingo-oophorectomy with staging is appropriate. This is also true for the early-stage, low malignant epithelial and sex cord tumours, allowing for continuation of the pregnancy. The higher-risk malignancies will require chemotherapy, with the obvious dilemmas of teratogenicity.

Carcinoma of the vulva and endometrium

These are very uncommon in pregnancy.

SUMMARY

- Cervical smears are an effective screening technique for cervical carcinoma.
- Cervical carcinoma is the second commonest female cancer after breast carcinoma, followed by ovarian and then endometrial.
- Uterine fibroids are the commonest benign tumours of the female genital tract.
- Ovarian cysts are common and management has been improved with the development of ultrasound and tumour markers.
- Ovarian carcinoma usually presents late and is therefore the main cause of mortality from gynaecological cancer.

Uterovaginal prolapse and urinary incontinence 8

CHAPTER CONTENTS

UTEROVAGINAL PROLAPSE

In the majority of women the uterus is said to be in a position of anteversion (the fundus directed forwards) and anteflexed (the body of the uterus bent forward over the cervix) – retroversion and retroflexion are the converse of these and occur in approximately 20% of cases. The main structures that hold the uterus in position are the uterosacral and transverse cervical ligaments. The normal uterus is mobile and is, therefore, able to adjust its position in the pelvis as a result of any pelvic mass or distension of the bladder or rectum. The secondary support of the uterus is the muscular pelvic floor.

Definition

Uterovaginal prolapse is defined as descent of a pelvic organ or structure into and sometimes outside the vagina. 'Prolapse' can be taken as meaning pelvic organ prolapse, urogenital prolapse, genital prolapse, rectocele/cystocele/urethrocystocele, vaginal vault prolapse and uterine descent (Fig. 8.1).

Incidence

The incidence of prolapse in the female population is difficult to define as many women do not seek medical attention and clinical examination does not necessarily correlate with symptoms. It is estimated that a woman has an 11% lifetime risk of having an operation for prolapse by the age of 80 and that 30% of these patients will require further prolapse surgery.

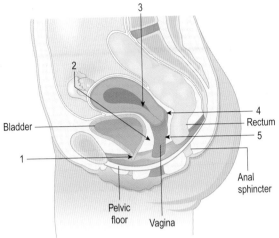

Figure 8.1 Areas of potential prolapse. (1) Urethrocele; (2) cystocele; (3) apical (uterus/vault); (4) enterocele; (5) rectocele.

Anatomy of the pelvic floor

Prolapse is caused by a failure of the supporting structures of the genital tract and it is, therefore, important to have an understanding of this anatomy. The pelvic floor consists of muscular and fascial structures that support the abdominopelvic cavity and the external openings of the vagina, urethra and rectum. The uterus and vagina are suspended from the pelvic side walls by endopelvic fascial attachments that support the vagina at three levels or anatomical sections:

- Level 1 (upper third of the vagina) support consists of endopelvic fascial tissue that condenses laterally as the cardinal (transverse cervical) ligaments and posteriorly as the uterosacral ligaments.
- Level 2 (middle third of vagina) support attaches the middle portion of the vagina to the arcus tendineus and fascia of the levator ani muscles.
- Level 3, the lower vagina, is supported predominantly by connections to fibres of the pelvic diaphragm and the perineal membrane.

Most of the endopelvic fascia fibres attach to the vaginal wall, but a few pass from one side to the other and are recognized as the rectovaginal septum separating the vagina and rectum. Damage at the different levels of vaginal support causes different types of prolapse. Level 1 support failure results in vaginal vault or uterine prolapse, whereas loss of level 2 support leads to development of cystocele and rectocele, and level 3 disruption results in any of the above (as it acts as an anchor for all the supports) and a deficient perineum.

Types of prolapse

Anterior vaginal wall prolapse may have bladder or urethra above it and this is known as a cystocele, urethrocele or a combination of the two. Posterior wall prolapse can contain a part of the rectum (rectocele) or higher up on the posterior wall when the pouch of Douglas containing small bowel can herniate through the posterior fornix (enterocele). An enterocele is usually associated with uterine prolapse, but is also known to be a late complication of previous colposuspension procedures.

Uterine prolapse is descent of the cervix and uterine body into the vagina and three types are recognized:

1. First-degree, in which there is descent of the cervix into the vagina but not as far as the introitus.
2. Second-degree, in which the cervix reaches the introitus.
3. Third-degree, in which the cervix and body of the uterus lie outside the introitus (this is also known as procidentia).

Vault prolapse is eversion of the vault of the vagina that can occur after hysterectomy.

Aetiology of prolapse

Congenital

The connective tissue is known to play an important role in pelvic organ support and collagen is the main provider of tensile strength. Deficiencies in collagen metabolism have been shown to be associated with stress urinary incontinence and prolapse.

Childbirth

Vaginal delivery and factors such as prolonged second stage, instrumental delivery and large birth weight of the infant have all been shown to be associated with disruption of the anatomical relations and possible denervation of the pelvic floor.

Menopause

The incidence of prolapse is known to increase with age and it is thought that this is due to the deterioration of collagenous connective tissue that occurs following oestrogen withdrawal.

Iatrogenic

Hysterectomy involves division of the uterosacral ligaments, which are important in level 1 support of the vagina. The cumulative risk of prolapse is 1% 3 years after hysterectomy, rising to 5% 15 years after.

Chronic predisposing factors

Prolapse is aggravated by any chronic increase in intra-abdominal pressure and, therefore, factors such as obesity, chronic cough secondary to smoking or respiratory tract conditions, heavy lifting at work or in the home and constipation.

Clinical assessment

Prolapse is often asymptomatic, but patients may complain of any or a combination of the symptoms outlined below.

There may be a dragging sensation in the pelvis or a feeling of 'something coming down' through the vagina. Patients may feel a swelling at the vagina that gets worse as the day progresses and describe difficulty with intercourse (dyspareunia).

Anterior wall prolapse can be associated with urinary symptoms, in particular leakage of urine with increased intra-abdominal pressure, e.g. on coughing or sneezing, or incomplete emptying of the bladder resulting in high residual volumes of urine that may lead to urinary tract infections. Patients may also complain of frequency, nocturia or urgency with or without incontinence, which could be due to cystitis or because of a coexisting overactive bladder.

Posterior wall prolapse may be associated with difficulty in defecation to the extent that many patients may need to attempt digital reduction of the prolapse to ease defecation. Procidentia may result in vaginal bleeding or discharge, as an erosion or decubitus ulcer may form on the exposed prolapsed uterus. Rarely, procidentia may result in ureteric obstruction causing chronic renal failure.

History

Ascertaining the degree of impairment of quality of life or daily activities will influence management. Specific questioning on urinary and bowel function as well as sexual function should be included. A full obstetric and gynaecological history as well as medical and surgical history will guide the practitioner as to the suitability of conservative or surgical management options. Specific instruments, for example, the King's Health Questionnaire, are available and are routinely used to measure quality of life.

Examination

Abdominal examination should always be performed to exclude any masses or organomegaly. The woman should first be examined in the dorsal position when she is asked to bear down, strain or cough, during which inspection of the introitus should reveal any obvious second- or third-degree prolapse; stress incontinence may be demonstrated and atrophy may be apparent. Examination is then performed with the patient in the Sims' position (patient in left lateral position with chest at 45°∞ to the examining couch, the left leg straight, the right hip extended and knee flexed) with a Sims' speculum, which allows full inspection of the uterine prolapse and vaginal walls (Fig. 8.2). The blade of the Sims' speculum is inserted along the posterior wall of the vagina and retracted in order to display the anterior wall, with the patient bearing down. The anterior wall can be supported with sponge forceps to assess for apical descent (cervix or vault) and then the anterior vaginal wall is supported in order to assess the posterior wall, with the patient bearing down. Vaginal examination is performed in the usual manner with assessment of the uterus and adnexae as previously outlized and any obvious descent of the cervix or prolapse of the vaginal walls noted. In the research setting and increasingly in specialist centres, a system called pelvic organ prolapse quantification (POPQ) can be utilized. This is a complex nine-point assessment of uterovaginal prolapse, which describes four stages of pelvic organ descent relative to the hymenal ring.

Urodynamics

Subtracted cystometry and flow studies should always be considered in women with genital prolapse and urinary symptoms before offering surgery. Stress urinary incontinence can be masked by prolapse and these patients may also have chronic voiding dysfunction.

Treatment

The choice of treatment depends on the patient's wishes, general health and desires regarding future sexual function. Conservative or surgical options are available and a combination of the two is ideal. Management will depend on the severity of symptoms and suitability for anaesthesia.

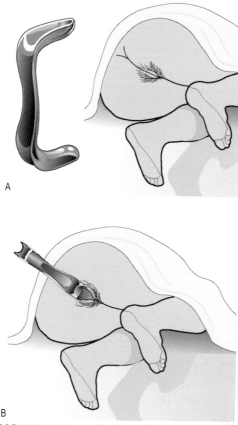

A

B

Figure 8.2 Patient in left lateral position for use of Sims' speculum.

Conservative measures

Many types of pessaries have been developed for vaginal and uterine support, although surgical correction should be considered whenever possible. A typical plastic ring pessary should comfortably rest between the posterior fornix and the symphysis pubis, thereby supporting and stretching the vaginal wall, preventing vault prolapse and directly supporting any cystocele present (Fig. 8.3). Pessaries need to be replaced 6-monthly to avoid infection or ulceration of the vagina. Pelvic floor re-education or strengthening is best achieved under the direction of a trained continence advisor or by a physiotherapist using directed muscle exercises or weighted vaginal cones that the woman must try to retain within the vagina. Sometimes this can be combined with electrical stimulation of the pelvic floor muscles, which has also been shown to be of benefit.

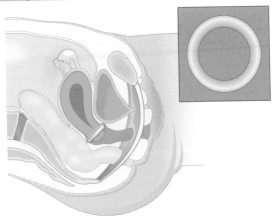

Figure 8.3 Placement of vaginal ring pessary for first- and second-degree uterovaginal prolapse.

Surgical procedures

The choice of procedure depends on the patient and the type of prolapse that exists – the 'site-specific' repair. Factors that influence the type of surgical procedure include fitness of the patient and suitability for anaesthesia, whether the patient is sexually active and the surgeon's preference.

Anterior repair (colporrhaphy) is a procedure that repairs fascial defects in the anterior vaginal wall and removes the excess vaginal skin that results from the prolapse (Fig. 8.4). This can also include the use of a

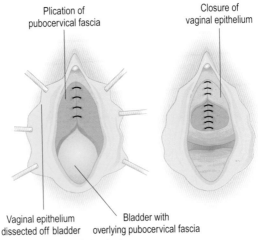

Plication of
pubocervical fascia

Closure of
vaginal epithelium

Vaginal epithelium
dissected off bladder

Bladder with
overlying pubocervical fascia

Figure 8.4 Anterior repair/colporrhaphy.

supporting suture (buttress) under the urethra. Complications are uncommon, although postoperative voiding difficulties may occur and recurrence of prolapse occurs in up to 50% of patients.

Posterior colpoperineorrhaphy is a repair of the posterior wall prolapse, which involves repair of rectovaginal fascial defect and approximation of the levator ani muscles medially to support the rectum with removal of the excess vaginal skin (Fig. 8.5).

Vaginal hysterectomy can be performed with the above procedures in cases where there is significant uterine descent, especially if the patient is postmenopausal or if there are significant menstrual problems.

To preserve the uterus, e.g. for women who may still wish to become pregnant, it is possible to combine the anterior and posterior colpoperineorrhaphy with partial amputation of the cervix (which is often elongated in prolapse) and approximation of the transverse cervical ligaments in the midline for support. This is called a Manchester (or Fothergill) repair.

Sacrohysteropexy is another procedure that can be performed if the patient wishes to preserve her uterus. It is an abdominal procedure that involves using a synthetic mesh placed between the cervix and the sacrum to support the uterus and this is increasingly being performed laparoscopically or robotically.

Vault prolapse can be corrected via either an abdominal (sacrocolpopexy) (Fig. 8.6) or vaginal (sacrospinous ligament fixation) procedure. The latter involves suturing the vault to the sacrospinous ligament. Both these techniques are effective, but the vaginal route has less immediate postoperative morbidity. Both techniques of vault fixation can cause either posterior or anterior (respectively) wall prolapse in the long term.

It is worth noting that some anti-incontinence procedures, in particular a Burch colposuspension (Fig. 8.7), may also cure a cystocele, especially if done in conjunction with a paravaginal repair.

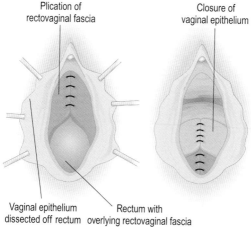

Plication of
rectovaginal fascia

Closure of
vaginal epithelium

Vaginal epithelium
dissected off rectum

Rectum with
overlying rectovaginal fascia

Figure 8.5 Posterior repair/colporrhaphy.

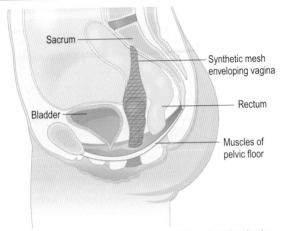

Figure 8.6 Abdominal sacrocolpopexy – fixation of the prolapsed vault using mesh attached to the sacral promontory.

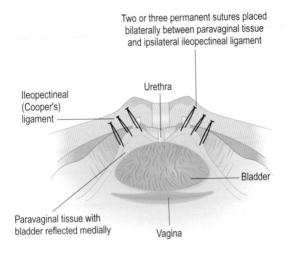

Figure 8.7 Burch colposuspension.

URINARY INCONTINENCE

Urinary incontinence is defined as the involuntary loss of urine that is a social and hygienic problem, and is objectively demonstrable. Urge (incontinence preceded by an urgent desire to void) and stress (incontinence during physical exertion, movement or any causes of increased intra-abdominal pressure) are the most prevalent forms of incontinence.

Physiology of micturition

The main function of the bladder is to convert the steady stream of urine produced by the kidney into a convenient intermittent process of evacuation. Therefore, the bladder must first act as a reservoir and, second, as an intermittent voluntary excretory organ that acts within socially acceptable restraints to allow voiding. This requires a complex neurological network, which coordinates sensory afferent input and motor efferent output in a reciprocal fashion.

Bladder innervation

Normal bladder function requires coordinated detrusor relaxation and urethral sphincter contraction during its filling phase and the converse during micturition. The detrusor muscle is innervated by parasympathetic cholinergic fibres derived from S2–4. These nerves are targeted by the anticholinergic medications to inhibit unstable detrusor contractions. It also has some sympathetic supply from the thoracic and lumbar segments T10–L2. Connections of the lower urinary tract to the central nervous system are extraordinarily complex and many discrete centres with influences on micturition have been identified.

Involuntary leakage of urine can only occur if the intravesical pressure exceeds the urethral closure pressure. Urethral sphincter contraction and detrusor relaxation are achieved by different mechanisms and so no simple drug effectively achieves both.

Assessment

History

A detailed history can often determine the cause of incontinence, differentiating between stress, urge or insensible loss. It is important to assess the effect of the problem on the patient's quality of life and daily routine. One specifically needs to ask about:

- Incontinence – how often does it occur, is it a daily problem, what is its impact on quality of life? Attempt to quantify leakage in terms of pad usage per day which, although subjective, is useful as an outcome measure of treatment
- Stress incontinence – leakage on exercise, walking, lifting or coughing. Establish which of these manoeuvres provoke incontinence
- Urgency or urge incontinence
- Frequency of micturition
- Nocturia (night-time voiding, in particular waking from sleep to void)
- Dysuria, bladder pain or haematuria
- Voiding dysfunction, e.g. poor stream, incomplete emptying
- Symptoms of prolapse
- Urinary tract infections
- Bladder stimulants, e.g. caffeine, alcohol, medications
- Past history – obstetric history, age at menopause, medical problems, surgery.

Examination

- General examination, including weight and urinalysis
- General gynaecological – evidence of excoriation as a result of chronic urinary leakage, atrophic vaginal changes and evidence of demonstrable stress incontinence during Valsalva manoeuvres
- Prolapse – careful evaluation of prolapse as outlined earlier, including use of a Sims' speculum. In particular, a large cystocele may actually

kink the urethra during Valsalva, preventing stress incontinence, but give rise to overflow incontinence or overactive bladder symptoms as a result of voiding difficulty. Also, a large rectocele may occlude the urethra during Valsalva, so that correction of this or the large cystocele may unmask a tendency to stress incontinence (occult stress incontinence)

- Local neurological examination, in particular, assessing for deficit in the areas innervated from the S2–4 nerve roots.

Investigation of urinary incontinence

Patients should be given a fluid chart or micturition diary to complete a week prior to the consultation so that a clear pattern of fluid intake and voiding can be established. At the same time a quality-of-life questionnaire can be completed to assess the extent of impact of symptoms on the patient's daily activities. This will provide a baseline against which the effects of treatment may be assessed.

Measurement of urinary flow rate can be performed on the patient who attends with a full bladder. This is performed with an intravesical pressure catheter, which can measure bladder pressures during voluntary voiding into a special commode that can measure the flow rate. This will differentiate poor flow as a result of an obstructed urethra as opposed to a poorly functioning detrusor muscle. While inserting the catheter, a specimen of urine can be collected to exclude urinary infection.

Subtracted cystometry is a urodynamic test that measures the intravesical pressure during artificial filling of the bladder and then during voiding. This can then determine the presence or absence of involuntary detrusor contractions and, therefore, diagnose detrusor instability if present.

Videocystourethrography is a test that can be performed at the same time as cystometry, using a radiopaque fluid as the filling medium. X-ray imaging of the full bladder can be performed to assess for ureteric reflux, bladder diverticulum, bladder descent or urinary leakage whilst the patient coughs. This is also a useful test if a vesicovaginal fistula is suspected.

OVERACTIVE BLADDER

Urinary urgency is a common problem, with a significant impact on patients' quality of life. Over 200 million people worldwide experience problems associated with urinary incontinence and an estimated 50–100 million people suffer from overactive bladder. The terms 'overactive bladder' and 'detrusor overactivity' have previously been used interchangeably to describe a condition in the bladder that results in the symptoms of urinary frequency, nocturia, urgency and urge incontinence. Detrusor overactivity is in fact a urodynamic diagnosis that can only be applied after patients have been investigated by cystometry; it is defined as 'a disorder of bladder filling and urine storage characterized by the presence of involuntary detrusor contractions while the patient is attempting to inhibit urination'. This definition subdivides detrusor overactivity into two subtypes, based on results obtained from cystometric (urodynamic) testing. These are detrusor hyperreflexia (caused by neurologic disease, e.g. spinal cord injury, multiple sclerosis, stroke or Parkinson's disease) and detrusor overactivity in the absence of neurologic disease. The latter is further subdivided into the idiopathic variety or that caused by bladder outlet obstruction (e.g. post bladder neck surgery for stress incontinence). Regardless of the cause or type, the condition is characterized by the symptoms of frequency (emptying the bladder more than eight times during the daytime), urgency (the sudden strong desire to micturate) or urge incontinence (the involuntary loss of urine that occurs after the sensation of impending leakage), either singly or in combination.

Management

Establishing an accurate diagnosis of the cause of urinary symptoms is important and requires invasive urodynamic investigation. However, treatment can be instigated prior to urodynamic assessment provided there is no contraindication and in the absence of the following: urinary tract infection, haematuria, neuropathy, uropathology, voiding difficulty, previous surgery or if uncertainty of the cause of the urinary symptoms exists. In these situations referral for further investigation is mandatory.

Women with mild overactive bladder symptoms may only require reassurance or advice on conservative measures such as reducing fluid intake, abstinence from caffeine drinks and alcohol, change of voiding habits, and alteration of medications, e.g. diuretics. However, the mainstay of treatment is drug therapy (anticholinergics) and bladder retraining or bladder drill:

- Propantheline is an inexpensive drug that is useful, but prone to the anticholinergic side effects of constipation, dry mouth and blurred vision. Propiverine is a newer alternative.
- Oxybutynin has both anticholinergic and smooth-muscle relaxant properties and is now available in a once-daily extended-release preparation or as a transdermal patch.
- Tolterodine may be better as it has been shown to reduce significantly the number of micturitions in 24 hours and also the number of incontinence episodes, as well as having fewer of the anticholinergic side effects. A newer variant is now available, called fesoterodine, that bypasses hepatic metabolism. Solifenacin is an alternative anticholinergic.
- Imipramine is particularly useful for the treatment of nocturia, nocturnal enuresis and intercourse incontinence.
- DDAVP is useful in the treatment of nocturia and enuresis. It is given intranasally by spray at night. Recently a tablet form has become available.

The main purpose of drug therapy is to overcome the initial overactive bladder symptoms so that simple measures like bladder retraining have a greater impact in the long term. If symptoms are completely unresponsive to conservative and medical treatments, surgery can be offered. Sacral nerve implants for neuromodulation and intravesical Botox therapy have been shown to be effective in patients with intractable overactive bladder symptoms.

STRESS INCONTINENCE

Stress urinary incontinence is a symptom whilst urodynamic stress incontinence (USI) is urodynamic diagnosis. It describes the involuntary loss of urine when the intra-abdominal pressure increases, e.g. with the patient coughing. USI is defined as the involuntary loss of urine when the intravesical pressure exceeds the maximum urethral pressure in the absence of a detrusor contraction.

Aetiology

The maximum urethral pressure is compromised as a result of pregnancy, childbirth and related trauma, and ageing, especially following the menopause. The symptom of stress incontinence is exacerbated by obesity, chronic cough, constipation and prolapse.

Management

Conservative measures include general advice regarding fluid restriction, weight loss, avoiding bladder irritants and changing medications (e.g. diuretics). All patients should attempt pelvic floor re-education and urodynamic investigation must be performed before any surgery is considered.

Surgery is performed when conservative measures have failed and the patient's quality of life is compromised. The options depend on the patient's fitness for anaesthesia and whether any other prolapse exists. Burch colposuspension was the gold-standard procedure, with a success rate of 85–90%. The retropubic space is entered through a small suprapubic incision and two or three permanent sutures are placed on either side of the bladder neck to the corresponding ileopectineal ligament (see Fig. 8.7). This procedure can also be performed laparoscopically. There are a variety of 'sling' procedures that can be performed abdominally or vaginally, with rectus sheath, fascia lata or synthetic materials. The commonest type is the tension-free vaginal tape (TVT) procedure (Fig. 8.8), which has the advantage that it can be performed under local anaesthesia. It has success rates of between 80 and 90% and has taken over from the Burch procedure as the gold-standard treatment for USI. An alternative method of placing the mid urethral sling is via the obturator foramen and this technique is also proving an effective alternative to TVT. Anterior colporrhaphy with bladder buttress is rarely performed for stress incontinence as it has cure rates of less than 50%.

Injectables or bulking agents are appropriate if previous surgery has failed or in very elderly patients. Various compounds may be used, including collagen, with success rates of 50%.

Complications for all these procedures include postoperative voiding difficulty, bleeding, infection, de novo detrusor overactivity and suture or mesh erosion (in the 'sling' procedure).

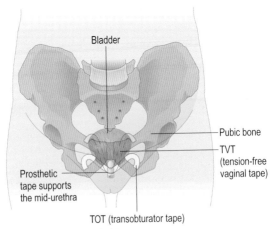

Bladder

Pubic bone

TVT (tension-free vaginal tape)

Prosthetic tape supports the mid-urethra

TOT (transobturator tape)

Figure 8.8 Position of midurethral tape.

Overflow incontinence

This is the frequent involuntary loss of small volumes of urine. There are often other associated voiding problems such as poor stream or a feeling of incomplete emptying.

Causes

Obstruction to urinary flow

1. Pelvic organ prolapse
2. Previous incontinence surgery
3. Pelvic mass such as fibroids
4. Constipation
5. Urethral stenosis
6. Postoperative, epidural anaesthesia.

Detrusor dysfunction

1. Medications with anticholinergic side effects
2. Neurogenic, e.g. spinal cord injury or multiple sclerosis.

Management

Accurate history and examination will usually elicit the cause. The following investigations should be performed:

- Midstream specimen of urine – these patients often have a urinary tract infection because of large urinary bladder residuals, which may require prophylactic antibiotic treatment.
- Intravenous pyelogram (IVP) – ureteric reflux may result from the bladder hypotonia.
- Urodynamics – flow studies will show a reduced flow rate with a strain or interrupted sinusoidal pattern. Cystometry will show a delayed first sensation, reduced detrusor pressure during voiding in hypotonia, or conversely, a high detrusor pressure with urethral obstruction.

Treatment

Patients may need to be taught intermittent self-catheterization or may need an indwelling catheter if unable to self-catheterize. If urethral obstruction is the cause, then consider urethral dilatation or urethrolysis, which involves either a vaginal or abdominal procedure to free up the urethra.

Detrusor hypotonia may be treated with cholinergic medication and severe cases may require a urinary diversion procedure.

TRUE INCONTINENCE

This is continuous urinary leakage, most commonly due to a fistula between the urinary tract and the pelvic organs. In the developing world this is commonly a result of obstructed labour. In the developed world these fistulae are usually caused by surgery or radiotherapy.

Assessment

- Enquire about a history of traumatic delivery, previous pelvic surgery or radiotherapy.
- Ask about a history of continuing urinary leakage from the vagina.
- Examination in Sims' position may reveal a fistula.
- Consider IVP, micturating cystourethrogram or cystoscopy.

Management

Often fistulae secondary to obstetric trauma may heal spontaneously. Otherwise surgical repair may be required. Surgical repair of a fistula can be performed vaginally or abdominally. When the fistula tract has been exposed it is repaired in a layered fashion and may require use of a graft (e.g. labial fat – Martius graft) to reinforce the repair.

SUMMARY

- Take a careful history of uterovaginal prolapse, bladder and bowel functions, and sexual activity.
- Accurate history and examination are crucial to making a correct diagnosis and assessing impact on quality of life so that an appropriate treatment strategy is commenced.
- Urodynamic investigation must be performed prior to any anti-incontinence surgery.
- Conservative management should always be offered and predisposing factors such as obesity, chronic cough, constipation and pelvic masses should be improved if possible.
- Great care should be taken in selecting the appropriate surgery for each individual patient. Remember that stress incontinence can be unmasked following surgical correction of prolapse.
- Careful counselling of patients prior to surgery regarding complications and success rates should be given.

Family planning and sexual health

CHAPTER CONTENTS

SEXUAL HEALTH

The World Health Organization defines sexual health as a state of physical, emotional, mental and social well-being related to sexuality. Sexual health requires positive and respectful approaches to sexuality and safe sexual experiences free of coercion, discrimination and violence. In such a way a woman can enjoy sex without putting herself or others at risk of physical or emotional harm.

In practice, sexual health means effective contraception, prevention of sexually transmitted infections (STIs), appropriate psychosexual help for sexual problems and support after sexual assault.

FAMILY PLANNING

Over 70% of women of reproductive age use some form of regular contraception. The decision on which method of contraception to use should be tailored to the individual's social, gynaecological and medical history. Whichever form is chosen, it is vital to give adequate education about how the method should be used and what to do if there is a failure in usage such as a missed pill or split condom. A trained nurse commonly performs this in a family planning or general practitioner setting. However, gynaecologists often need to advise on, prescribe or deal with problems relating to contraception.

The Pearl index

The Pearl index is used to rate the effectiveness of a contraceptive method and is defined as the number of women who will become pregnant if 100 women use that form of contraception properly according to instructions for 1 year (or the percentage of women experiencing an unwanted pregnancy in 1 year of use). This is distinct from the actual failure rate, which is found with 'typical use' rather than 'perfect use' of the method. Table 9.1 shows the Pearl index for the different contraceptive options.

Poor compliance and incorrect use apply particularly to condoms, contraceptive pills and natural family planning, where the actual failure rates are 14%, 5% and 25%, respectively. Long-acting reversible contraceptives

Table 9.1. Pearl index (the number of unwanted pregnancies per 100 women after 1 year of 'perfect' use of the following)

No contraception	80–90
Male condom	2
Female condom	5
Diaphragm and cap	4–8
Combined oral contraceptive pill	<1
Progesterone-only pill	1
Injectable progestogens	<1
Progestogen implants	<1
Contraceptive patch	<1
Intrauterine contraceptive device	1–2
Levonorgestrel-releasing intrauterine system (LNG-IUS)	<1
Natural family planning	2–6
Urinary hormone kit	6
Female sterilization	0.5
Male sterilization	0.05

(LARCs) are encouraged for those women who need reliable contraception and where compliance with remembering to use a contraceptive may be poor. LARCs include the contraceptive implant and injection as well as the intrauterine contraceptive device (IUCD) and system.

History

The important factors to be considered in the history are:
- Age
- Previous contraceptive history and side effects or failures with contraception
- Gynaecological problems: heavy or painful periods, ectopic pregnancy or functional ovarian cysts
- Current or previous STIs and pelvic inflammatory disease (PID)
- Medical problems: arterial or venous disease, liver disease, diabetes, mechanical heart valves, hypertension
- Current medications: enzyme inducers and some broad-spectrum antibiotics affect the efficacy of contraceptive pills
- Smoking
- Likely compliance with tablets or reliable use of barrier methods
- Need for protection from STIs
- Wishes for future fertility
- The importance to the woman of not becoming pregnant
- The male partner's willingness to take responsibility for contraceptive use.

The decision about contraception is always made between the doctor and the patient after explanation of:
- How the contraceptive is used
- Efficacy
- Risks
- Side effects
- Future fertility intentions.

Barrier methods

Male condom

This is a latex rubber or polyurethane sheath, often coated with spermicidal lubricant. It is used by 18% of couples in the UK.
- **Mode of action:** A condom acts as a physical barrier to prevent sperm entering the vagina.
- **How to use:** The condom is placed over the erect penis before contact with the female genitalia. After ejaculation it is removed with all ejaculate inside and checked for any defects.
- **Benefits:** Benefits are its use only during sexual intercourse, protection from viral and bacterial STIs, ready availability (free on the National Health Service (NHS)) in different sizes and colours and absence of hormonal side effects.
- **Disadvantages:** Disadvantages are interruption of love-making, some reduction in sensitivity for the male partner, occasional allergy of the man or woman to the latex or spermicide used and reliance on the male partner being motivated to use a condom on all occasions. If allergy occurs, polyurethane, low-allergy or non-spermicidal condoms should be tried. Failure occurs from damage to the condom from fingernails, jewellery or oil-based lubricants and from the condom slipping off or splitting. Pregnancy can also occur if the penis is in contact with the vagina when the condom is not in place (before or after ejaculation).

Female condom

This polyurethane sheath is inserted to line the vagina and act as a barrier to sperm reaching the cervix. It can be inserted at any time before intercourse. It has similar advantages and disadvantages to the male condom, but is not a commonly used contraceptive.

Diaphragm and cap

A diaphragm is a dome-shaped rubber device. The three types of diaphragm are flat, coil and arcing spring, depending on the amount of vaginal support. Contraceptive caps (Vimule, vault or cervical) are much smaller rubber or silicone devices that attach to the cervix by a suction effect.

- **Mode of action:** Both devices are used with spermicidal gel or cream and act by creating a spermicidal barrier, preventing motile sperm reaching the cervix.
- **How to use:** Two strips of spermicidal cream or gel are placed on either side of the diaphragm (caps should be one-third filled) and the device is inserted downwards and backwards into the vagina. The position is checked to ensure it is covering the cervix. It can be inserted up to 3 hours prior to sexual intercourse and extra spermicide is needed if it is more than 3 hours between insertion and sexual intercourse or if having sex for a second time. It must be left in the vagina for at least 6 hours after intercourse (up to 30 hours), then removed and washed in soapy water and stored in its plastic box. It is replaced every 2 years or earlier if damaged. Pelvic examination in the clinic is used to estimate the appropriate size of diaphragm (between 5 and 10 mm diameter).
- **Benefits:** Advantages are no interruption to sexual intercourse, use only when needed, no loss of sensation for either partner, some protection against STI and a slight reduction in cervical cancer.
- **Disadvantages:** Disadvantages are that a doctor or nurse is needed to fit the device, the technique needs to be learnt, occasional allergy occurs to rubber or spermicide and the man may be aware of the device. It is not a common form of contraception and offers little protection against most STIs. Side effects include recurrent urinary tract infections, which may be relieved with a smaller device. Diaphragms also need to be refitted if there is more than 3 kg weight change and after childbirth.
- **Contraindications:** Contraindications to use are unwillingness to touch the genitalia, inability to reach and identify the cervix, poor pelvic floor support to hold the device in place, history of toxic shock syndrome, recurrent urinary tract infection and allergy to rubber or spermicide.

Hormonal methods

Combined oestrogen and progesterone contraceptives

Seventy per cent of women aged 20–24 and 25% of all women aged 15–45 use a contraceptive pill in the UK.

Combined oral contraceptive pill

Combined oral contraceptive pills (COCPs) contain ethinyloestradiol (except Norinyl-1, which contains mestranol) and a progestogen.

- **Mode of action:** The main mode of action of the COCP is the inhibition of ovulation, but thickening of the cervical mucus and thinning of the endometrium also occur.
- **Types of combined oral contraceptive pill:** Different ethinyloestradiol strengths are suitable for different groups:
  - Low-strength (20 µg): suitable for women with circulatory risk factors, such as venous thrombosis or arterial disease risks.

- Standard-strength (30 or 35 μg): suitable for most women.
- High-strength (50 μg) (no longer licensed): previously used in obese women, those with breakthrough bleeding or on enzyme-inducing medication.

The progestogens are classed as 'second-generation' (e.g. norethisterone and levonorgestrel) or 'third-generation' (e.g. desogestrel and gestodene). The third-generation pills have a small increased risk of thrombosis, but may still be more suitable for women with acne, hirsutism, breast tenderness, weight gain and breakthrough bleeding on other preparations.

Monophasic COCP preparations are generally used, with all tablets in the pack containing the same quantity of oestrogen and progestogen. Biphasic and triphasic pills vary in the dose of progestogen and/or oestrogen during the pill cycle and can be used to obtain better cycle control in those with breakthrough bleeding (bleeding starting outside the normal pill-free interval) or in those who do not have a withdrawal bleed on monophasic preparations. 'Everyday' pill packs contain 21 active pills and seven placebo pills instead of the normal pill-free interval.

- **How to use:** Standard packs contain 21 pills which are taken continuously, followed by a 7-day break during which time a withdrawal bleed commences. The next pack of pills is then started on the 8th day, regardless of whether the bleed has finished.
- **When to start:** The first packet should be started in the first 7 days of the cycle, in which case it is effective immediately. In an amenorrhoeic or oligomenorrhoeic woman the COCP can be started at any time, but pregnancy must first be excluded and additional contraception should be used for the first 7 days. Women undergoing termination of pregnancy (TOP) should start on the day of the operation and the COCP can be commenced immediately after a miscarriage. Postnatally it should be avoided for 6 weeks due to the higher thrombosis risk and possible irregular bleeding.
- **Benefits of the combined oral contraceptive pill:** Benefits of the COCP are control of painful, heavy and irregular periods, a reduction in ovarian cancer (50% reduction if taken for more than 5 years; effect lasts after stopping pill) and endometrial cancer (40% reduction if taken for more than 5 years), less benign breast disease, reduction in functional ovarian cysts, improvement in premenstrual tension and endometriosis, control of fibroids and improvement in acne and hirsutism. The effect of the pill disappears immediately on stopping the pill (there is no evidence for the 'post-pill amenorrhoea' theory) – women are just as likely to become pregnant whether or not they have just finished the COCP.
- **Disadvantages of the combined oral contraceptive pill:** Disadvantages are the need to remember to take a pill everyday, lack of protection against STIs and an increase in cervical cancer (though this may relate to the lack of barrier protection against human papillomavirus (HPV)). The increased risk of breast cancer is still under investigation.
- **Side effects:** Serious side effects are thrombosis, hypertension and migraine. The pill should be stopped if these are suspected. More minor side effects include irregular bleeding in the first few cycles, weight gain or loss, reduced libido, nausea, bloatedness, breast tenderness, headache and mood change. Most of these symptoms do not persist after the first 3 months of use.

Essentials of Obstetrics and Gynaecology

- **Contraindications:** Contraindications include pregnancy, hypertension (>160/100 mmHg), severe migraine, previous history or high risk of thrombosis, ischaemic heart disease, cardiovascular accident, liver disease, porphyria, diabetes, smokers over 35 years and unexplained irregular vaginal bleeding. The COCP is contraindicated with breastfeeding as it may impair milk production.

- **Drug interactions:** Drug interactions must be avoided. Enzyme inducers such as antiepileptics and griseofulvin increase metabolism of the COCP and a high-strength pill should be used if there is no suitable alternative contraceptive. However, with rifampicin and rifabutin the enzyme-inducing effect is too potent and the COCP should not be used at all until 8 weeks after stopping. Some broad-spectrum antibiotics such as ampicillin and doxycycline interfere with COCP absorption. The COCP antagonizes the effects of many antihypertensives, diuretics, warfarin, antidepressants and diabetic drugs. Corticosteroid concentrations are increased by the COCP.

- **Missed pills:** A 'missed pill' is one that is either completely forgotten or taken more than 12 hours after the normal time. It should be taken once remembered and the rest of the packet continued, with a barrier method of contraception used in addition for 7 days. If the pack ends within those 7 days then the next pack should be started straightaway, without a break. The '7-day rule' is a helpful guide: it takes 7 days of continuous pills for ovulation to be suppressed and 7 days without pills for ovarian activity to resume.

  If vomiting or severe diarrhoea occurs within 3 hours of taking the pill, extra precautions should be taken, as for a missed pill.

  Women taking some antibiotics (e.g. ampicillin or doxycycline) should continue to take the pill but use a barrier contraceptive until 7 pill-taking days after completing the course of antibiotics. The exception is long-term antibiotics, such as those for acne, where the barrier method needs only to be used for the first 3 weeks until the gut flora adjusts.

- **Thrombosis risk with the combined oral contraceptive pill:** The risk of thrombosis is increased by COCP use, but is far less than the risk of thrombosis in pregnancy. The rate of thrombosis per 100 000 women per year is shown in Table 9.2.

  The risk of thromboembolic events also depends on age, weight, smoking history and family history of thrombosis, so the risk of the COCP needs to be individually assessed. Women should be counselled about any individual increased risk and a joint decision can then be made with the doctor about starting, after considering other methods of contraception. A thrombophilia screen should be performed before starting the COCP for women with a family history of thrombosis.

Table 9.2. Rate of thrombosis per 100 000 women per year of combined oral contraceptive use

Previously healthy non-pregnant, non-pill-taking woman	5
Woman taking second-generation COCP	15
Woman taking third-generation COCP	25
Pregnant woman	60

COCP, combined oral contraceptive pill.

Contraceptive patch

The contraceptive patch contains oestrogen and progesterone and the mode of action is as for COCP. It is applied on the first day of the period and changed on the 8th and 15th days (once a week). It is removed on day 21 and a withdrawal bleed starts during the patch-free week. Benefits, disadvantages and side effects are similar to those with the COCP.

Progesterone-only pill

The progesterone-only pill (POP) is also known as the mini-pill.

- **Mode of action:** POPs thicken the cervical mucus to inhibit sperm entry through the cervical canal. They also thin the endometrium and in a few women inhibit ovulation.
- **How to use:** POPs are taken as a continuous preparation, in 28-day packs, with no break between packs. The POP must be taken at the same time each day and, if taken more than 3 hours late, contraceptive efficacy is immediately reduced. Similarly, diarrhoea and vomiting also impair absorption (and therefore efficacy) of the pill. Missed pills (or those taken late or with diarrhoea or vomiting) should be managed as for COCP.

  The dose is doubled (two pills daily) in women over 70 kg.

  Most women continue to menstruate, though some may have lighter periods and a few become amenorrhoeic. Heavy or irregular bleeding can occur in the first few months.
- **When to start:** As for the COCP, they are started in the first 7 days of the cycle, on the day of TOP, immediately after miscarriage or at any time in an oligomenorrhoeic or amenorrhoeic woman as long as pregnancy has been excluded and extra precautions are used for 7 days. They can be started immediately postpartum.
- **Benefits of progesterone-only pill:** POPS are beneficial when there are concerns regarding potential side effects of oestrogen-containing pills or if the COCP is contraindicated, for example in older women, smokers, immediately postpartum, whilst breastfeeding, and when there is a risk of deep venous thrombosis, hypertension, migraine or diabetes. They may also help with premenstrual syndrome.
- **Disadvantages of progesterone-only pill:** Disadvantages are reduced efficacy compared with the COCP and the close time interval for taking the pills.
- **Side effects:** Side effects are an increase in functional ovarian cysts and a higher risk of ectopic if pregnancy occurs. Acne, headache, breast tenderness, nausea and irregular bleeding tend to settle after a few months. Weight change occurs in a few. There is a small increase in breast cancer diagnosis.
- **Contraindications:** Contraindications are pregnancy, previous ectopic pregnancy, problematic functional ovarian cysts, severe arterial disease (myocardial infarction or cerebrovascular accident, active liver disease, porphyria, undiagnosed irregular vaginal bleeding and breast cancer.
- **Drug interactions:** Enzyme-inducing drugs, but not broad-spectrum antibiotics, interfere with the effectiveness of POPs. Management with enzyme-inducing drugs is as for the COCP.

Injectables and implants

- **Injectables:** Medroxyprogesterone acetate (12 mg) and norethisterone enantate (200 mg) are the two available forms of injectable contraceptives, given by intramuscular injection into the buttock every 12 and 8 weeks, respectively.

- *Mode of action* - Injectables act by inhibiting ovulation, and also thickening cervical mucus and thinning the endometrium. Norethisterone enantate is used as a short-term contraceptive only (maximum two doses). They are given initially on day 1–5 of the cycle, or within 5 days of parturition, but should be delayed until 6 weeks in breastfeeding women.

  Irregular bleeding is normal in the first few months and most women become amenorrhoeic thereafter. After the last injection fertility may return immediately or be delayed by up to 18 months.

- *Benefits* - Benefits are high efficacy, no need to remember to take a pill, no interference with intercourse and use where oestrogens are contraindicated. They also do not have the increased ovarian cysts or ectopic risk of oral progesterone-only preparations because they reliably inhibit ovulation.

- *Disadvantages* - Disadvantages are the possible delayed return of fertility and side effects of weight gain, progestogenic side effects and persistent irregular bleeding. There is a possible increased risk of osteoporosis with long-term medroxyprogesterone acetate use and current recommendations suggest that prescribers re-evaluate suitability of treatment after 2 years.

- *Contraindications* - Contraindications are pregnancy, undiagnosed vaginal bleeding, severe arterial disease and liver disease. The effect of norethisterone entantate (but not medroxyprogesterone acetate) is diminished by enzyme-inducing drugs and should not be used in conjunction with these.

- Implants: The etonogestrel-releasing implant is the only implant currently available and is a progestogen rod (40 × 2 mm) inserted subdermally into the upper inner arm under local anaesthetic. Another implant, the levonorgestrel-releasing subdermal system (Norplant), consisting of six subdermal rods, has been discontinued, but a few women may still present to have the rods removed.

  - *Mode of action* - The etonogestrel-releasing implant thickens cervical mucus, thins the endometrium and, in a few women, ovulation is inhibited.

  - *How to use* - The etonogestrel-releasing implant can be inserted in the first few days of the cycle or immediately after childbirth, TOP or miscarriage. Twenty per cent of women become amenorrhoeic and 26% have irregular spotting, which usually settles within the first year. No failures have been reported. It should be replaced after 3 years or 2 years if the body mass index is greater than 35 kg/m². The implant is removed fairly easily and periods and fertility return to normal immediately.

  - *Benefits* - Benefits are that it is extremely effective, causes no interference with sexual intercourse, has some protection against PID and endometrial cancer, can be used with breastfeeding, and is useful when oestrogen-containing products are contraindicated or cause side effects.

  - *Disadvantages* - Disadvantages include progestogenic side effects in some women (headache, breast tenderness, weight gain, mood disturbance) and most women experience irregular bleeding within the first year, which then settles. Some, however, are then amenorrhoeic or have persistent irregular bleeding. There is an increase in functional ovarian cysts and possible increase in depression. Occasionally, bruising, itching or infection occurs at the site of the implant.

- *Contraindications* - Contraindications are the same as for injectables, but also include severe depression. The implant should not be used with enzyme-inducing drugs.

Levonorgestrel-releasing intrauterine system

This is a flexible intrauterine rod on a T-shaped frame, which releases 20 μg levonorgestrel every 24 hours. It is shown in Figure 9.1.

- **Mode of action:** It thickens the cervical mucus and thins the endometrium, with inhibition of ovulation in some cycles for some women.
- **How to use:** The LNG-IUS is fitted in the first 7 days of the cycle, or later if another contraceptive is used for 7 days after fitting. It can be inserted immediately after TOP or miscarriage and 6 weeks postnatally. Antibiotic cover is needed for insertion, as for other intrauterine devices. The intrauterine system should be changed after 5 years.

  Most women have very light or absent bleeding after 2–3 months of irregular bleeding. Fertility returns immediately on removal. The LNG-IUS should be removed if pregnancy does occur as there is a theoretical teratogenic risk.

- **Benefits:** Benefits are a reduction in bleeding, reduced dysmenorrhoea and reduced incidence of PID. There is also a significantly reduced ectopic risk and few progestogenic side effects, due to the local action. There is no significant effect of enzyme-inducing drugs.
- **Disadvantages:** Disadvantages are irregular bleeding in the first 3 months (the commonest reason for early removal), increased risk of functional ovarian cysts, risks of expulsion and perforation. If progestogenic side effects do occur, they usually resolve within the first few months.

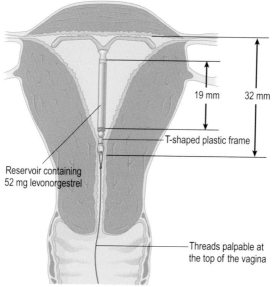

19 mm

32 mm

T-shaped plastic frame

Reservoir containing
52 mg levonorgestrel

Threads palpable at
the top of the vagina

Figure 9.1 The levonorgestrel-releasing intrauterine system.

Essentials of Obstetrics and Gynaecology

- **Contraindications:** Contraindications are pregnancy, undiagnosed irregular bleeding, active liver disease, severe arterial disease, mechanical heart valves, untreated STI and a history of ovarian or endometrial carcinoma. Nulliparity is not a contraindication, though fitting may be less well tolerated.

Intrauterine devices

Used by about 5% of women, IUCDs are copper-containing devices on a T-shaped frame. They have two threads attached to the lower end, which protrude from the ectocervix and curl around the lips of the cervix and are grasped for removal. A frameless device is also available, which is attached to the uterine fundus by a knot.

- **Mode of action:** Copper is spermicidal and toxic to the early embryo. The device also creates an inflammatory response in the endometrium to prevent implantation.
- **How to use:** IUCDs are inserted into the uterine cavity via the cervix in the outpatient setting, under local anaesthetic if needed. Women should be screened first for STIs or given antibiotic cover with azithromycin 1 gram (single dose) or doxycycline 100 mg daily for 7 days. IUCDs are usually inserted in the first 7 days of the cycle, but can be inserted up to day 19 (the earliest predicted implantation date). Otherwise they are fitted immediately after miscarriage or TOP or 6 weeks postpartum.

  The threads should be checked by a doctor or nurse after the first month and subsequently on palpation by the woman after each period.

  If PID occurs, this is most likely in the first 20 days after insertion, and the IUCD should be removed unless the infection is mild and resolving with antibiotic treatment.

  Removal of IUCDs should be in the first 7 days of the cycle. If removed midcycle, emergency contraception should be given if sexual intercourse has occurred within the last 5 days.

Pregnancy with an intrauterine contraceptive device in situ

If pregnancy occurs with the IUCD in situ then there is an increased chance that it will be an ectopic pregnancy and an urgent scan is needed to confirm the pregnancy location. The coil should be removed if the pregnancy is intrauterine as the risk of midtrimester complications outweighs the risk of miscarriage from removal in the first trimester.

- **Benefits:** Benefits are the long-term efficacy and lack of hormonal side effects.
- **Disadvantages:** The main disadvantage is that copper IUCDs increase menorrhagia. There is also an increased PID risk. Perforation can occur at fitting and expulsion is most likely with the first period.

  Actinomycosis can occur in women with an IUCD in place. It is very rare in women without an IUCD. The infection is often found incidentally on a cervical smear. If pelvic pain or a mass is present then the IUCD must be removed and the infection treated with penicillin for several months.

- **Contraindications:** Contraindications to the IUCD are pregnancy, undiagnosed irregular vaginal bleeding, untreated STI or high risk of infection, heavy or prolonged periods, anaemia, previous ectopic, previous uterine scarring and mechanical heart valves. Wilson's disease and copper allergy are also contraindications.

Lost coils

If the threads cannot be identified on speculum, gentle exploration with a coil hook will retrieve them from the cervical canal. If the threads are not found then an urgent scan should be arranged to confirm that the coil has not been expelled and hysteroscopic removal should be arranged in the outpatient clinic. Pregnancy should be excluded in women with a lost coil and alternative contraception prescribed, unless the scan confirms correct positioning of the coil at the fundus. Rarely, the coil is located outside the uterus and is identified on X-ray or ultrasound before laparoscopic removal.

Natural family planning

Sperm may survive for up to 7 days after intercourse and eggs survive for approximately 24 hours after ovulation. Therefore, the fertile period lasts for about 8 days. Natural family planning involves identification of the timing of ovulation to prevent contact between the egg and viable sperm during this time.

Natural family planning is only effective in women who have been properly taught the technique and have a regular cycle. Three methods are used, often in conjunction with each other, to identify the fertile time during which intercourse is avoided or a barrier contraceptive is used: (1) basal body temperature; (2) cervical mucus; and (3) time in cycle.

Basal body temperature

The temperature is taken daily, with a narrow-range fertility thermometer, before getting out of bed and having anything to eat or drink. Ovulation is followed by a basal temperature rise of approximately 0.5°C. By identifying where in the cycle ovulation occurs, the woman can avoid intercourse for 7 days before this and for 1–2 days after the temperature rises.

Cervical mucus

The cervical mucus becomes moist, sticky and white preovulation and then clear, copious and stretchy (spinnbarkeit) at the most fertile time.

Time in cycle

Ovulation occurs 12–16 days before a period.

Pain from ovulation and breast changes are less reliable indicators of fertility.

Advantages

The advantages of natural family planning are the absence of chemicals or hormones, the absence of side effects, and cultural and religious acceptability.

Disadvantages

Disadvantages are that both partners need to be committed to abstinence or condoms during the fertile period (8–9 days in each cycle) and that cycles are altered by stress, illness and travel.

Lactational amenorrhoea

The lactational amenorrhoea method is the reliance on amenorrhoea during breastfeeding as contraception. It is effective in 98% of women who use the method. However, efficacy reduces as soon as:

- The mother menstruates
- The first supplementary milk or 'solids' feed is given
- The baby is more than 6 months old.

Urinary hormone kit

A commercial kit uses urinary hormone changes to predict the fertile period. It is expensive, takes several cycles to be reliable and is not as effective as other contraceptive methods.

Emergency contraception

Indications

Emergency contraception is indicated where no contraception has been used, where compliance with the usual method has been poor (e.g. missed pill) or when the usual method has failed (e.g. split condom). The two licensed methods are levonorgestrel and the IUCD. Ten per cent of women have used emergency contraception in the preceding 2 years.

Levonorgestrel

This is a progesterone-only regime consisting of 1.5 mg levonorgestrel as a single dose.

- **Mode of action:** The precise mode of action is unknown, but probably involves inhibition of egg transport, ovulation and implantation.
- **Efficacy:** The overall pregnancy risk after a single act of sexual intercourse on any day in the cycle is 2–4%. This increases to 30% in the days around ovulation. Levonorgestrel prevents 95% of expected pregnancies if given within 24 hours of unprotected intercourse and efficacy reduces thereafter to 58% at 72 hours, but there may still be benefit up to 5 days after intercourse.
- **How to use:** Levonorgestrel 1.5 mg is given as soon as possible after intercourse. If vomiting occurs within 3 hours, a replacement dose can be given with an antiemetic (ideally domperidone) or an IUCD inserted. Women should be advised:
- Their next period may be early or late.
- To have a pregnancy test if the next period is more than 7 days late.
- To seek medical help immediately if severe abdominal pain occurs, due to risk of ectopic pregnancy.
- **Side effects:** Side effects include nausea, irregular bleeding and occasional abdominal pain.
- **Interactions:** Levonorgestrel emergency contraception can be used in conjunction with other hormonal methods and the only contraindication is porphyria. In women taking enzyme-inducing drugs, 1.5 mg levonorgestrel should be given or an IUCD fitted instead.

The Yuzpe method or PC4 involved two doses of ethinyloestradiol 100 mg and levonorgestrel 500 mg 12 hours apart and has been discontinued due to excessive vomiting compared with levonorgestrel (20% versus 5%).

Postcoital intrauterine contraceptive device

- **Efficacy:** Insertion of a copper IUCD within 72 hours of intercourse prevents 98% of expected pregnancies.
- **How to use:** It is usually 5 days from ovulation to implantation so the IUCD can be inserted up to 5 days after intercourse or at any time before day 19 in the cycle if intercourse has also occurred earlier in the cycle. If there is a chance of pregnancy from earlier intercourse and the woman presents after day 19 then the IUCD should not be fitted, as implantation may have already occurred (and, therefore, the IUCD may cause very early termination of pregnancy).

Antibiotic cover is needed, as for other IUCD fitting.

The coil can be kept in or removed after the next period. Pregnancy must be excluded if the next period is more than 7 days late, very light or short, or if abdominal pain occurs.

Permanent methods

Surgical sterilization (of the woman or her partner) is reported as the method of avoiding pregnancy in 23% of women in the UK. Approximately 45 000 tubal occlusions and 65 000 vasectomies are performed in England each year.

Advantages

The advantages are that it is relatively simple (especially vasectomy), permanent, has no hormonal side effects and does not interfere with intercourse.

Disadvantages

Disadvantages are the small failure rate, complications from the procedure, irreversibility and no protection from STI.

Laparoscopic sterilization

A clip or ring is applied to the mid-portion of each fallopian tube by laparoscopic control under general anaesthetic as a day case. This prevents fertilization of the oocyte by preventing contact with the sperm.

All women need careful counselling prior to the procedure and surgical risk needs to be assessed (e.g. high body mass index, previous operations, medical problems). Ten per cent regret the procedure, especially if they were under 25 years of age at the time of sterilization, had no children or were not in a relationship at the time. However, there is no place for a blanket lower age limit for sterilization. The commonest reason for requesting reversal is a new partner.

Reversal is often unsuccessful (pregnancy rates 55–90%) and depends on the length of time since the procedure, the number of clips applied to each tube and their position. There is also a 5% ectopic pregnancy risk after reversal procedures.

Before arranging sterilization, all women must be informed of the following:

- How the procedure is performed.
- Operative risks: infection, bleeding or visceral damage (bowel, bladder, vessel injury) occurs in 6 in 1000 cases.
- Mini-laparotomy: sterilization by mini-laparotomy if the laparoscopic approach is technically difficult should be agreed to and included on the consent form.
- The lifetime failure rate of 1 in 200 (or two to three pregnancies per 1000 women over 10 years).
- Increased ectopic risk if pregnancy occurs.
- Need for contraception until the next period starts.
- Permanence: the procedure should be viewed as irreversible as reversal is technically difficult, not available on the NHS and has poor success.
- Regret: ask about what the woman would feel if any existing children died or she had a new partner.
- Alternatives: has the woman considered alternative methods? The LNG-IUS is more effective, easily reversible and less invasive. Vasectomy has fewer operative risks and a lower risk of failure.
- There is no effect on periods in the long term – some women report heavier periods, but this probably relates to age and to stopping hormonal contraception.

Laparoscopic sterilization is contraindicated in women with surgical risks or those uncertain about their desire for future fertility.

Vasectomy

Vasectomy is safe and very effective (failure rate 1 in 2000 after confirmation of azoospermia). It involves bilateral division of the vas deferens, usually under local anaesthetic by a urologist, as a day case. A scrotal support and analgesia are needed in the first postoperative days.

Azoospermia needs to be confirmed on semen analysis at 2 and 3 months; two azoospermic samples are required before alternative contraception is abandoned.

Advantages are efficacy, avoidance of general anaesthetic and permanence.

Disadvantages are the need for motivation for the procedure, the need for alternative contraception until at least 3 months following the procedure and possible side effects, including infection, bruising, haematoma, pain and sperm granuloma (extravasation of sperm from the cut vas causing a painful mass).

Failure may occur early, in which case azoospermia is never confirmed, or late, with recanalization of the vas deferens.

Contraception in teenagers

In the UK, the Fraser rules or Gillick criteria allow for contraception to be prescribed to girls under the age of 16, without parental consent, as long as the doctor is satisfied that:

- The girl understands the advice, including the implications of having sex and the contraception method.
- He/she has tried to persuade the girl to talk to her parents or other responsible adult about having sex and contraceptive use.
- The girl intends to have sex whether contraception is given or not and, therefore, the risk to her mental or physical health of not giving contraception outweighs the risk of giving contraception.
- The girl is giving proper consent to sexual intercourse.

Barrier contraception should be encouraged, often as well as hormonal, to prevent STI.

The age of the partner should be ascertained, as it is illegal to have intercourse with a girl under the age of 16. However, this law is generally only applied when the intercourse is non-consensual or the male partner is significantly older.

Contraception around the menopause

Fertility diminishes with age (10–20 pregnancies per 100 women over 45 years of age compared with 80–90 under 40 years). However, pregnancy in older women is more complicated, with much higher rates of termination, fetal abnormality, miscarriage and pregnancy complications, including maternal and fetal mortality. Therefore, effective contraception should be used for 2 years after the last period if the woman is under 50 years, or 1 year after the last period if she is over 50 years. The trend is towards greater use of sterilization as age increases.

The risks of oestrogen-containing pills increase with age. The POP is, therefore, commonly used after the age of 40 (or earlier in smokers). An IUCD inserted after the age of 40 years can be left in situ until 50 years old, as the risk of pregnancy is low.

Contraception and operations

Oestrogen-containing contraception increases the risk of postoperative thrombosis. It should be stopped 4 weeks before elective major or lower-limb operations and an alternative method used. For minor procedures, such as laparoscopy, it can be continued as long as prolonged immobilization does not occur. For emergency operations, the pill should be stopped on admission and extra thromboprophylaxis should be prescribed.

The COCP can be restarted 2 weeks after full mobilization.

PSYCHOSEXUAL MEDICINE

Definitions

Female sexual problems are classified as:

- Loss of desire (hypoactive sexual desire disorder): reduced or absent spontaneous interest in sex with or without difficulty with arousal.
- Poor arousal (impaired sex drive): inability to respond to sexual feelings by becoming physically aroused.
- Anorgasmia: failure to achieve orgasm.
- Dyspareunia: pain with sexual intercourse or stimulation, which may be superficial or deep.
- Vaginismus: involuntary spasm of the muscles of the pelvic floor, triggered by attempted penetration, such that it is difficult or impossible to achieve full penetration.

Prevalence

Forty per cent of women experience some form of sexual dysfunction; 80% of these women complain of a loss of desire; and 12% of women do not experience orgasm. Of those who do, 25% of women achieve orgasm with penetrative sex and 75% need extra clitoral stimulation.

Aetiology

The aetiology of sexual problems is poorly understood, but psychological and physical factors may be involved. Table 9.3 outlines the main causes.

Clinical presentation

Women may present in a variety of ways, either directly with a problem or commonly by using another excuse for the consultation such as difficulty with contraception or dyspareunia. There is often difficulty discussing sexual problems both with partners and with health professionals.

Sexual problems may be situational, partner-dependent or occur all the time. They may be primary (since first sexual intercourse) or secondary (developed later). Some problems may not be perceived as a problem; for example, many women who never achieve orgasm still become aroused during sex and find it pleasurable and intimate.

Sexual difficulty can occur at any stage of the normal sexual response process, which involves sexual desire, arousal and orgasm, followed by a resolution phase. These physiological phases are independent of each other so, for example, a woman with loss of desire may still become fully aroused and achieve orgasm with sexual stimulation.

History

Setting

It is important to avoid embarrassment as far as possible by using appropriate body language and arranging chairs so there is no physical barrier (such as a desk) between the doctor and patient. Privacy should be ensured and the woman should be assured that the consultation is confidential. In general, women will find it easier to discuss sexual problems if the doctor approaches the problem in a matter-of-fact, but non-judgemental, manner.

Table 9.3. Causes of psychosexual problems

Psychological:
Stress
Life changes
Secondary to sexual assault
Changes in self-image relating to becoming a mother, hysterectomy, loss of reproductive ability at the menopause or loss of a partner (some increase their sex drive once the concern about becoming pregnant has gone)

Physical:
Physiological
Premenstrual, postnatal or perimenopausal
Fatigue
Depression

Hormonal:
Androgen insufficiency, e.g. after TAH and BSO or chemotherapy
Hyperprolactinaemia
Low oestrogen level means longer to become aroused, vaginal dryness, tiredness, mood changes, less sensitive genitalia and breasts

Neurological:
Diabetes
Multiple sclerosis

Cardiovascular:
Cardiovascular disease

Social:
Alcohol excess

Drugs:
Antiandrogens (cyproterone acetate, GnRH analogues)
Antioestrogens (COCP, tamoxifen)
Antidepressants (especially tricyclics)
Anticonvulsants (especially carbamazepine and phenytoin)
Hypertensives
Diuretics
Anticholinergics

TAH, total abdominal hysterectomy; BSO, bilateral salpingo-oophorectomy; GnRH, gonadotrophin-releasing hormone; COCP, combined oral contraceptive pill.

Sufficient time must be available for the consultation, with deferment to another appointment if necessary.

In addition to a gynaecological history, a sexual and social history should be taken.

Sexual history
- Problem:
- What is the problem?
- How long has it been present? Does it relate to time, place or partner?
- Was there an event or trigger for the problem?
- Does it relate to desire for sex, arousal or orgasm, or is there pain superficially or deep during intercourse?

- Does the problem occur just with penetrative sex or also with masturbation?
- For vaginismus and dyspareunia, is the woman able to use tampons and tolerate smear examinations?
- Is there history of recent or former sexual assault or abuse?
- Partner:
- Is there a current partner? How long has she been with this partner?
- When was the last partner before this one?
- Does she still find her partner attractive?
- How often do they have sex?
- Is she worried about him, for example because of his health?
- Are there other relationship difficulties, for example is either partner having an affair?
- Psychological factors:
- Does the woman feel depressed, anxious or angry?
- What is her self-image? Does she feel attractive?
- If she has had a hysterectomy or become menopausal, does she feel less of a woman?
- Has her self-image changed as a result of childbirth?
- Is there a fear of pregnancy or infection?
- Social factors:
- Does either partner hold religious or cultural views about sex (for example, about contraception or sex after the menopause)?
- Is there excessive alcohol intake?
- Are there stress factors, such as financial or employment difficulties or concerns about children or dependants?
- Medical factors:
- Depression and psychotic illness cause loss of desire. Hypothyroidism is associated with low desire and poor arousal.
- Pelvic trauma or operations may interrupt the innervation to the genitalia. Other medical problems such as pain from arthritis or immobility from stroke can interfere with sexual activity.
- Is there vaginal atrophy from postmenopausal hypo-oestrogenization?
- Has there been a recent STI?
- Drugs:
- Are medications being taken that may reduce desire or arousal?

Examination

In many situations an examination is not necessary in the assessment of sexual problems. However, in some cases a full general examination is vital to exclude neurological or endocrine problems that may be suggested by the history. Genital examination is also useful in cases of dyspareunia, to diagnose any physical and treatable cause, and reassure the woman if the findings are normal. The reason for the examination must be carefully explained and it can be necessary to defer the examination if the woman feels nervous or uncomfortable at the first consultation. Occasionally, examination is performed under anaesthetic, for example where vaginismus is very severe and pathology has not been excluded.

Particular attention must be made to ensure privacy and a chaperone should be used for both male and female doctors.

General examination

- Does the woman appear depressed? Is she confident with her body? What is her general mobility? Can she easily reach the couch and bend her legs for examination?

- Look for signs of hyperandrogenism (acne, hirsutism) or thyroid disease and check pulses and blood pressure.
- Check for neurological deficit by examining gross sensation, power and reflexes.
- Perform an abdominal examination for masses or tenderness.

Genital examination

- Check the labia for infection (herpes simplex virus (HSV), HPV) or atrophy. Is the introitus scarred by episiotomy, tears or other vaginal surgery? Is the perineum deficient? Perform a speculum examination for signs of infections such as *Candida* and bimanual examination for tenderness or masses.
- Vaginismus may be noted as muscle spasm and pain on attempting to insert the speculum or finger for examination.

Investigations

Urinalysis for glycosuria should normally be performed. Vaginal and cervical swabs should be sent where infection is suspected. Otherwise investigations are only indicated by findings in the history or examination.

Management

General

Treatment of any underlying physical cause of the problem is vital. Gynaecologists trained in counselling can deal with some psychosexual problems but many women will need to be referred for more specialist counselling, cognitive behavioural approaches or sex therapy. Sex therapy may be with the woman alone, or with the partner, where the relationship itself is seen as the 'patient'. Sensate focus, established in the 1970s by Masters and Johnson, involves a programme of abstinence from all sexual activity with a gradual reintroduction of sexual contact over a period of weeks once fear has gone and trust between the couple has been re-established. Cognitive behavioural therapy is a relatively short programme aiming to analyse negative thinking patterns and teach more positive thinking and behaviour.

Individual problems

- **Loss of desire:** Any medical problems should be treated and causative medications changed where alternatives are available. A cognitive behavioural approach and sex therapy, often with the couple together, are helpful. The couple should be encouraged to talk through the problem and learn new love-making techniques, explore the sexual expectations and needs of each other, and encourage acceptance of each other's positions.
- **Impaired sex drive:** These women should be screened carefully for medical problems, particularly thyroid disease.
- **Anorgasmia:** Women should be taught about the body and taught to talk about feelings, such as fear of losing control over feelings and behaviour. Discussion should cover how comfortable the woman feels with herself and her partner. Sex therapy, either individually or in groups, can address issues of self-exploration, masturbation, use of vibrators and resolution of fears.
- **Dyspareunia:** The cause may be underlying pelvic pathology or relate to a psychological problem. Lack of lubrication, vaginismus, vestibulitis, *Candida*, genital herpes and sensitivity to condoms are all potentially treatable causes of superficial dyspareunia. Simple lubrication may

help dryness and topical oestrogens should be used for atrophy. Endometriosis, PID, infections (e.g. *Candida*) or tumours causing deep dyspareunia should be treated.

Counselling may still be necessary if the initial problem (e.g. *Candida*) has been treated, but sex has come to be associated with pain.

- **Vaginismus:** This is a conditioned response from the association of sex with pain or fear and management is focused on this, after any current physical causes (e.g. infection) have been appropriately treated.

Reassurance is helpful, after examination, that there is no physical cause for the problem. Cognitive behavioural therapy and a relaxation programme, with the use of vaginal trainers, gradually increase the woman's tolerance of penetration and allow her to regain her confidence, with a very high success rate.

Rape and sexual assault

Up to 20% of women experience some form of rape or sexual assault during their lifetime. Rape by a stranger is rare (less than 20%) and the perpetrator is usually a partner or ex-partner, friend, acquaintance or family member. Women often do not want police involvement and may present to a gynaecologist at any time after the event. However, any allegation should be treated as a potential legal case. Documentation by the doctor should include 'what you heard, what you saw and what you did'. Diagrams are very useful for annotation of any injuries to the general body or genital region, though there are often no signs of rape, especially if the woman is premenopausal, sexually active and parous. In most areas an examination by a forensic-trained doctor can be arranged, but a woman may decline this and the examination will need to be performed by the general gynaecologist.

Girls under the age of 14 should never be examined by a gynaecologist in a suspected assault case and should be referred to an appropriately trained community paediatrician. Between 14 and 16 years, it may occasionally be appropriate for a gynaecologist to perform the examination if a forensic-trained doctor is not available and the girl has been previously sexually active.

- Management:
- Treat any immediate injuries, referring to Accident and Emergency if necessary.
- Perform a full examination to identify any injuries to the head, body or limbs.
- Examine the genitalia for bruises, bleeding, tenderness, tears or foreign bodies.
- Give appropriate contraception – levonorgestrel or the emergency IUCD – after excluding pregnancy.
- Perform an STI screen and repeat after 3 weeks, to allow for incubation periods.
- Consider prophylactic antibiotics for *Chlamydia*, gonorrhoea and *Trichomonas*.
- Store serum for virology and repeat the sample for human immunodeficiency virus (HIV), hepatitis B and hepatitis C after 3 months.
- Depending on the assailant details, give hepatitis B immunoglobulin and initiate an accelerated vaccination course. Postexposure prophylaxis for HIV is indicated in rare situations.
- Arrange counselling.
- Encourage reporting of the incident to the police.
- Ensure the woman has a safe place to stay or arrange a place of refuge.

SEXUALLY TRANSMITTED INFECTIONS

Incidence

One in 10 women under the age of 25 in the UK have *Chlamydia* (3–5% of the total female population of reproductive age) and most STIs are becoming more common, with double the incidence of gonorrhoea and six times the incidence of syphilis in the last 6 years.

Age

STIs occur most commonly in the 18–25-year age group.

Presentation

Women with STI may complain of symptoms or an infection may be found incidentally during investigation for pelvic pain or irregular bleeding. Alternatively, a woman may have been given a 'contact slip' by a partner who has been diagnosed with an STI. Many women attend genitourinary medicine (GUM) clinics for regular sexual health screens.

Clinical features

Presenting features for STIs in symptomatic women are vaginal discharge, postcoital bleeding, intermenstrual bleeding, itching, dyspareunia, abdominal pain, vulval irritation or blisters.

History

Women may find the sexual history or symptoms embarrassing, but they are more relaxed if the doctor is matter of fact in approach. In addition to a general gynaecological and obstetric history the sexual history must include:

- Presenting complaint:
  - nature, onset, site, severity, duration, trigger factors
  - colour, consistency and odour of any vaginal discharge
  - postcoital or intermenstrual bleeding (which may occur with any vaginal or cervical infection)
  - dyspareunia (superficial is common with *Candida*; deep suggests PID from *Chlamydia* or gonorrhoea)
  - abdominal pain
  - lumps or blisters suggestive of herpes or warts
  - any recent interventions such as IUCD insertion, TOP or evacuation of retained products of conception?
- Sexual history:
  - does she have a current partner (male or female)?
  - how long has she been with this partner? Does he have any symptoms?
  - when was the last time she had sex with another partner? How many partners have there been in the last 3 months?
  - does she have anal sex or oral sex?
  - has she (or her partner) had any previous STIs?
- Contraception:
  - what contraception is used?
  - if condoms are used, what is compliance like?

Examination

Abdominal examination should be performed to check for tenderness or masses and for inguinal lymphadenopathy. The external genitalia may show signs of blisters (HSV), warts (HPV), excoriation or inflammation. Rarely, a syphilitic chancre or tropical ulcer may be identified.

Speculum findings may include discharge (note the amount, consistency and any odour), cervicitis (inflamed reddened cervix, possibly 'strawberry cervix' of *Trichomonas*), contact bleeding or vaginal warts. Bimanual examination should always be performed for cervical excitation, adnexal tenderness or pelvic mass suggestive of a possible abscess.

Examination findings are often unremarkable with *Chlamydia* and gonorrhoea, the commonest bacterial infections.

Investigations

Swabs

The technique of swab-taking is very important to the diagnosis of infection, particularly *Chlamydia* and genital herpes.

- **Vaginal and cervical swabs:** The following 'triple swabs' (Fig. 9.2) should all be taken for women suspected of any STI:

1. High vaginal for *Candida, Trichomonas* and bacterial vaginosis: swab gently in posterior fornix.
2. Endocervical swab for gonorrhoea: insert microbiology swab 1 cm into the endocervical canal and rotate gently to collect cellular material.
3. Endocervical for *Chlamydia*: swab must be inserted 1 cm into the endocervical canal and vigorously rotated (for about 10 seconds) to ensure cellular material is collected. The collection of discharge on the swab should be avoided by removing secretions first. The swab is transported in a specific medium.

Urethral swab for gonorrhoea and *Chlamydia* may pick up a few more cases, but is poorly tolerated and generally not carried out.

Women who have anal or oral sex should have additional rectal and throat swabs for gonorrhoea.

- **Viral swab:** HSV is diagnosed by viral culture from a swab of the blister. It should be taken vigorously to obtain viral particles from the vesicle and base and the patient should be warned that this procedure is painful. The swab must be sent in viral culture medium.

Serum

Serological tests for HIV, hepatitis B and hepatitis C, and syphilis may be carried out after appropriate counselling. Serological tests for HSV and *Chlamydia* are not of practical help.

Ultrasound scan

Ultrasound scan should be arranged if a pelvic collection or mass is suspected from clinical examination.

Management

Women diagnosed with STIs should be encouraged to attend a sexual health or GUM centre with appropriate facilities for diagnosis and follow-up. Health advisors are specially trained in counselling and sexual health education. They can help with the anxiety associated with the diagnosis of a STI and help the woman to inform sexual contacts of any infection.

Women diagnosed with one STI must be screened for others, as co-pathology is common: up to 40% of women with gonorrhoea have coexistent *Chlamydia* infection.

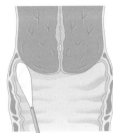

Figure 9.2 (A) High vaginal swab for *Candida*, *Trichomonas* and bacterial vaginosis. Endocervical swabs for gonorrhoea (B) and *Chlamydia* (C).

Posterior   Anterior

A   Swab gently in posterior fornix

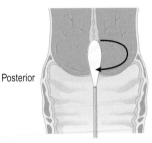

Posterior   Anterior

B   Insert microbiology swab 1 cm into endocervical canal and rotate gently

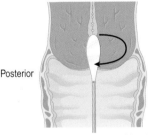

Posterior   Anterior

C   Remove debris and mucus with cotton bud. Insert *Chlamydia* swab 1 cm into endocervical canal and rotate vigorously (for about 10 s) to ensure collection of cellular material

Women should not have intercourse during treatment or until the cure has been confirmed and not until their partner has also been treated, to prevent reinfection.

Persistent positive tests for infection after treatment often represent reinfection rather than failure of the treatment, and this relates to sexual intercourse during treatment or failure of the partner to be treated.

Chlamydia

Chlamydia trachomatis is an intracellular bacterium that infects the endocervix and urethra. Factors associated with high risk of infection are age of less than 25 years, new sexual partner, lack of barrier contraception, women undergoing TOP and use of the COCP. Seventy per cent of women (and 50% of men) are asymptomatic, but symptoms may include discharge, lower abdominal pain, irregular vaginal bleeding or dyspareunia.

Examination may be normal or may show discharge, cervicitis, contact bleeding or adnexal tenderness.

Diagnosis can be made by culture, direct fluorescent antibody or enzyme immunoassay, from endocervical or urethral swab or enzyme immunoassay of a urine sample.

Antibiotic treatment for uncomplicated infection is governed by local guidelines and usually involve a combination like:

- Azithromycin 1 gram orally in a single dose

or

- Doxycycline 100 mg twice daily for 7 days

or

- Erythromycin 500 mg four times a day for 7 days.

In pregnancy or breastfeeding doxycycline is contraindicated, but azithromycin and erythromycin are not known to be harmful.

As erythromycin is less effective (<95%), a test of cure should be performed 3 weeks after treatment is completed in these women.

Complications of *Chlamydia* infection are PID (10–30%), ectopic pregnancy (*Chlamydia* is responsible for about 40% of ectopic pregnancies), chronic pelvic pain and infertility (half the cases of tubal infertility have positive chlamydial serology).

In pregnancy the prevalence of *Chlamydia* is around 6%. There is an associated risk of preterm delivery (odds ratio (OR) 1.6) and fetal growth restriction (OR 2.5) and low birth weight, with increased neonatal morbidity (conjunctivitis and pneumonia) and mortality.

The new national screening programme may help to reduce this risk.

Gonorrhoea

Neisseria gonorrhoeae is a Gram-negative diplococcus, which infects the mucous membranes of the endocervix, urethra, rectum, eye and throat. Fifty per cent of women are asymptomatic but the commonest symptoms are discharge, lower abdominal pain, irregular bleeding and dysuria.

Clinical findings may include discharge, cervicitis, contact bleeding or pelvic tenderness.

Diagnosis is by culture from an endocervical swab (swab, rotated 1 cm inside endocervical canal). In 90% of women the cervix is the only site of infection so urethral, rectal and throat swabs should be taken only if the symptoms or sexual history indicate.

Treatment involves:

- Ciprofloxacin 500 mg as a single dose

or

- Ampicillin 2 grams orally as a single dose.

However, sensitivity from culture should be checked to be sure the organism is not resistant.

In pregnancy or breastfeeding, ampicillin 2 grams orally or ceftriaxone 250 mg intramuscularly may be used.

A test of cure should be performed at least 3 days after treatment.

Trichomonas

Trichomonas is a flagellate protozoon that infects the vagina, urethra and paraurethral glands. Ninety per cent of women with vaginal infection also have urethral infection. Up to 50% of women are asymptomatic, but common symptoms are an offensive odour, itching, profuse discharge and dysuria.

Clinical findings are vulval excoriation, vulvovaginal inflammation, a profuse frothy yellow offensive discharge and 'strawberry cervix' (red and inflamed).

Diagnosis is made by high vaginal swab, with direct observation of flagellates on a wet smear at microscopy. Alternatively, swab culture detects 95% of *Trichomonas* infections. The diagnosis is sometimes made on midstream specimen of urine microscopy or as an incidental finding on cervical smear.

Twenty per cent of infections spontaneously resolve without treatment. However, treatment should always be given if the diagnosis is made:

- Metronidazole 2 grams orally as a single dose

or

- Metronidazole 400 mg twice daily for 5 days.

If metronidazole is ineffective, a single dose of tinidazole 2 grams orally may be used.

Metronidazole and tinidazole are not recommended in early pregnancy and the high-dose metronidazole regime is not recommended at all in pregnancy, though there is no clear evidence of harm. Pregnant women should generally be treated with the 5-day metronidazole course, after the first trimester.

A test of cure is only needed if symptoms persist.

Complications

Preterm delivery and low birth weight are both associated with maternal *Trichomonas* infection. Neonatal *Trichomonas* occurs in 5% of babies of untreated mothers.

Genital herpes

Genital herpes is caused by HSV type 1 or 2. After primary infection the virus is latent in the local sensory ganglia and may reactivate, causing infectious viral shedding with or without symptoms. It usually presents with multiple small blisters around the labia, often associated with dysuria and vaginal discharge. The first (primary attack) is the most severe, often with general malaise, fever, anorexia and lymphadenopathy. Secondary attacks, if they occur, may be as frequent as every few weeks, or occur at times of stress, such as exams. Secondary attacks are generally minor and may be virtually unnoticed.

Multiple small labial blisters and lymphadenopathy may be present on examination.

Diagnosis is by viral swab from the base of a lesion. This involves vigorous rubbing over the lesion to de-roof it and is very painful.

Treatment involves general measures such as saline bathing, analgesia and topical anaesthetic agents. Admission is occasionally needed for systemic symptoms, urinary retention or meningism.

Genital herpes is usually self-limiting, but aciclovir (200 mg five times a day) or famciclovir (250 mg three times a day) for 5 days can be started within 5 days of the attack, to shorten the duration and severity, though it has no impact on the likelihood of recurrence.

Prophylactic aciclovir or famciclovir can be used for 6–12-month periods in women with more than six recurrences per year.

Counselling in a GUM clinic should be arranged to deal with the anxiety around the diagnosis of genital herpes and recurrences. Women can be infectious during recurrences and asymptomatic viral shedding is common in the first year. Condoms do not fully protect against transmission.

Pregnant women who develop a primary attack of HSV within 4 weeks of delivery should be advised to have a caesarean section as the risk of neonatal herpes infection is 50%. For those with recurrent attacks in pregnancy there is no evidence for caesarean section. Those with a recurrent attack and lesions present at the time of delivery have a very small risk of neonatal infection (0.25–3%) as the baby is generally protected by transplacental immunoglobulin G (IgG) from the mother. In this case the risks of caesarean section to the mother should be weighed against the risk of infection in the fetus.

In pregnancy there is no clear evidence of harm from aciclovir and it can be considered from 36 weeks to prevent recurrence around the time of delivery.

Complications

Complications include urinary retention, aseptic meningitis and, very rarely, encephalitis (usually in the immunocompromised).

Genital warts

Clinical warts affect 1% of the population, most commonly involving HPV types 6 and 11. Lesions occur on the vagina, cervix, urethral meatus and anus. The lesions are usually painless, but unsightly and embarrassing.

On examination single or multiple irregular lesions may be seen, either broad-based or pedunculated, from 1 to 20 mm in size. Diagnosis is usually clinical, though biopsy is indicated if the lesion is pigmented, to exclude other pathology.

Treatment depends on the site, size and nature of the lesions, with various treatments available. All treatments have a high recurrence rate and expectant management is an option for non-troublesome warts. Options include:

- Podophyllin, podophyllotoxin or trichloroacetic acid: local treatments applied in the clinic or at home in cycles

or

- Cryotherapy with liquid nitrogen or a cryoprobe

or

- Excision under local or general anaesthetic

or

- Electrocautery or laser treatment.

In pregnancy, local pharmacological treatments are contraindicated because of the risk of teratogenicity.

Florid warts are common in pregnancy and reassurance should be given that spontaneous resolution usually occurs postnatally. Rarely, caesarean section is indicated in women with gross cervical or vaginal warts where haemorrhage at delivery is a potential problem.

Laryngeal papillomatosis is a very rare neonatal complication of maternal genital warts.

Molluscum contagiosum

Molluscum, caused by a poxvirus, is transmitted by direct skin contact. It is a common benign skin problem in children, with spontaneous resolution. In adults, genital infection from sexual contact occurs with multiple discrete pearly white smooth lesions up to 5 mm diameter, with an 'umbilicated' centre.

There are no symptoms except for cosmetic concerns. Diagnosis is based on the clinical appearance.

The lesions regress spontaneously over a few months, but treatment can be given for cosmetic indications:

● Cryotherapy
● Piercing with a phenol or iodine-soaked orange stick.

Scabies

Sarcoptes scabiei is a mite that burrows under the skin to lay eggs. Infection causes intense itching. Clinical features are silvery lines of burrowing tracks and signs of excoriation, either genitally or between fingers.

Permethrin 5% cream or malathion 0.5% aqueous lotion is applied to the whole body and washed off after 12 hours, though the itch may persist for several weeks after treatment. Household contacts and partners should all be treated simultaneously.

Crabs (pubic lice)

Crabs are 2-mm crab-shaped lice found in pubic hair. The female lays tiny white eggs, which are seen tightly adherent to the hair shafts. Transmission may be by close physical as well as sexual contact. The predominant symptom is itching, but women may note the eggs or lice themselves, or find tiny brown specks in underwear (louse droppings). The diagnosis is usually clinical on identifying lice or eggs (confirmation under microscope is possible).

Malathion 0.5% aqueous liquid or permethrin 5% dermal cream is applied to all coarse hair (pubic and underarm) and left for 12 hours. The treatment is repeated after 7 days to kill any lice emerging from surviving eggs. Other sexual and family contacts should be screened and treated if infected.

Syphilis

Syphilis is caused by *Treponema pallidum*, a spirochaete. It is transmitted by sexual contact and has an incubation period of up to 90 days.

Classification

Syphilis is classified according to the timing of presentation and clinical features.

● Primary syphilis: Clinical features are typically a single painless indurated exudative genital ulcer (chancre) with regional lymphadenopathy. However, syphilitic ulcers can mimic those of other infections such as herpes, chancroid or lymphogranuloma.
● Secondary syphilis: This occurs within 2 years of infection and features include malaise, fever and arthralgia with a polymorphic rash, condylomata lata (warty plaque-like lesions in moist areas such as perianally), generalized lymphadenopathy or mucocutaneous lesions.
● Latent syphilis: This term refers to positive serology with no clinical features.

- **Tertiary syphilis:** Late syphilis involves gummatous (chronic granulomatous lesions), neurological and cardiovascular features.
- **Congenital syphilis:** Early congenital syphilis (less than 2 years) involves a rash (condylomata lata), snuffles, haemorrhagic rhinitis, osteochondritis, hepatosplenomegaly, lymphoadenopathy, neurological involvement, haematological involvement, ocular involvement and renal problems.

    Late congenital syphilis (later than 2 years) may present with interstitial keratitis, Hutchinson's incisors, Clutton's joints, saddle-nose deformity, frontal bossing and deafness.

Presentation
Women may present with a genital ulcer or features of secondary syphilis. Otherwise diagnosis is made after screening in pregnancy, screening at a GUM clinic or contact with an infected partner.

Incidence
The incidence of syphilis is increasing, especially in socially deprived and immigrant groups.

The diagnosis of syphilis is made by demonstration of *Treponema pallidum* from the ulcer or lymph nodes by dark-field microscopy, direct fluorescent antibody or polymerase chain reaction. Alternatively, serological testing may detect the disease:

- Specific tests:
  - treponemal enzyme immunoassay (EIA)
  - *Treponema pallidum* haemagglutination test (TPHA)
  - *T. pallidum* partical agglutination assay (TPPA)
  - fluorescent treponemal antibody absorption test.
- Non-specific tests:
  - Venereal Diseases Research Laboratory (VDRL) carbon antigen test
  - rapid plasma reagin test (RPR).

Generally, treponemal EIA or VDRL/RPR or TPHA/TPPA is used for screening tests. VDRL, although non-specific, is also useful for assessing response to treatment.

Lumbar puncture and chest X-ray are used for suspected late syphilis.

Treatment
- Procaine penicillin G 750 mg intramuscularly daily for 10 days

or

- Doxycycline, azithromycin or ceftriaxone if penicillin-allergic.

Patients should be warned about the possibility of the Jarisch–Herxheimer reaction to treatment (acute fever, myalgia and rigors).

In all, 70–100% of babies of infected mothers will have congenital syphilis, with 30% resulting in stillbirth, so treatment should be initiated as soon as possible in pregnant women. If they have documented treated syphilis in the past and reinfection is excluded by testing the partner, then treatment can be omitted if the VDRL or RPR titre is negative or very low. All babies of women with current or former syphilis should be checked serologically and clinically for signs of neonatal syphilis.

Partners of pregnant women diagnosed with syphilis are infected in 45–60% of cases and all partners should, therefore, be treated.

VDRL or RPR should be repeated for 1 year to ensure effective treatment and no reinfection. Specific antibody tests are likely to remain positive for life.

Tropical genital ulcers

Lymphogranuloma venereum (lymphogranuloma inguinale)

Lymphogranuloma venereum is caused by *Chlamydia trachomatis*. The primary lesion is a painless pustule on the vulva, vagina or cervix, with secondary lymphadenopathy. The tertiary phase involves a disfiguring chronic inflammatory response of the vulva. Diagnosis is made by a combination of clinical features with isolation of *C. trachomatis* from the lesions. Treatment is with doxycycline 100 mg twice daily for 21 days.

Chancroid

Haemophilus ducreyi is a very common cause of genital ulceration in Africa and Asia.

The clinical appearance is of single or multiple painful non-indurated necrotic-based ragged-edged ulcers with contact bleeding. They usually occur at the fourchette and painful lymphadenopathy is common. Diagnosis is by isolation of the organism from scrapings of lesions, generally by culture. Treatment is with a single dose of azithromycin 1 gram orally or ceftriaxone 250 mg intramuscularly.

Donovaniasis

Calymmatobacterium granulomatis causes single or multiple papules that develop into friable ulcers or hypertrophied lesions that gradually increase in size and are not particularly painful. Lymphadenopathy occurs with abscess formation over the inguinal skin. Identifying Donovan bodies from scrapings or biopsy makes the diagnosis. Multiple treatment options are available, including azithromycin or erythromycin. Complications include genital and inguinal lymphoedema and mutilation, squamous cell carcinoma, haematogenous spread to bones or viscera, and neonatal infection.

Hepatitis B

Hepatitis B is caused by a DNA virus that is carried by up to 20% of people in South-East Asia. In the UK prevalence is 0.01–0.04% of the general population, but >1% in homosexual men and drug users. Infection is sexual, parenteral (e.g. needle-sharing or blood products) or congenital. The incubation period is 40–160 days and infectivity is from 2 weeks prior to the onset of jaundice, if it occurs, until the surface antigen is negative.

Clinical features

The infection is asymptomatic in 10–50%. Symptoms of acute infection include a prodromal illness with flu-like symptoms, followed by jaundice, anorexia and fatigue, which may last a few weeks. Chronic infection may have no signs, or there may be features of chronic liver disease. Examination may reveal jaundice, tender hepatomegaly and dehydration.

Fulminant hepatitis occurs in fewer than 1% of infections, but chronic infection (lasting more than 6 months) occurs in 5–10%.

Diagnostic tests

Hepatitis B surface antigen is positive in all cases of infection. Hepatitis B e antigen indicates high infectivity and IgM antibody represents acute infection. Women with chronic low infectivity and resolved infection may continue to carry anti-e antibody. Vaccination is confirmed by the presence of anti-hepatitis B surface antibody.

Liver function should be checked for active or chronic infection.

Treatment

Treatment is supportive, except for chronic infection, where interferon-α and antiviral agents can be considered. Immunoglobulin may be offered within 48 hours of a sexual contact with a possible hepatitis B carrier. The accelerated vaccination course can be given to close contacts of those with hepatitis B.

Serology should be checked 6 months after acute infection to assess chronic infection or carrier status.

Pregnancy

The prevalence of hepatitis B infection in pregnancy is 0.5–1%, and much higher in Asian women. If e antigen is positive, then 90% of babies will be infected. If e antigen is negative, 10–30% are infected. Most infected babies become chronic carriers with the chance of long-term morbidity from hepatocellular carcinoma and cirrhosis. Vaccination and immunoglobulin at birth reduce transmission by 90%. Breastfeeding does not increase the risk of vertical transmission.

Hepatitis C

Hepatitis C is caused by an RNA virus. It is found in 0.06% of blood donors and 60% of intravenous drug users. Transmission is generally parenteral, from shared needles, but 2–11% of long-term sexual partners will become infected.

Clinical features

Eighty per cent of infections with hepatitis C are asymptomatic, but 20% develop acute hepatitis 4–20 weeks after infection. Signs are as for hepatitis B. Of those infected, 50–85% go on to become asymptomatic chronic carriers, of whom liver disease occurs in 35%.

Diagnosis is by screening antibody test followed by specific confirmation of the virus if positive. Treatment is similar to that for hepatitis B.

Pregnancy

The prevalence of hepatitis C in pregnancy is 0.14–0.8%. Vertical transmission is 3–5% and no specific measures are known to reduce the risk. There is no evidence as to whether breastfeeding increases the risk and avoidance should be considered, especially in those with symptoms or a high viral load.

HIV

HIV is an RNA retrovirus. It is transmitted, as for hepatitis B, by sexual contact, blood (e.g. shared needles, blood products prior to 1990) and vertical transmission. The incubation period is up to 3 months.

Incidence

Currently about 50 000 people in the UK (60 million worldwide) have HIV. In the UK 33% of infections overall and 57% of new diagnoses are through heterosexual spread. Vertical transmission to the fetus is transplacental, during delivery and through breastfeeding. Three hundred infected women in the UK give birth each year.

Age

The commonest age for diagnosis is 25–35 years, though infection may have occurred some time previously.

Clinical features

In the obstetrics and gynaecology setting women are generally diagnosed after antenatal screening. However, they may be diagnosed secondarily to admission for a severe illness. The acute seroconversion illness involves flu-like symptoms and lymphadenopathy. HIV illnesses from reduced immunity include oral *Candida*, tuberculosis and respiratory or gastrointestinal tract infections. Acquired immunodeficiency syndrome (AIDS)-defining illnesses include *Pneumocystis carinii* pneumonia and Kaposi's sarcoma.

Diagnosis

Antibody tests (enzyme-linked immunosorbent assay or Western blot) are used for screening and diagnosis. Any positive test is repeated for confirmation.

Investigations

CD4 count and viral load are useful indicators of the disease process.

Treatment

Combination antiretroviral drugs are the mainstay of treatment, with very good success rates for survival. In addition, *P. carinii* prophylaxis is indicated when the CD4 count is less than 200 cells/mm^3. Specific complications, such as fungal infections, are treated as indicated.

Pregnancy

Screening for HIV in pregnancy is now recommended for all women. On diagnosis, a multidisciplinary team approach must be adopted immediately, with good counselling as well as medical and obstetric input.

In combination, the following four factors reduce the incidence of neonatal HIV from about 24% to <5%:

1. Elective caesarean section.
2. Intravenous antiretroviral therapy for 4 hours immediately preceding delivery.
3. Oral antiretroviral therapy to the baby for the first 6 weeks.
4. Avoidance of breastfeeding.

In addition, oral antiretroviral therapy aims to reduce the viral load to an undetectable level during the pregnancy.

If spontaneous labour occurs in an HIV-positive woman, then artificial rupture of membranes and invasive procedures such as fetal blood sampling and fetal scalp electrode must be avoided. Delivery should be expedited as soon as possible after spontaneous rupture of membranes.

PELVIC INFLAMMATORY DISEASE

Definition

PID is infection of the pelvic organs almost invariably from ascending infection through the genital tract. Infection is most common in the fallopian tubes (salpingitis), but endometritis, parametritis, oophoritis, tubo-ovarian abscess and pelvic peritonitis also occur.

Incidence

The incidence of PID is unknown because non-specific or absent symptoms and signs mean that the diagnosis is probably often missed.

Age

PID is most common in 18–25-year-olds, but may occur earlier or even much later.

Aetiology

The commonest organism found is *Chlamydia* (50%), but PID can also be caused by gonorrhoea (14%), bacterial vaginosis and atypical anaerobes. Tuberculosis (TB) is a rare but important cause. In most cases a causative organism is not isolated.

Pathophysiology

Infection is largely by sexual contact. PID is very rare in non-sexually active women. The infection may be asymptomatic for some time (up to years) and be activated spontaneously or after instrumentation of the uterus.

Risk factors

Risk factors for PID include those for other STIs (see *Chlamydia*, above), insertion of an IUCD and smoking.

Clinical features

Abdominal pain is the main presenting feature of PID and women with acute infection are often systemically unwell with fever, vomiting, anorexia and malaise. Dyspareunia, postcoital or irregular bleeding, menorrhagia or dysmenorrhoea, discharge or back pain may also occur. Many women are asymptomatic, but have evidence of PID at later laparoscopy, for example for infertility.

Examination

General examination should be performed for temperature, pulse, blood pressure and signs of dehydration. Abdominal palpation typically reveals tenderness (usually bilateral). Peritonism is relatively common.

Speculum may show discharge and abnormal bleeding and typically bimanual examination reveals cervical excitation (pain on moving the cervix from side to side) and adnexal tenderness. Occasionally, a pelvic mass (e.g. tubo-ovarian abscess) may be palpable.

Investigations

A pregnancy test should always be performed to exclude the important differential diagnosis of ectopic pregnancy.

High vaginal and endocervical swabs (high vaginal for *Trichomonas vaginalis*, *Candida* and bacterial vaginosis, endocervical for gonorrhoea and endocervical for *Chlamydia*) should be taken, paying attention to using the correct technique.

Midstream specimen of urine should be sent for microscopy and culture.

Full blood count and C-reactive protein are important if the woman is systemically unwell, and urea and electrolytes should be analysed if she is vomiting.

Ultrasound scan will exclude a large tubo-ovarian collection, but is usually normal with PID except for possible free peritoneal fluid, which is a non-specific finding.

Laparoscopy is indicated if the diagnosis is unclear or there is no response to treatment after 48 hours.

Differential diagnosis

Other gynaecological causes of abdominal pain include ectopic pregnancy, miscarriage, ovarian cyst torsion, rupture or haemorrhage, endometriosis, fibroid degeneration and ovulation pain.

Non-gynaecological causes include adhesions, appendicitis, urinary tract infection or pyelonephritis, constipation, irritable bowel syndrome, inflammatory bowel disease and gastroenteritis. The pain may also be functional, often after a previous diagnosis of PID.

Management

The importance of education and advice is generally overlooked in gynaecological settings. The woman must be advised verbally and with clearly written advice:

- PID is an infection of the pelvic organs and is generally sexually transmitted. However, the organism is often not identified and may have been asymptomatic in either partner for some time so the diagnosis does not necessarily imply recent infidelity by either partner.
- Her partner(s) will need testing and empirical treatment at a genitourinary clinic (50% will have *Chlamydia*, 40% gonorrhoea) and she should be provided with a letter for him to take to explain her illness.
- She should not have sex until both she and her partner have completed their courses of treatment because of the risk of reinfection.
- The treatment is prolonged, but symptoms generally improve within a few days of starting treatment.
- She should be seen after treatment has been completed for a full STI screen to exclude any resistant infection.
- There is an increased risk of chronic pelvic pain after PID.
- Ectopic pregnancy is more likely and she should have an early scan (5 weeks) when pregnant, to confirm intrauterine gestation.
- Subfertility is more common after PID (1% tubal infertility after a mild episode and 21% after a severe episode) because of tubal damage, but she should continue to use contraception as most women with treated PID can still become pregnant.
- Barrier contraception will protect her against reinfection.

Treatment involves analgesia, fluids and antibiotics. As the causative organism is not usually isolated, *Chlamydia*, gonorrhoea and anaerobic organisms must all be covered by treatment, and there should be a low threshold for treatment in view of the serious sequelae of untreated disease. Antibiotic regimens vary, but some recommended outpatient schedules are:

- Azithromycin 1 gram orally as a single dose, or doxycycline 100 mg twice daily for 2 weeks

and

- Ciprofloxacin 500 mg orally as a single dose or amoxicillin 2 grams orally as a single dose

and

- Metronidazole 400 mg twice daily for 2 weeks.

Criteria for admission for intravenous antibiotics and fluids are:

- Vomiting
- Temperature >38°C
- Severe pain, not controlled with simple oral analgesia
- Inability to tolerate oral antibiotics
- No improvement after 48 hours of oral antibiotics.

A suitable intravenous antibiotic regime is:

- Cefuroxime 750 mg twice daily for 5 days

and

- Metronidazole 500 mg three times daily for 5 days

and

- Azithromycin 1 gram intramuscular as a single dose or doxycycline 100 mg orally twice daily for 2 weeks once tolerating tablets.

The intravenous treatment can be discontinued and changed to oral after 24 hours of systemic improvement and apyrexia.

Urgent laparoscopy is indicated where ovarian pathology (such as torsion) cannot be excluded or no improvement occurs after 48 hours of intravenous antibiotics. Infected tubes appear red, inflamed, congested and exudative. Laparoscopy can also be performed electively for persistent pain after treatment and may show peritubal adhesions and perihepatic adhesions (Fitz-Hugh–Curtis syndrome).

Tubo-ovarian abscess can be managed conservatively initially, but drainage by laparoscopy or laparotomy is indicated where there is no improvement after 48 hours or the patient is systemically unwell.

An IUCD should be removed if it has been inserted recently or if the infection is severe, as it may act as a focus of infection. However, possible pregnancy risk must be considered and emergency contraception given if necessary or the woman counselled about the risk of pregnancy if she has had intercourse in the last 5 days.

Complications

These include:

- Tubo-ovarian abscess (usually with anaerobic infection)
- Fitz-Hugh–Curtis syndrome (10–20%) (perihepatitis resulting in perihepatic adhesions)
- Tubal infertility (21% after a severe episode)
- Ectopic pregnancy (10%)
- Chronic pelvic pain (24–75%).

Pregnancy

PID is extremely uncommon in pregnancy, probably due to the mucous cervical plug and the pregnancy itself impeding passage of organisms into the fallopian tubes. In pregnancy or breastfeeding, penicillin or ceftriaxone can be used instead of ciprofloxacin. Erythromycin should be used instead of doxycycline or azithromycin, although azithromycin is not known to be harmful.

Follow-up

Women treated as outpatients should be reviewed after 72 hours to ensure improvement and for their microbiology results. This may be in a GUM clinic if the woman is given an appropriate referral letter and details. Further review is indicated 2 weeks after completing treatment to check response to treatment, check compliance with antibiotics, ensure partner(s) have been tested and treated and perform a full STI screen.

OTHER VAGINAL INFECTIONS

Candida (thrush)

Candida albicans is a very common cause of abnormal vaginal discharge, occurring at any age, more often during reproductive years. A total of 10–20% of women of reproductive age have asymptomatic *Candida*. It is more common in pregnancy, diabetes, after antibiotics and possibly with combined oral contraceptive use.

Pathophysiology

Ninety per cent of vulvovaginal candidiasis is caused by *C. albicans*. Other varieties, such as *C. glabrata*, are rare and the features and antifungal sensitivities are usually the same.

Clinical features

Candida typically presents with white, grey or blood-stained, lumpy (curd-like) or smooth discharge. Other symptoms are itching, vulval pain, dysuria or superficial dyspareunia. The infection is very often asymptomatic. Signs of vulval excoriation and inflammation may be seen and speculum reveals discharge and vaginal erythema. Speculum or bimanual examination may be superficially painful.

Investigations

Diagnosis is usually by microscopy showing spores and pseudohyphae. Culture and sensitivity are only needed in cases resistant to treatment.

Treatment

Treatment is only indicated in symptomatic cases. Conservative measures include avoiding tight-fitting clothes, wearing cotton underwear and avoiding irritants (bath additives, commercial 'hygiene' sprays, soap, douching). Live yoghurt is reported to be successful if eaten or used vaginally.

The mainstay of treatment is antifungals such as clotrimazole pessary 500 mg as a single dose, 200 mg for 3 nights or 100 mg for 7 nights. Alternatives are nystatin, econazole and fenticonazole. Pessaries should be put in at night; bathing and showering should be avoided for at least 12 hours and a discharge should be expected the following day.

Topical clotrimazole cream also helps symptoms. Oral fluconazole and itraconazole are available, but are no more effective than pessaries.

Pregnancy

Both asymptomatic and symptomatic candidiasis is increased in pregnancy. Oral preparations are contraindicated, but pessaries and cream are safe and may need to be given in more prolonged courses.

Recurrent *Candida*

Women with immunodeficiency, steroid use, repeated antibiotics and diabetes are more prone to recurrent *Candida*. Diabetes should be excluded and sensitivity of the yeast checked. Weekly pessaries or oral preparations reduce the recurrence, but 50% of women relapse after treatment is stopped. Recurrent infection may respond to fluconazole 100 mg weekly for 6 months. The partner may be treated, especially if he is symptomatic, but there is no clear evidence that reinfection from a partner is the cause of recurrent symptoms.

Bacterial vaginosis

Bacterial vaginosis is caused by an overgrowth of anaerobic organisms within the vagina, particularly *Gardnerella vaginalis*, *Mycoplasma hominis* and *Mobiluncus* species. It occurs and resolves spontaneously, though may occur more after sexual intercourse.

Incidence

The condition is very common, affecting 12–30% of women, both sexually active and non-sexually active. It is extremely embarrassing and recurrent infection is common.

Pathophysiology

The overgrowth of anaerobic organisms causes eradication of the normal lactobacilli and an increase in the vaginal pH to up to 7 (normally <4.5). The condition is commoner in smokers, IUCD users and in black women.

Clinical features

Fifty per cent of women are asymptomatic. Others complain of an offensive ('fishy') smell or profuse creamy discharge. Pain or irritation does not occur. A thin smooth white discharge is seen within the vagina on speculum.

Diagnosis

Diagnosis is based on Amsell's criteria, where three of the four following are found:

1. Thin creamy discharge.
2. Clue cells (epithelial cells coated with bacilli) at microscopy.
3. The sniff test (fishy odour on adding 10% potassium hydroxide to the discharge on a slide).
4. Vaginal fluid pH >4.5.

In practice, microscopy alone is often relied upon.

Treatment

Conservative measures include avoidance of vaginal douching, bath additives and soap. Oral metronidazole 400 mg twice daily for 5 days or metronidazole 2 grams as a single dose can be used or intravaginal clindamycin cream (2%) daily for 7 days or 0.75% intravaginal metronidazole gel daily for 5 days.

Recurrent bacterial vaginosis can be treated with repeated oral or topical preparations. Alternatively, an acetic acid vaginal jelly preparation can be tried to restore the normal vaginal pH. Some women have fewer recurrences with condom use as they are protected from the alkaline environment of seminal fluid.

Pregnancy

Bacterial vaginosis is associated with an increased risk of mid-trimester loss, preterm prelabour rupture of membranes, preterm delivery and postnatal endometritis. However, large randomized trials have failed to show an improvement in outcome from treating asymptomatic bacterial vaginosis carriers in pregnancy. Metronidazole is not known to be harmful in pregnancy and can be considered for treatment of symptomatic infection in pregnancy. PID is more common following termination in women with bacterial vaginosis and metronidazole should be given prophylactically to all undergoing the procedure.

SUMMARY

- Contraceptive failure is generally user failure rather than method failure and contraceptive teaching is vital to safe and effective use.
- Women requesting sterilization should have clear counselling about complications of the procedure, failure rates, irreversibility, the risk of future ectopic pregnancy and alternative methods of contraception.
- The levonorgestrel-releasing IUD is an effective and reversible alternative to female sterilization.
- Female sexual dysfunction is underreported and women may initially present with an indirect symptom such as dyspareunia.
- Privacy, confidentiality and time are essential for a psychosexual consultation.
- Women who report sexual assault need to have injuries, infection, contraception, counselling and police involvement addressed.

- STIs are increasing and often poorly treated in the gynaecology setting.
- Partner tracing, advice about abstinence during treatment, encouragement of compliance with treatment and follow-up are essential for women with suspected or confirmed STIs.
- A low threshold for antibiotic treatment for suspected PID reduces the long-term complications of chronic pain, ectopic pregnancy and subfertility.

Bleeding in early pregnancy 10

CHAPTER CONTENTS

Vaginal bleeding in the first trimester is a common event, occurring in up to 30% of all pregnancies, and about one-half of these will eventually miscarry by 12 weeks' gestation. More than 90% of spontaneous miscarriage occurs in the first trimester.

Causes of bleeding in the first trimester include spontaneous abortion, physiological bleeding of a normal pregnancy, ectopic pregnancy, trophoblastic disease and non-obstetrical causes such as cervical lesions, e.g. polyps, ectropion or carcinoma.

MISCARRIAGE

Definition

Miscarriage (abortion) is the involuntary loss or termination of pregnancy prior to 24 weeks' gestation. Other definitions include the loss of pregnancy before viability. The World Health Organization definition is 'expulsion or extraction of an embryo or fetus weighing 500 g or less from its mother'. However, this weight criterion corresponds to a gestational age of 20–22 weeks, the irreducible age for fetal viability. An empty sac (formerly known as blighted ovum or anembryonic pregnancy) occurs when an embryo has failed to develop although there is an identifiable gestational sac and placental tissue. This is, in fact, an early form of missed miscarriage.

Types of miscarriage (Fig. 10.1)

- Threatened – uterine bleeding without dilatation of cervix or passage of products of conception (POC). The fetus is still viable and the uterus is the expected size for dates. Only one-quarter of these will go on to miscarry.
- Inevitable – heavy bleeding with cervical dilatation, but without passage of POC. The fetus may still be alive, but miscarriage will occur.
- Incomplete – bleeding with cervical dilatation and passage of some, but not all, POC.
- Complete – bleeding which diminishes with complete passage of POC. Pain and bleeding ease, uterus returns to normal size and cervix is closed.
- Missed – fetal death, bleeding or pain; the fetus or embryo has been dead for some weeks, but no tissue has been passed. This is often not recognized until bleeding occurs, the patient complains that she feels 'less pregnant than before' and an ultrasound has been performed confirming fetal demise.
- Septic – any of the above that becomes infected, resulting in endometritis and often parametritis and peritonitis.

Pathophysiology

Up to 50% of spontaneous miscarriages are the result of a major genetic abnormality, e.g. trisomy. The remainder have been linked to other factors such as uterine abnormalities (such as fibroids or müllerian duct abnormalities), cervical incompetence (usually mid-trimester loss),

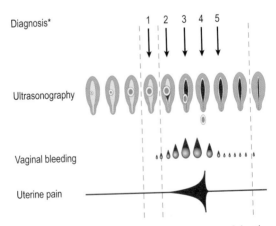

*1. ultrasonography shows early anembryonic pregnancy (missed miscarriage); 2. vaginal bleeding occurs (threatened miscarriage); 3. open cervical os (inevitable miscarriage); 4. miscarriage (products of conception are expelled, and cramps and bleeding soon subside); 5. utlrasonography may show uterine contents – decidua, blood, and some villi.

Figure 10.1 Stages of miscarriage.

maternal systemic disease, progesterone deficiency in the luteal phase of the cycle and immunological factors.

Once the woman has a positive pregnancy test and the pregnancy fails, there is usually a cessation of the symptoms of pregnancy and the serum human chorionic gonadotrophin beta-subunit (βhCG) levels plateau or fall. Eventually, she will begin to bleed and after hours or weeks of bleeding in varying amounts she will experience lower abdominal cramping or back pain. At this point the eventual outcome is recognized even if the pregnancy failed weeks previously. The final event in this sequence is the passage of POC as the body attempts to evacuate the contents of the uterus, and this is often associated with severe pain, bleeding and often symptoms and signs of shock if products remain in the cervix.

This sequence of events is often mimicked by ectopic pregnancy and, therefore, this must always be excluded. Both entities have positive pregnancy tests, variable symptoms of pregnancy, vaginal bleeding and pelvic pain. However, a ruptured ectopic pregnancy will produce signs of shock and signs of a haemoperitoneum, such as rebound tenderness, rigid abdomen or shoulder-tip pain (caused by diaphragmatic irritation).

Assessment

When a patient presents with first-trimester bleeding, begin with an accurate history including careful questioning on the sequence of events, symptoms, menstrual history, method of contraception, previous obstetrical, gynaecological, surgical and medical history. Attempting to establish estimated/expected gestation of the pregnancy is imperative.

General examination including vital signs and cardiovascular status must be performed. An abdominal examination is important, particularly if one suspects an ectopic pregnancy, assessing for signs of a haemoperitoneum. A speculum examination will eliminate any local cause of vaginal bleeding and will reveal any cervical dilatation, and at this stage POC can be removed with a sponge holder if seen in the cervix. A bimanual examination may be necessary if the speculum examination is normal and this will allow assessment of uterine size, cervical dilatation, cervical excitation – pain on movement of the cervix (an indicator of a possible ectopic or pelvic infection) – and the presence of an adnexal mass.

Investigations

- Full blood count, blood group and consider serum βhCG assay
- Ultrasound scan of pelvis.

Management

- Conservative
- Uterine curettage (evacuation of retained POC – ERPC) if incomplete or non-viable pregnancy
- Anti-D immunoglobulin if patient is Rhesus D-negative.

The management of bleeding in early pregnancy will depend on clinical, ultrasound and biochemical factors.

Clinical

If the clinical picture suggests complete, incomplete or threatened miscarriage, an ultrasound scan should be arranged for the patient. If the clinical picture suggests an ongoing ectopic pregnancy, or if the vaginal bleeding is dangerously heavy, the patient will need to be admitted.

Ultrasound assessment

The patient undergoes an ultrasound scan, usually transvaginally. There are several likely outcomes, outlined below with the appropriate management.

If the pregnancy is intrauterine and continues to be viable, reassure the patient and arrange either a booking or follow-up antenatal appointment within 2 weeks.

If viability is uncertain, usually because the pregnancy may be too early for proper assessment, a rescan should be booked in 1–2 weeks' time.

In a case where there are no retained products, the patient needs to be reviewed and the certainty of the previous diagnosis of pregnancy re-evaluated. If an intrauterine pregnancy has not previously been confirmed, then serial hCG monitoring is needed to ensure that it is decreasing consistent with a miscarriage.

In a case where there is suspicion of an ectopic pregnancy there should be an empty uterus, possible fluid in the pouch of Douglas and an adnexal mass. A heart beat may be apparent within this adnexal mass.

In incomplete/inevitable miscarriages, the majority of women can be managed conservatively in the first instance and this should be discussed with the patient. Expectant management of miscarriage in selected cases is successful in approximately 80% of women. When there is a missed miscarriage, or significant retained products, complete miscarriage is less likely. If there is any suspicion of molar pregnancy, then the patient is not suitable for expectant management and should be referred for an ERPC so that histology is obtained.

Medical management of miscarriage involves administration of prostaglandins, often preceded by mifepristone, and antiprogestogen. This is suitable for women who choose this option.

All women who miscarry should be warned of the signs and symptoms of pelvic infection so that they can seek treatment promptly.

If the patient opts for conservative management, she should return in 1 week's time for repeat scan. If there are still retained products on the repeat scan, or it appears on initial assessment that ERPC is likely to be required, the patient can have an elective ERPC arranged.

Biochemical

βhCG is a very sensitive marker of pregnancy. Levels in the blood will generally double within 48 hours with a viable intrauterine pregnancy, unlike an ectopic pregnancy, which is discussed later.

Complications

- Haemorrhage or infection if tissue is retained
- Uterine perforation at time of ERPC with possible bowel trauma
- Later problems can include Asherman's syndrome (with recurrent or overzealous curettage) or cervical incompetence.

Follow-up

All patients should be adequately counselled and assured that this was an unfortunate outcome that could not have been prevented. The emotional reaction of patients may require bereavement counselling and the Miscarriage Association is a patient-organized group which many patients and their partners find useful.

THERAPEUTIC ABORTION

Definition

Therapeutic termination of pregnancy is defined as medical or surgical termination of pregnancy before 24 weeks' gestation. However, in the UK, 90% of terminations are performed before 12 weeks' gestation.

Legal aspects of pregnancy termination

In 1967 the Abortion Act was passed in England and Wales; this allowed termination of pregnancy to be carried out by a medical practitioner in a licensed institution. Two medical practitioners must agree with the patient's request and sign the consent form (certificate A). The grounds for termination are stated in certificate A and must be indicated by the consenting practitioners. These grounds are that continuation of the pregnancy will:

A. Endanger the life of the woman
B. Endanger the physical or mental well-being of the woman
C. Endanger the physical or mental well-being of the children of the pregnant woman
D. Involve substantial risk that the child would suffer physical or mental handicap.

The vast majority of terminations are performed for reason B.

Assessment

All patients requesting termination of pregnancy should be fully counselled to ensure that their decision is definite and that they are committed to proceeding with the surgery. Usually these patients will have seen their family doctor for this, but all clinics should provide a support service.

History and examination should include menstrual history for pregnancy dating and suitability for anaesthesia. Ultrasound scan should be performed to confirm gestation. A full blood count should be taken and group and antibody status ascertained.

Methods of termination

1. Suction curettage is most commonly performed prior to 12–14 weeks' gestation. The cervix must be dilated and often in nulliparous patients the cervix is 'ripened' prior to the procedure with a prostaglandin pessary for ease of dilatation.
2. Antiprogesterone tablets (RU486) are effective up to 9 weeks' gestation when taken in conjunction with a prostaglandin pessary so that anaesthesia can be avoided.
3. Dilatation of the cervix and evacuation of the uterine contents can be performed after 12 weeks' gestation until 16–20 weeks. This involves dilatation of the cervix and destruction of the fetal parts followed by evacuation of the uterine contents.
4. Prostaglandin induction is used after 14–16 weeks' gestation and an oxytocin infusion may also be necessary to expedite what can sometimes be a long, arduous and painful process. Antiprogesterone tablets can be administered 48 hours beforehand to improve the efficacy of this procedure.

Complications

The complications of surgical evacuation of the uterus include those of anaesthesia, bleeding, infection and uterine perforation with its association of possible bowel damage. Longer-term complications related to the surgery include Asherman's syndrome and cervical incompetence.

RECURRENT MISCARRIAGE

Definition

Recurrent miscarriage is defined as the loss of three or more consecutive pregnancies before 24 weeks' gestation.

Prevalence

Between 12% and 15% of clinically recognized pregnancies miscarry. This implies that the risk of three consecutive pregnancy losses occurring by chance alone is around 0.3%. However, the incidence quoted for couples experiencing recurrent miscarriage is accepted to be 1%. The fact that the observed frequency of recurrent miscarriage is significantly higher than that expected by chance alone implies that in some women there is a persistent underlying cause to account for their pregnancy losses.

Aetiology

This will depend on the gestation at which the miscarriage occurs.

First trimester

Polycystic ovaries (PCO) are found more commonly in women with recurrent miscarriage (58%) than the general population (22%), and 56% of women with PCO hypersecrete luteinizing hormone (LH). An association with this raised or hypersecretion of LH and recurrent miscarriage has been implicated, although the mechanism of pregnancy failure is unclear.

Women with a history of recurrent miscarriage tend to lose fetuses that have a normal karyotype. However, a parental chromosome abnormality is found in 3–5% of couples with recurrent miscarriage. It is, therefore, essential that blood karyotyping is performed on both partners in order to identify those couples with a genetic cause for their pregnancy losses. These couples should be referred for genetic counselling in order that they may be given a prognosis for future pregnancies and prenatal diagnosis should be offered in ongoing pregnancies.

Recurrent miscarriage has been shown to be associated with antiphospholipid antibodies – lupus anticoagulant and anticardiolipin antibodies – in up to 15% of women. The primary antiphospholipid syndrome (APS) is the association between either recurrent miscarriage and/or thrombosis with antiphospholipid antibodies. Recurrent miscarriage is also thought to be associated with other thrombophilic defects, including deficiencies of antithrombin III and factor XII deficiency, and low levels of the naturally occurring anticoagulants protein C and protein S. Activated protein C resistance, a recently identified thrombophilic defect, is found in 20% of women with a history of second-trimester miscarriage where fetal loss is associated with placental thrombosis. As well as accounting for recurrent first-trimester loss, these abnormalities are associated with second-trimester loss and poor obstetric outcome.

The alloimmune theory, that the genetic dissimilarity between the mother and fetus may give rise to a rejection mechanism causing recurrent miscarriage, has not been proven.

Second trimester

Up to 10% of patients with recurrent miscarriage have some uterine abnormality. These include intracavity fibroids and congenital structural abnormalities such as bi/unicornuate uteri. Cervical incompetence is a recognized cause of recurrent mid-trimester miscarriage and patients classically give a history of a painless pregnancy loss after 16 weeks' gestation. The role of cervical cerclage in these patients is still controversial, but each patient should be considered individually.

Any severe infection may cause a sporadic miscarriage but to be responsible for recurrent loss the infection must persist (often asymptomatically) in the genital tract for a long period of time. Bacterial vaginosis is one such organism that may play a part in the aetiology of recurrent miscarriage and also in preterm delivery.

Assessment

A full history and examination should include a detailed background of the pregnancy losses, at what gestation they occurred and whether an ultrasound scan was performed, pain/bleeding preceding the loss, same partner, cycle length and ease of conception. Is there a history of systemic disease or thrombosis, surgery to the cervix, family history of miscarriage or thrombosis?

Investigations

- Blood – LH, follicle-stimulating hormone, testosterone on day 5–8 of cycle (PCO syndrome (PCOS) screen)
- Antiphospholipid antibody, anticardiolipin antibody and lupus anticoagulant for APS or systemic lupus erythematosus screening
- Chromosomes of both partners
- Ultrasound scan to exclude PCOS or uterine abnormality.

Management

These patients and their partners are often distressed and require a great deal of psychological support. Often the investigations are negative and few treatments are of proven value. Once a pregnancy has been achieved then support with regular ultrasound reassurance is vital and has been shown to be of value.

Patients with systemic lupus erythematosus and APS should be referred to a specialist centre. Recent studies suggest that these patients have a better outcome when treated with low-dose aspirin 75 mg daily and heparin 5000 IU subcutaneously throughout pregnancy.

ECTOPIC PREGNANCY

Definition

An ectopic pregnancy is when the embryo implants outside the uterine cavity. The most common site is in the fallopian tube, although implantation can occur in the cornua of the uterus, the cervix, ovary or abdominal cavity (Fig. 10.2). These sites are unable to contain the growing trophoblast and embryo, so rupture may occur, leading to catastrophic bleeding.

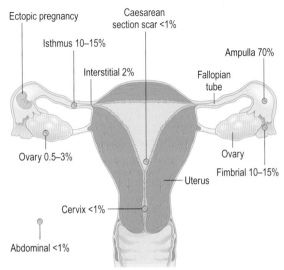

Figure 10.2 Sites of ectopic pregnancies.

Incidence

This is now becoming more common in the UK, representing 4% of direct and indirect maternal deaths in 1997–99. Its incidence has doubled over the last 30 years (from 4.9 to 9.6 per 1000 pregnancies or 1 in 100 pregnancies). In the USA, deaths due to ectopic pregnancy comprised 9% of all maternal deaths in 1992 and its incidence has apparently increased fourfold (from 4.5 to 20 per 1000 pregnancies) between 1970 and 1992. The mortality, however, has decreased 10-fold in the USA and fivefold in the UK during these timeframes, indicating improved diagnosis and management.

Aetiology

In many cases the cause is unknown. Ectopic pregnancy is often very difficult to diagnose as the clinical presentation can vary from vaginal spotting to haemoperitoneum and shock. Risk factors are present in 25–50% of patients with an ectopic pregnancy and include:

- Previous pelvic inflammatory disease (PID) (increases the risk of ectopic pregnancy 10-fold). The recent increase in PID is thought to have contributed to the increased incidence of ectopic pregnancy.
- Previous tubal surgery, including reconstruction and sterilization (increases the risk of ectopic pregnancy 4½-fold).
- Previous ectopic pregnancy (10-fold). Even if a tube has been previously removed, the initial causative pathology is often bilateral.
- Assisted reproductive techniques (in vitro fertilization or gamete intrafallopian transfer).
- Intrauterine contraceptive device (IUCD). This is a risk if pregnancy occurs whilst in situ. Most current contraceptive methods protect against ectopic pregnancy except when the method fails. However

modern copper-bearing IUCDs (Copper T 380, Multiload Cu 375) and the levonorgestrel-releasing intrauterine system (Mirena) are extremely effective contraceptives with failure rates of around 1 in 100 after 5 years of use, making them acceptable contraceptive choices for women with a previous history of ectopic pregnancy.

- The progesterone-only contraceptive pill.

Assessment

The diagnosis is often difficult clinically (accuracy of 50%), but should always be considered in a woman of childbearing age with amenorrhoea, abnormal bleeding, abdominal pain or collapse. It is a diagnosis of exclusion in any such women and has been made simpler with advances in early diagnostic techniques, in particular the quantitative measurement of βhCG, transvaginal ultrasonography and dedicated early pregnancy assessment clinics. Assessment includes:

- A history of pain, irregular scanty bleeding and amenorrhoea
- General examination of vital signs, evidence of acute abdomen, cervical excitation with a bulky uterus and a tender adnexae on vaginal assessment
- Checking for the presence of βhCG, which is detected in the urine as early as 14 days postconception or in the serum 5–9 days postconception by sensitive assays. Between 2 and 4 weeks after ovulation serum βhCG levels double approximately every 2 days in a normal intrauterine pregnancy; a lesser increase (<66% over 48 hours) is associated with ectopic pregnancy and spontaneous abortion. In order to increase the sensitivity of quantitative βhCG, a discriminatory zone has been described whereby a titre of 1000–1500 IU/l (international reference preparation) will be associated with the presence of an intrauterine sac on transvaginal ultrasound
- Transvaginal ultrasound: positive signs of an intrauterine pregnancy on ultrasound scan include a gestation sac (at approximately 4 weeks' amenorrhoea), the double decidual sign (at 5 weeks), the yolk sac (5–6 weeks) and, finally, the fetal heartbeat (7 weeks). Ectopic pregnancy should be suspected if there are ultrasonic appearances of an empty uterus, an intrauterine pseudosac, evidence of a tubal swelling or ring sign with a fetal heartbeat, or fluid in the pouch of Douglas. Demonstration of a viable intrauterine pregnancy does not exclude the possibility of heterotopic pregnancy (frequency 1/30 000–40 000 spontaneously to 1–3% after assisted reproduction), i.e. a coexisting ectopic and intrauterine pregnancy.

Management

If an ongoing ectopic is suspected, the patient should be admitted to hospital for further investigation, with blood taken for crossmatching and intravenous access (Fig. 10.3).

Acute presentation

The patient is resuscitated and arrangements made for immediate laparoscopy/laparotomy with salpingectomy of the affected tube, if the other tube appears normal.

Subacute presentation

Women in whom an ectopic pregnancy is visualized should be managed surgically or medically as described below. Where the location of the pregnancy cannot be initially confirmed ('pregnancy of uncertain location'),

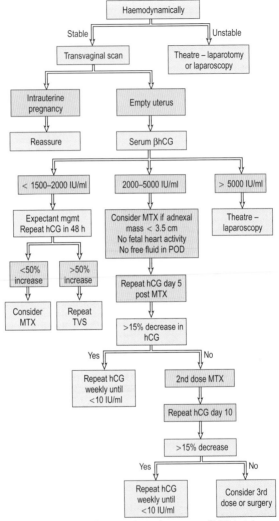

Figure 10.3 Management of suspected ectopic pregnancy. βhCG, beta human chorionic gonadotrophin; POD, pouch of Douglas; MTX, methotrexate; TVS, transvaginal scan.

then serial hCG monitoring should be established, with clear advice to the woman to reattend urgently if she develops pain. Where a woman has significant pelvic pain or echogenic free peritoneal fluid suggestive of haemoperitoneum, then laparoscopy should be considered, even in the absence of positive ultrasound visualization of an ectopic pregnancy.

Surgical treatment

Laparoscopic treatment of ectopic pregnancy will depend on the patient's physical condition, the location, size and state of the ectopic pregnancy, the experience of the surgeon, and the availability of equipment. The advantages of the laparoscopic approach have been well documented in terms of shorter hospital stay, quicker return to normal routine, fewer postoperative analgesic requirements, as well as reduced costs. The laparoscopic approach is also superior compared with laparotomy in terms of subsequent rate of intrauterine pregnancy and recurrent ectopic. The operation of choice for ectopic pregnancy is controversial, but clear guidelines are now available from bodies such as the Royal College of Obstetricians and Gynaecologists:

- Linear salpingotomy can be performed for an ampullary ectopic and fimbrial expression for an ectopic that is extruding from the fimbrial end. Salpingotomy is a reasonable approach when there is only one tube, but is associated with a 20% rate of further ectopic.
- Salpingectomy is preferred to salpingotomy when the contralateral tube is healthy as it is associated with a lower rate of persistent trophoblastic tissue, lower subsequent ectopic pregnancy and a similar subsequent intrauterine pregnancy rate. Salpingectomy is also indicated in the presence of uncontrolled bleeding, a second ectopic in the same tube, a severely damaged tube and occasionally when childbearing is complete.
- If patient is haemodynamically compromised or the surgeon has little experience in laparoscopic surgery, then a laparotomy is a reasonable approach.

Medical treatment

Early diagnosis has made medical management of ectopic pregnancy an option in centres with relevant expertise. It is appropriate in patients that are haemodynamically stable, reliable and compliant (as careful follow-up is important), with an ectopic pregnancy within the tube, measuring 3.5 cm or less in its greatest diameter, and with no evidence of rupture or significant bleeding. The advantages of this are that surgery and anaesthesia are avoided, there is less tubal damage, it is cost-effective and future fertility potential is maintained. Methotrexate has been used by single or multiple intramuscular doses or by injection directly into the ectopic pregnancy with good success.

GESTATIONAL TROPHOBLASTIC DISEASE

This is a general term used to describe hydatidiform mole, invasive mole, placental-site tumour and choriocarcinoma. It occurs when trophoblastic tissue, which is part of the blastocyst and normally invades the endometrium to form the placenta, proliferates abnormally and aggressively. The incidence in the UK is approximately 1 in 2000 pregnancies, compared with 1 in 200 in Asia.

Definitions

A hydatidiform mole is a benign tumour of the trophoblast and can be either partial or complete.

Partial mole

This is the commonest type: fetus or fetal tissue is present, cells are triploid derived from two sperm and one egg, and rarely become malignant.

Complete mole

This is much less common: no fetus is present, the cells are entirely paternal in origin, usually occurring when a sperm fertilizes an empty egg and then undergoes mitosis so that the cells are diploid, usually 46,XX; there is a 5–10% risk of malignant change.

Invasive mole

This is a tumour-like process invading the myometrium with metastatic potential. It usually follows a complete mole and may resolve spontaneously as it is less aggressive than a true cancer.

Choriocarcinoma

This is a carcinoma arising from the trophoblast after a mole, a miscarriage or even following a normal pregnancy.

Assessment

Moles usually present with bleeding in early pregnancy. They are associated with grossly elevated βhCG levels and so symptoms of pregnancy are exaggerated, such as excessive hyperemesis. Patients may present with early-onset pre-eclampsia or hyperthyroidism.

The uterus is large for dates and ultrasound may show a 'snowstorm' appearance due to the presence of the hydropic 'grape-like' vesicles within the uterine cavity.

Serum βhCG is grossly elevated. Chest X-ray should be performed to exclude metastases.

Management

Suction curettage with oxytocin infusion should be performed by an experienced surgeon as there is significant risk of incomplete evacuation or perforation. Hysterectomy may be considered if the patient's family history is complete.

Urgent histological analysis of tissue must be carried out and anti-D immunoglobulin must be administered if appropriate. The patient should be registered with the regional specialist centre.

Follow-up

All patients with molar pregnancy should be registered with a centre for trophoblastic disease. These patients require detailed follow-up that will be arranged by these centres. Serum βhCG samples should be obtained at 2-weekly intervals postevacuation until normal levels are reached. Following these, urinary βhCG samples are requested at 4-weekly intervals until 1 year postevacuation, then every 3 months in the second year of follow-up. Further serum samples are only requested if subsequent βhCG becomes abnormal. If the patient's βhCG values reach normal range within 8 weeks of evacuation, follow-up will be limited to 6 months. Adverse sequelae have not so far been observed in these patients. The majority of patients with partial hydatidiform mole, and patients with lesions suspicious of hydatidiform mole, fall into this short-term follow-up group. It also includes some patients with complete hydatidiform mole. Patients in the 6-month follow-up group may consider starting a new pregnancy at the end of that 6-month period.

Patients who do not have normal βhCG values within 8 weeks of evacuation should have 2-year follow-up. If these women are keen to pursue a further pregnancy it is only advisable after βhCG levels have been normal for 6 months. In this group the risk of choriocarcinoma occurring is 1 in 286.

Further estimations of βhCG 6 and 10 weeks after any future pregnancy are recommended because of the small risk of choriocarcinoma developing in such patients. In some cases the choriocarcinoma arises from the new pregnancy.

Hormonal preparations taken for contraceptive or other purposes between evacuation of a mole and the return to normal βhCG levels appear to increase the risk of choriocarcinoma developing. It is suggested that these be avoided until βhCG has become undetectable in serum.

Prognosis

The diagnosis of malignancy is usually made from persistently elevated or rising βhCG levels, persistent vaginal bleeding or evidence of metastatic spread to the lungs. The tumour is highly malignant, but also very chemosensitive, with 5-year survival rates of 95%. The mortality from trophoblastic disease is six to eight women per year in the UK.

SUMMARY

- Detailed history and examination are vital in the assessment of early-pregnancy bleeding.
- Transvaginal ultrasound assessment is a key part of the assessment of early-pregnancy complications.
- Ectopic pregnancy should always be considered, as the presentation is highly variable and the consequences can be devastating if diagnosis is missed.
- Pregnancy loss is highly emotive and psychological support should always be offered.
- Patients with recurrent pregnancy loss must be fully investigated, as causes such as APS can be managed successfully.
- Cases of gestational trophoblastic disease must be registered at regional centres, as follow-up of these patients is vital.

Section 3

Obstetrics

Prepregnancy counselling, prenatal diagnosis and antenatal care 11

CHAPTER CONTENTS

PREPREGNANCY COUNSELLING

Many pregnancies are unplanned but some women will request prepregnancy advice from their general practitioner (GP). At other times the discussion may take place opportunistically, for example during a routine gynaecology appointment or in counselling after a miscarriage. It is very important that women with specific medical problems such as diabetes, epilepsy and heart or renal disease are referred for prepregnancy assessment and management by a specialist obstetrician or physician. The aim of prepregnancy counselling is to optimize the outcome of the pregnancy for the fetus and to minimize the effect of pregnancy on any medical problems in the mother.

History

A detailed gynaecological, obstetric and medical history should be taken. Previous pelvic pathology or infection may affect the likelihood of conception and risk of ectopic pregnancy. Previous miscarriages may suggest investigations for recurrent miscarriage are indicated. In the obstetric history women should be questioned about previous fetal abnormalities (e.g. neural tube defects) or medical problems (e.g. deep-vein thrombosis), which may need to be addressed prior to a new pregnancy. A family history will also highlight any increased risk of inherited fetal abnormalities or gene disorders (such as haemoglobinopathies, muscular dystrophy or cystic fibrosis), which indicate referral for genetic counselling.

Women should be asked about any medications, whether prescribed or over-the-counter, as these may have an effect on either fertility or the development of the fetus. A social history should include smoking, alcohol and recreational drug use.

General advice

Timing of intercourse
Women are most likely to become pregnant by having intercourse two to three times per week. The most likely conception is by intercourse during the 6 days prior to ovulation (days 8–14 in a regular 28-day cycle).

Smoking
Smoking is associated with intrauterine growth restriction, prematurity, respiratory disease in infants and cot death. Women should stop smoking and be offered counselling support if necessary. Partners should also stop because of the risks of passive smoking. As smoking in men reduces sperm count this should also encourage cessation if there is a history of fertility problems.

Alcohol
Excessive alcohol in pregnancy causes fetal alcohol syndrome (fetal growth restriction, neurological impairment and facial deformities). Moderate alcohol intake causes an increased spontaneous miscarriage rate and lower birth weight and is associated with abruption and preterm labour. No adverse effects are known to occur with intake less than 15 units per week but, in practice, many women choose to avoid alcohol completely in pregnancy.

Recreational drugs
Marijuana itself does not affect pregnancy outcome, though it is often associated with tobacco smoking or the use of other harmful drugs. Ecstasy may be associated with heart and limb defects in the fetus. Both cocaine and crack cocaine lead to prematurity, stillbirth, abruption and growth restriction. Opiates (including methadone) cause growth restriction, premature delivery and stillbirth as well as neonatal addiction. Women using these drugs should be carefully managed with the local drug addiction team, to limit drug use prior to and during pregnancy. They should consider preconceptual human immunodeficiency virus (HIV), hepatitis B and hepatitis C testing as these cause infection in the baby in utero, at delivery and during breastfeeding.

Weight
Women should maintain their body mass index (BMI) (weight (kg)/height (m)^2) between 20 and 25. Women who are underweight may not be able to conceive due to hypothalamic anovulation and putting on weight to maintain their BMI above 18 will usually cause periods and fertility to return. Overweight women (especially if BMI is greater than 30) should be advised to lose weight before pregnancy, as obesity is a major risk factor for pre-eclampsia, gestational diabetes, thrombosis and infection (especially urinary tract infection and wound infection). Obesity is also associated with macrosomia and difficulty in monitoring the growth of the baby. Overweight women who are having difficulty conceiving often have polycystic ovarian syndrome and relatively small amounts of weight loss (1–2 stone or 6–13 kg) will normally restore ovulation.

Exercise

Excessive exercise inhibits hypothalamic function and causes hypothalamic hypogonadotrophic anovulation. Moderate exercise is not harmful in pregnancy and activities such as swimming and walking are recommended. High-impact sports and some racket sports should be avoided from early pregnancy if they are more likely to cause falls and trauma, with a consequent risk to the fetus.

Diet

A healthy diet is low in salt and saturated fat, high in fibre, fresh fruit and vegetables, with more white meat and fish than red meat.

Some foods need to be avoided in pregnancy due to the risk of listeriosis, salmonella and toxoplasmosis. These include:

- Unpasteurized milk and cheese
- Pâté and uncooked or poorly cooked meat
- Shellfish
- Raw eggs.

Women should wash their hands before cooking, and wash fruit and vegetables to reduce the risk of contamination. Liver should not be eaten, as high doses of vitamin A are associated with congenital abnormality.

Vitamins

Folic acid (vitamin B_9) reduces the risk of neural tube defects in the fetus by up to 75%. It is advised that 400 µg (available over the counter) should be taken daily from 12 weeks prior to conception until 12 weeks' gestation. This is increased to 5 mg daily for women on antiepileptic medication and those with a family or previous obstetric history of a neural tube defect. Other vitamin supplements are not needed with a normal diet and excessive vitamin A intake should be avoided.

Medications

- **Drugs associated with subfertility:** Many antipsychotics and antidepressants cause infertility by antagonizing dopamine, thus inducing hyperprolactinaemia and inhibiting ovulation. These may need to be reviewed prior to attempting pregnancy. Newer drugs such as clozapine and olanzapine and serotonin-specific reuptake inhibitors do not have this effect.

- **Drugs in pregnancy:** The National Teratology Information Service and individual drug data sheets give information on harmful effects of drugs in pregnancy. Many common drugs such as paracetamol, penicillins and cephalosporins are safe in pregnancy. Non-steroidal anti-inflammatory drugs should be avoided because of their likely link with miscarriage in the first trimester and oligohydramnios and patent ductus arteriosus later in pregnancy.

  Women on warfarin therapy should be converted to heparin, preferably low-molecular-weight, before pregnancy occurs in view of the association between warfarin and congenital abnormality, and this is an important point in prepregnancy counselling. This risk occurs between 6 and 12 weeks' gestation. However, women with artificial heart valves, in whom the risk of stopping warfarin is very significant, should be seen by the haematologist prior to pregnancy to plan anticoagulation management, weighing the risk of thrombosis and stroke from suboptimal anticoagulation against teratogenicity and fetal or maternal haemorrhage from warfarin.

Antiepileptic medications are associated with congenital malformations and should be reviewed prepregnancy to reduce the number of different drugs, thus reducing the risk to the fetus.

Angiotensin-converting enzyme inhibitors can cause skull defects, oligohydramnios and renal complications in the fetus. Diuretics should be avoided, as they are teratogenic in animal studies. Beta-blockers may cause growth restriction, hypotension and neonatal bradycardia in the fetus and are generally avoided. Calcium channel antagonists, hydralazine and labetalol are not known to be harmful but methyldopa has been used most safely in pregnancy and a plan should be made to convert most women on other hypertensives to methyldopa or labetalol once pregnancy is confirmed.

Rubella

Most women have now been immunized against rubella in childhood, but the antibody level can be checked prepregnancy as some women will have low-level or absent antibodies and should have a further vaccination. Care must be taken to ensure that the woman is not pregnant at the time of administration as the vaccine is live and there is a theoretical risk of infection of the fetus (although no cases of congenital rubella syndrome have been reported from inadvertent vaccination during pregnancy).

Fetal abnormality and genetic disorders

Parents with a family history or previous personal history of a baby with a fetal structural abnormality (e.g. neural tube defect), chromosomal disorder (e.g. trisomy 21) or gene disorder (e.g. muscular dystrophy, cystic fibrosis or haemoglobinopathies) have an increased risk of future pregnancies being affected. Details of prepregnancy and antenatal tests for such conditions should be explained. Prior to pregnancy these may include karyotyping or DNA analysis of both parents, and possibly extended-family members. In pregnancy, early scans and diagnostic tests, such as chorionic villous sampling (CVS) and amniocentesis, are available to diagnose many disorders.

Couples must be allowed to choose the investigations they would like and at what stage. Many parents choose to decline all preconceptual and prenatal testing for fetal abnormality.

For some specific disorders steps may be taken to reduce the chance of a fetus being affected. For example, women with a high risk of neural tube defect in their fetus should take a higher dose of folic acid preconceptually (5 mg daily).

Preimplantation genetic diagnosis

Preimplantation genetic diagnosis is a new technique used for families with serious genetic problems (sex-linked conditions such as Duchenne muscular dystrophy, single-gene disorders such as cystic fibrosis and chromosomal abnormalities). In vitro fertilization is used to produce multiple embryos. These are allowed to develop to the 8-cell stage (day 3) when a cell is removed from each embryo for genetic analysis. Affected embryos can thus be identified and discarded, with only 'healthy' embryos transferred back into the uterus.

The technique can only be used where the disorder has been characterized genetically and when it causes significant effects on the child.

Specific medical conditions

Women with the following medical problems should have specialist review of their management prior to pregnancy.

Diabetes

Good glycaemic control significantly reduces the incidence of fetal abnormality. Diabetic retinopathy should be treated before conception to reduce the risk of deterioration with pregnancy. Prepregnancy assessment also allows for screening for nephropathy, which is a strong predictor of pre-eclampsia and worsening renal function in pregnancy. Many units now manage these patients in specialized joint clinics with endocrinology.

Epilepsy

The risk of fetal abnormality increases with the number of different anti-convulsant medications being taken and women considering pregnancy should, therefore, have the number minimized.

All epileptics on medication should also be given 5 mg folic acid daily from 3 months preconception to counteract the folate-antagonist effect of the drugs and thus reduce the chance of a neural tube defect in the fetus. It should also be emphasized that antiepileptic medication should be continued in pregnancy as the threshold for fits is likely to reduce and the risk to the mother of having fits outweighs the teratogenic risk of the medication.

It is worth considering stopping all medication prior to conception if a woman has had no fits for 2 years.

Cardiac disease

Women with severe cardiac disease, specifically Eisenmenger's syndrome (right-to-left shunt as a result of fixed high pulmonary vascular resistance), pulmonary hypertension from any cause and uncorrected tetralogy of Fallot should be strongly advised not to become pregnant as there is a significant maternal mortality (50% for Eisenmenger's syndrome). There is also a very high chance of extreme prematurity in the fetus and a high perinatal mortality rate.

Women with moderate- to high-risk cardiac disease such as mitral stenosis, aortic stenosis, Marfan's syndrome and coarctation of the aorta should all be assessed by a cardiologist before pregnancy. This will allow for assessment of the risk of becoming pregnant and treatment to improve the outcome of pregnancy, such as repair of coarctation or mitral valve surgery.

Low-risk heart diseases such as atrial and ventricular septal defects, patent ductus arteriosus, and mitral or tricuspid valve regurgitation are well tolerated in pregnancy and generally these women do not need prepregnancy assessment.

Hypertension

Women with raised blood pressure should be assessed before pregnancy to rule out any underlying cause for the hypertension such as renal disease, coarctation of the aorta or endocrinological disorders. Their renal function should also be checked as raised creatinine would indicate a higher risk of pre-eclampsia and deterioration of renal function.

Renal disease

Renal disease is likely to be worsened by pregnancy and women with high creatinine levels (greater than 125 μmol/l) are at particular risk. If the creatinine level is above 250 μmol/l then they should consider avoiding pregnancy as up to 50% would develop long-term deterioration of their kidney function.

Women undergoing renal dialysis have impaired fertility and rarely become pregnant. However, they should still be advised to use contraception as pregnancy would be unlikely to have a successful neonatal outcome and would cause major problems in dialysis management. Women who have had a renal transplant, and in whom the renal function is stable, may consider pregnancy 2 years posttransplant, as their likely long-term prognosis is good.

PRENATAL DIAGNOSIS

Prenatal diagnosis refers to the diagnosis of fetal abnormalities in utero. The abnormalities may be minor or severe. If severe they may not be compatible with life or may be likely to cause long-term serious morbidity or handicap. Some abnormalities may require therapy in utero or a plan made for postnatal management. Screening programmes focus on the commonest chromosomal abnormality, Down's syndrome (trisomy 21), though both the ultrasound and serum tests often detect other chromosomal and structural abnormalities. There is an important distinction between screening tests and diagnostic tests.

Screening tests

Screening tests give an estimate of risk for that particular pregnancy. Age alone, for example, is a risk factor for Down's syndrome; in the baby of a woman aged 20 the risk is 1 in 1500, whereas at age 40 it is 1 in 50. Paternal age has no effect on fetal chromosomal abnormality.

Serum screening

The triple test, quadruple test and integrated test use combinations of serum markers (alpha-fetoprotein (AFP), oestriol, human chorionic gonadotrophin beta-subunit, inhibin A and pregnancy-associated plasma protein A) combined with the age of the mother and confirmed gestation of the pregnancy to give a calculated estimate of risk of Down's syndrome. The tests can usually be performed from 14 to 20 weeks' gestation and the results are generally available within 2 weeks. The false-positive rate depends on the test but is around 5% and the tests detect 85–90% of babies with Down's syndrome.

Ultrasound scan

The nuchal translucency test or NT is performed between 11 and 14 weeks' gestation, when the fetus has a crown–rump length of between 45 and 84 mm. It involves measuring the thickness of the fold of skin over the back of the fetus' neck and size of the baby and combining this with the mother's age and gestation of the pregnancy to estimate the risk of Down's syndrome. A higher risk of Down's syndrome is found with a greater nuchal translucency. The test detects 85% of babies with Down's syndrome with a false-positive rate of about 5%. A high NT is also found with many other chromosome abnormalities, especially trisomy 18, 13 and Turner's syndrome.

In the second trimester, specific ultrasound markers for Down's syndrome can be identified such as brachycephaly, venticulomegaly, atrial septal defect, duodenal atresia, echogenic bowel, hydronephrosis and short limbs. The risk of Down's syndrome increases with the number of abnormalities detected.

Combined tests

Some tests use both NT and biochemical markers to calculate a risk of Down's syndrome.

All of the above tests involve calculation of an estimated risk of Down's syndrome for that particular fetus. Generally, a positive result is given if the risk is greater than 1 in 250 and those couples are then offered a diagnostic test such as amniocentesis or CVS. Prior to the introduction of serum screening and nuchal translucency, all women over the age of 35 were considered high-risk and offered amniocentesis. Most women over 35 are now reassured by low-risk NT or serum screening test results and therefore avoid unnecessary invasive tests.

Limits of screening tests

- **Pretest counselling:** All women who undergo a screening test should have the test fully explained prior to the procedure. The concept of risk, however, is often poorly understood and, therefore, informed consent can be difficult to obtain.
- **False positives and unnecessary tests:** Both serum screening and nuchal translucency measurement have a false-positive rate of about 5%. This causes anxiety and unnecessary invasive tests. Most women who have a positive screen result will not in fact have an affected fetus.
- **False-negative results:** As the tests are screening rather than diagnostic tests, some Down's syndrome babies will be born to women with low-risk results.

   Ethnicity, diabetes and bleeding in early pregnancy affect the serum marker concentrations, making the test less reliable in some groups.
- **Twins:** Serum screening cannot be used effectively for multiple pregnancies, though nuchal translucency is still possible.

Screening tests to detect other abnormalities

Other than Down's syndrome, screening tests may suggest a high risk of other abnormalities and indicate referral to a fetal medicine unit for further scans or invasive tests.

- **AFP:** Raised AFP alone, found incidentally at serum screening, is associated with neural tube defects and anterior abdominal wall defects as well as Patau's syndrome (trisomy 13). In the absence of structural abnormality, increased AFP is associated with intra-uterine growth restriction and so regular ultrasound assessment is recommended
- **Increased NT:** In women with a high-risk NT but no chromosomal abnormality, there is an association with multiple abnormalities, including congenital heart disease, exomphalos, diaphragmatic hernia and skeletal defects.

Structural abnormalities

The commoner minor abnormalities found at second-trimester scan include equinovarus (talipes or club foot), cleft lip and palate, renal pelvis dilatation, echogenic foci in the heart and mild hydronephrosis. These cases should all be referred to the fetal medicine unit to confirm the abnormality, look for other associated abnormalities and determine any further prenatal investigation. Depending on the abnormality, postnatal management can be planned, such as surgery for cleft defects, antibiotics for hydronephrosis or physiotherapy for talipes. Major abnormalities such as cardiac defects will involve a multidisciplinary approach and consideration of delivery in a hospital with a specialized neonatal unit.

Diagnostic tests

Diagnostic tests give a couple a definite answer that their baby does or does not have a disorder. They may be performed after a positive Down's syndrome screening result or may be requested by the woman instead of a screening test. They are also used where the pregnancy is known to be at high risk of a single-gene disorder or chromosomal abnormality other than Down's syndrome.

Amniocentesis

A fine needle is inserted transabdominally into the uterus under ultrasound control, after local anaesthetic infiltration. A few millilitres of amniotic fluid, which contains desquamated fetal skin cells, is aspirated and cultured. Chromosome analysis is then performed. The result takes about 2 weeks, but polymerase chain reaction techniques are increasingly being used when an urgent result is necessary as it can detect these chromosomal abnormalities within 2–3 days.

The test can be performed from 15 weeks' gestation and the risk of miscarriage from the procedure is about 1%. Earlier amniocentesis is avoided as it carries a higher risk of miscarriage and talipes.

Chorionic villous sampling

CVS uses ultrasound guidance to take a biopsy from the placenta for analysis. The risk of miscarriage is also about 1%. As CVS is performed at 11–14 weeks, it is often preferred to amniocentesis as the result is known earlier and decisions about termination can be made sooner. However, it has a higher rate of failed culture compared with amniocentesis. In a very small number of cases an inconclusive result is given due to placental mosaicism. In these cases amniocentesis will be needed at 16 weeks. CVS is only performed after 11 weeks as fetal limb abnormalities can occur if performed earlier.

Cordocentesis

Cordocentesis involves aspiration of fetal blood directly from the umbilical cord, again transabdominally under ultrasound control. It is used from 18 weeks, mostly when an in-utero transfusion may be required, such as with haemolytic disease or alloimmune thrombocytopenia. Other uses of cordocentesis include testing the fetus for infection, such as after maternal parvovirus infection, and for the investigation of fetal hydrops. The risk of miscarriage from the procedure is 1–2%.

Ultrasound in pregnancy

All pregnant women should be offered first- and second-trimester scans. The role of each is as follows.

First trimester (10–14 weeks)

- Establish viability: some pregnancies have failed by the time of the first-trimester scan and the diagnosis of missed miscarriage is made if crown–rump length >7 mm with no fetal heart detected. These women should be offered counselling and evacuation of retained products of conception (ERPC).
- Confirm gestation: up to 14 weeks, the estimated due date should be amended if there is more than 7 days' discrepancy between dates by

last menstrual period and by crown–rump length at scan. Beyond 14 weeks, the gestation should be estimated by biparietal diameter or head circumference, and estimated due date corrected if there is more than 14 days' discrepancy with menstrual dates. Correct dating is very important for planning induction if the woman does not go into spontaneous labour, but dating of pregnancy becomes less accurate with increasing gestation.

- Gross anatomy: major anomalies such as anencephaly, cystic hygroma, bladder outflow obstruction and major anterior abdominal wall defects can be detected at first-trimester scan.
- Multiple pregnancies: multiple pregnancies can be detected and chorionicity and amnionicity are most reliably determined in the first trimester.

Second trimester (18–24 weeks)

- Structural anatomy: the whole fetus should be examined (brain, face, heart, kidneys, abdomen, spine, hands and feet, genitalia, bladder) and referral made to a fetal medicine unit if any abnormalities are detected.
- Fetal growth: very rarely, often associated with pre-eclampsia, early-onset intrauterine growth restriction or oligohydramnios is detected at the second-trimester scan and indicates further follow-up in the fetal medicine department and close monitoring for pre-eclampsia.
- Fetal sex: this can be determined in the second trimester with 99% accuracy if parents wish it, though concerns over the misuse of this information by some cultural groups means that it is not offered in all units.
- Placental site: if the placenta encroaches into the lower segment of the uterus a further scan is arranged for 34 weeks to recheck its location and plan delivery accordingly.

Further scans

Further scans may be arranged for suspected growth restriction or abnormal liquor volume. They may also be needed to follow up any abnormality found at the second-trimester scan. Later in pregnancy ultrasound may also be used to assess fetal well-being by Doppler assessment of blood flow in the umbilical artery and other fetal vessels, or by biophysical profile (breathing movements, gross body movements, fetal tone, heart rate reactivity and amniotic fluid volume).

Other ultrasound screening tests

Fetal echocardiography

All women with a high risk of fetal cardiac abnormalities should be offered a second-trimester fetal echocardiography scan. This includes women with congenital heart disease, diabetes or epilepsy as well as those with a previous child with a congenital cardiac problem. A high-risk NT result and abnormal or inadequate views of the heart at routine second-trimester scan are other indications for fetal echocardiography.

Uterine artery Doppler

Many units use Doppler flow studies to assess the resistance in the maternal uterine arteries. High resistance at 20–24 weeks' gestation indicates a high chance of pre-eclampsia, abruption and growth restriction, so these women should be offered close blood pressure and fetal growth monitoring.

Cervical length

There is currently great interest in the transvaginal measurement of the cervical length to indicate risk of late miscarriage and extreme prematurity. If the cervix is short then there is some evidence that elective cervical cerclage in high-risk women may prolong the time to delivery.

ANTENATAL CARE

Antenatal care aims to optimize the health and well-being of mother and baby, and to detect and treat any abnormal events in pregnancy. The commonest significant disorder diagnosed is pre-eclampsia.

Antenatal care may be provided by the GP, midwife (in hospital or in the community) or the obstetrician team. The commonest is shared care between the midwife and GP, with referral for obstetric input when indicated.

Most women will not need to see an obstetrician unless factors in the booking or during the antenatal period indicate. Indications for referral at booking are shown in Table 11.1.

At all visits, the woman should be encouraged to discuss her concerns and any minor disorders of pregnancy, discuss tests and their results, and have her blood pressure and urinalysis checked. In the second trimester growth is assessed by measurement of symphysis–fundal height (SFH) and from 36 weeks, presentation is clinically assessed by palpation. Antenatal visits also provide an opportunity to discuss the forthcoming delivery and the woman's birth plan.

Women should keep their own obstetric notes, in which all the health professionals involved make their documentation, and all pregnancy results are filed. These are then stored with the main hospital records following delivery.

Table 11.1. Factors at booking indicating referral for obstetric or senior midwifery review

Age over 40 years or under 19 years
Body mass index ≥35 or <18
Grand multiparity (more than six pregnancies)
Conditions such as hypertension, cardiac or renal disease, endocrine, psychiatric or haematological disorders, epilepsy, diabetes, autoimmune diseases, cancer, human immunodeficiency virus (HIV)
Previous caesarean section or other uterine surgery
Previous postpartum haemorrhage
Severe pre-eclampsia or eclampsia
Previous pre-eclampsia or eclampsia
Three or more miscarriages
Previous preterm birth or mid-trimester loss
Previous psychiatric illness or puerperal psychosis
Previous neonatal death or stillbirth
Previous baby with congenital abnormality
Previous small for gestational age (SGA) or large for gestational age (LGA) infant
Family history of genetic disorder

Women with an uncomplicated first pregnancy would normally be seen 10 times during the pregnancy and parous women who have had previous uncomplicated pregnancies seven times.

Typical timing of antenatal visits, which might be with GP, midwife or obstetrician, for a nulliparous woman are outlined below.

Booking (6–12 weeks)

A medical, gynaecological, obstetric, family and social history should be taken. Drugs and allergies are recorded. Examination should include height and weight, and calculation of BMI. Booking blood pressure must be recorded. Breast or pelvic examination is not indicated and should never be performed in the antenatal setting without a specific indication and informed consent from the woman, with a chaperone present. One such indication for pelvic examination is in a woman with a history of female genital mutilation, who may need early referral to a specialist clinic for antenatal de-infibulation, and a management plan made for delivery.

First-trimester scan should be arranged to confirm dates and screen for Down's syndrome. If the woman presents after 14 weeks a scan should be arranged to confirm gestation (by biparietal diameter or head circumference) and serum screening for Down's syndrome offered. Urine should be checked for proteinuria and a midstream urine sample sent to screen for asymptomatic bacteriuria. Booking blood tests should be taken. The woman should be referred to an obstetrician if indicated from the previous history. Information should be given on diet, smoking, alcohol, exercise (see prepregnancy counseling, above) and antenatal care.

Booking blood tests
All the tests should be explained including the reasons why they are being taken and what action might be taken if the results are abnormal:
- Full blood count: to exclude anaemia.
- Group and antibody check: to detect Rhesus-negative women and atypical antibodies.
- Haemoglobinopathy screen: this may be checked in all women or used selectively for those of Afro-Caribbean, Mediterranean or Asian origin. Those with positive results should be offered counselling and partner testing followed by antenatal diagnosis for at-risk fetuses.
- Rubella: to check immunity and plan postnatal vaccination for those with low-level or no immunity. Such women must also be warned about avoiding exposure to the virus.
- Syphilis: to check for syphilis antibodies, which indicate a possibility of current infection in the mother and therefore risk of congenital abnormality in the fetus. Women with a positive result must be referred to a genitourinary medicine (GUM) clinic, though many will be false positives from pregnancy or previously treated disease.
- Hepatitis B: women with positive results should be referred to a gastroenterologist. Neonatal vaccination and immunoglobulin must be planned and interventions such as fetal scalp electrode and fetal blood sampling in labour should be avoided.
- HIV: HIV-positive women should be referred to GUM physicians, offered counselling and given antiviral agents prior to delivery. They should be advised to deliver by caesarean section and avoid breastfeeding.

16 weeks

All results from the booking visit should be given and explained. Anaemia should be treated if necessary. Blood pressure and urine should be checked.

25 weeks

The result of the anomaly scan should be reviewed. Blood pressure and urine should be checked and SFH recorded. Fetal movements should be asked about (usually felt at 18–20 weeks in nulliparous, 16–18 weeks in parous women). Fetal heart beat should be checked with Doppler or Pinnard stethoscope. Antenatal classes should be discussed.

28 weeks

Blood pressure, urine and SFH should be checked. Fetal movements should be asked about and fetal heart auscultated. Repeat screen for anaemia by full blood count, and an antibody screen should be sent (regardless of Rhesus status). Anti-D should be given to Rhesus-negative women.

31 weeks

Blood pressure, urine and SFH should be checked. Fetal movements should be asked about and fetal heart auscultated. Iron should be commenced if haemoglobin is less than 10.5 g/dl.

34 weeks

Blood pressure, urine and SFH should be checked. Fetal movements should be asked about and fetal heart auscultated. A second dose of anti-D should be given to Rhesus-negative women.

36 weeks

Blood pressure, urine and SFH should be checked. Fetal movements should be asked about and fetal heart auscultated. The position of the baby should be assessed clinically and external cephalic version recommended and arranged if breech. If the placenta was low at 20 weeks then the repeat scan should be reviewed for placental site.

38 weeks

Blood pressure, urine and SFH should be checked. Fetal movements should be asked about and fetal heart auscultated. Fetal position should be checked.

40 weeks

Blood pressure, urine and SFH should be checked. Fetal movements should be asked about and fetal heart auscultated. Fetal position should be checked.

41 weeks

Blood pressure, urine and SFH should be checked. Fetal movements should be asked about and fetal heart auscultated. The fetal position should be checked. Membrane sweep should be offered and recommended and a plan made for induction of labour by 42 weeks.

For parous women the 14-, 25- and 31-week visits can be omitted unless specific factors indicate that an extra visit is needed.

Obstetric-led care

Some women will need obstetric-led care and the timing of these visits should be tailored to the specific problem. For example, a diabetic woman may need to be seen by the hospital team every 2 weeks throughout the pregnancy, whereas a woman with a previous caesarean section who plans a vaginal birth in this pregnancy may see the obstetrician once and then be referred back to her midwife for the rest of her antenatal care.

Some women should have antenatal care within a multidisciplinary team. These would include those with diabetes, cardiac or renal disease.

Rhesus disease and other red-cell alloimmune antibodies

All women should have their blood sent for group and antibody screen at booking as 15% are Rhesus-negative (they do not carry the Rhesus D antigen on their red blood cells). These women are, therefore, at risk of developing anti-D antibodies to a Rhesus-positive fetus. This would not usually occur in a first pregnancy unless sensitization had occurred previously, for example from a blood transfusion. Potentially sensitizing events in the pregnancy include:

- Threatened miscarriage, miscarriage, ERPC or ectopic pregnancy
- Trauma to the abdomen, such as amniocentesis, CVS or road traffic accident
- External cephalic version
- Abruption or other antepartum haemorrhage
- Delivery, especially if multiple pregnancy or manual removal of placenta
- Spontaneous fetomaternal haemorrhage.

Haemolytic disease of the fetus involves anaemia and fetal hydrops, which can result in fetal death if not treated by intrauterine blood transfusion.

The rate of sensitization has reduced to 1.5% by the use of anti-D at delivery and at potentially sensitizing events. However, it is estimated that this rate will reduce to 0.3% if routine anti-D prophylaxis is given to all Rhesus-negative women at 28 and 34 weeks as well as at delivery.

A standard dose of 500IU anti-D antibody should be given by intra-muscular injection at 28 weeks and 34 weeks as well as 500IU within 72 hours of delivery (if the baby is Rhesus-positive), to prevent development of anti-D antibodies in a non-sensitized mother. Many units have not implemented this policy due to cost and, therefore, use the traditional strategy of giving anti-D antenatally after a potentially sensitizing event. In this case a Kleihauer test should be taken before giving the anti-D. This gives an indication of the volume of fetomaternal haemorrhage by estimating the number of fetal cells present in the maternal circulation. If the result is greater than 4ml then the anti-D dose needs to be increased accordingly, after liaison with the haematologist.

Women who already have anti-D antibodies, whether from previous pregnancy sensitization or from a blood transfusion in the past, should not be given anti-D prophylaxis, but have their anti-D titre monitored every 4 weeks from booking. If the antibody titre increases to 15IU/ml then fetal anaemia is likely and cordocentesis may be needed to estimate fetal haemoglobin and allow transfusion of the fetus if necessary.

Other antibodies

Other antibodies (often described as 'atypical') may be detected at booking and may have an effect for the mother or the fetus.

Effect on the fetus

Apart from Rhesus (D) antibodies, the other common antibodies that cause severe haemolytic disease of the newborn are anti-c and anti-K. Anti-e, -Ce, -Fya, -Jka and Cw only rarely cause fetal haemolysis. Women with any of these antibodies should be followed up in the fetal medicine department as for women with anti-D antibodies.

ABO incompatibility between mother and fetus may cause neonatal jaundice, but rarely causes severe haemolytic disease of the newborn.

Effect on the mother

Atypical antibodies in the maternal blood may make crossmatch difficult, and liaison with a haematologist will determine whether any action needs to be taken around delivery to ensure maternal blood loss is minimized and blood can be available if needed. This may involve correcting any anaemia with antenatal iron supplements or arranging a crossmatch late in the third trimester for long-term storage in case of emergency.

Antenatal education

First-time mothers and their partners should be encouraged to attend antenatal classes. These provide information for couples on pregnancy, childbirth and parenting. Topics include the physical and psychological changes in pregnancy, the stages of labour, analgesia in labour, what can go wrong in labour, breastfeeding, the postnatal period and caring for a newborn baby. Classes are thought to reduce anxiety in parents and provide a social interaction with other parents-to-be, though evidence is lacking over whether there is any effect on birth outcomes.

Seat belts in pregnancy

Pregnant women should be advised to continue to wear seat belts, but to position the lap belt under the gravid abdomen, to minimize the impact to the fetus and placenta if an accident occurs.

Flying in pregnancy

Airline protocols vary on when women can fly in pregnancy and women should always check with their airline what their protocol is. Many airlines will carry women until 34–36 weeks' gestation, though they may request a letter of confirmation from the obstetrician regarding the pregnancy well-being. This should be provided as long as there are no specific risks. As pregnancy and probably flying both increase the risk of thrombosis, women should avoid sitting for too long, perform regular calf exercises and drink plenty of fluids. For long-haul flights antithrombotic stockings may be prescribed.

Insurance companies also need to be consulted when flying during pregnancy as they may have limited cover, especially for neonatal care in case of premature delivery abroad.

SUMMARY

- Prepregnancy counselling is vital for those with serious medical conditions such as diabetes, epilepsy and cardiac or renal disease to minimize the likely impact of pregnancy on the disease and of the disease (or medication) on the pregnancy.
- Women with high-risk cardiac disease or severe renal disease should be advised not to become pregnant.

- Antenatal screening for Down's syndrome should be offered early to all pregnant women, with clear counselling regarding screening versus diagnostic tests. The screening tests are also useful in predicting other abnormalities such as cardiac disease.
- Ultrasound in the first trimester will confirm gestation and viability, check for major abnormalities and determine chorionicity in multiple pregnancy.
- Second-trimester ultrasound will check the detailed anatomy of the baby, but also confirm the placental site and growth of the baby.
- Rhesus status must be checked at booking to ensure that Rhesus-negative women are given anti-D either routinely at 28 weeks, 34 weeks and delivery, or after sensitizing events.
- Other important antibodies in haemolytic disease of the newborn are anti-c and anti-K.
- Most women will have normal pregnancies and do not need to see an obstetrician antenatally, but those with obstetric or medical problems must have their care tailored accordingly, often within a multidisciplinary team.

Physiology of pregnancy and pregnancy problems **12**

CHAPTER CONTENTS

PHYSIOLOGY OF PREGNANCY

The major physiological changes occurring during pregnancy are outlined below. Many of the systemic problems associated with pregnancy, such as gestational diabetes, venous thromboembolism (VTE) and worsening cardiac disease, can be related to these physiological alterations.

Cardiovascular

Blood pressure falls in early pregnancy as a result of vasodilatation and reduced systemic vascular resistance. From the mid-trimester blood pressure rises again as cardiac output increases. Immediately after delivery blood pressure falls, but then increases to a maximum 3–4 days' postpartum.

Cardiac output increases by 40% (20% within the first 8 weeks) to compensate for the fall in systemic vascular resistance caused by peripheral vasodilatation. This is achieved by an increase in both stroke volume and heart rate. The maximum cardiac output is achieved at 20–28 weeks.

The heart rate increases by 10–20 beats per minute in pregnancy.

The gravid uterus impairs venous return in the supine position and cardiac output can, therefore, fall by up to 25% when a pregnant woman lies on her back.

Respiratory

In response to the increased oxygen demand, maternal ventilation increases by 50% in pregnancy. This is mainly achieved through an increase in tidal volume rather than a high respiratory rate.

$PaCO_2$ is reduced due to the increased ventilation, with a compensatory fall in serum bicarbonate. This causes a mild compensated respiratory alkalosis.

Haematological

A physiological hypercoagulable state develops in pregnancy and hence thrombophilia screening can be unreliable during and shortly after pregnancy. This involves increases in factors VIII, IX, X and fibrinogen, with decreased fibrinolytic activity, antithrombin III, protein C and protein S (endogenous anticoagulants). Routine coagulation tests, however, remain normal. These coagulation changes last until 6 weeks after delivery. The hypercoagulability and venous stasis in the legs from the gravid uterus predispose to thrombosis.

There is a threefold increase in iron requirement and 10–20-fold increase in folate requirement in pregnancy. However, although red cell mass increases, the expansion in plasma volume is such that haemoglobin, haematocrit and red cell count fall. The platelet count also falls, though in 95% of women the level still remains within the normal non-pregnant range.

Renal

Renal plasma flow increases by 60–80% in pregnancy and glomerular filtration rate also increases. The creatinine clearance increases by 50% and there is a fall in serum urea and creatinine. Urinary protein excretion increases to up to 300 mg per 24 hours in normal pregnant women. Eighty per cent of women develop oedema due to physiological sodium and water retention, especially later in pregnancy.

The renal collecting system becomes dilated because of ureteric smooth muscle relaxation (a progesterone effect) and compression from the gravid uterus. This is more pronounced on the right than the left.

Hepatic

Serum protein decreases in pregnancy because of the 20–40% fall in serum albumin concentration. This is a dilutional effect from the increase in plasma volume. Alkaline phosphatase concentration increases due to production from the placenta. Alanine transaminase and aspartate transaminase fall in pregnancy.

Gastrointestinal

Pregnancy is associated with delayed gastric emptying and delayed lower gastrointestinal transit.

Metabolic

Human placental lactogen, cortisol and glucagon from the placenta cause a physiological insulin resistance and glucose intolerance during pregnancy. Insulin production doubles in response to this, with glucose tolerance decreasing with advancing gestation. Glucose metabolism also alters such that postprandial glucose is increased, though preprandial glucose is reduced when compared with non-pregnant values.

The renal threshold for glucose falls and glycosuria occurs in most normal women at some point in pregnancy.

Endocrine

Total thyroxine (T_4) and triiodothyronine (T_3) increase in pregnancy in response to increased thyroid-binding globulin production by the liver. In the first trimester thyroid-stimulating hormone (TSH) falls due to the excess human chorionic gonadotrophin beta-subunit (βhCG), which has a similar structure and effect.

In the third trimester, TSH increases and free T_4 and free T_3 are reduced.

MINOR DISORDERS OF PREGNANCY

Nausea and vomiting

Incidence

Fifty per cent of pregnant women experience nausea or vomiting, which is excessive in 1% (hyperemesis gravidarum).

Pathophysiology

Nausea and vomiting occur probably due to βhCG secreted by the placenta, particularly in the first trimester. The problem is, therefore, exacerbated in multiple and molar pregnancies.

Clinical features of hyperemesis

Women may present with intractable vomiting, usually for weeks, and are often dehydrated and exhausted. Epigastric pain may occur secondary to prolonged vomiting and Mallory–Weiss tears occasionally cause haematemesis. Nutritional or electrolyte disturbances may occur, but there is rarely a detrimental effect on the fetus, unless maternal weight loss is significant. Most cases resolve between 12 and 14 weeks, and 90% have resolved by 20 weeks.

Psychological effects are commonly experienced relating to interference in relationships with other children, time off work and exhaustion. Some women feel anger or resentment towards the pregnancy and even consider termination.

Management

For mild to moderate symptoms, without ketonuria, women should be managed as an outpatient with support, oral fluids and small amounts of regular food. Oral or rectal antiemetics can be prescribed if needed.

Admission is indicated for severe hyperemesis. Full blood count (FBC) should be checked to exclude anaemia, or a leukocytosis, which would suggest an infective cause for the vomiting. Urea and electrolytes and liver function tests should be checked for abnormalities.

Thyroid function tests to exclude thyrotoxicosis as a cause of vomiting should be sent, but treatment should depend on clinical signs and symptoms of thyroid disease, as abnormal biochemical markers of thyroid function are common in hyperemesis.

Urinalysis is performed to check for ketonuria and a midstream urine (MSU) sample sent for culture to exclude a urinary tract infection (UTI) as a cause of the vomiting.

Ultrasound scan should be arranged to exclude multiple or molar pregnancy.

Intravenous fluids

Saline or Hartmann's solution (0.9%) is used for rehydration. Sodium is important because of the hyponatraemia associated with hyperemesis. Dextrose should not be used (as it may precipitate Wernicke's encephalopathy). Depending on the serum potassium result, potassium should usually be added to the intravenous fluids.

Antiemetics

Cyclizine, prochlorperazine and metoclopramide are commonly used antiemetics in pregnancy. They have not been shown to be harmful in pregnancy, but can occasionally cause oculogyric crises. Initial treatment should be intravenous, followed by oral or rectal administration.

Corticosteroids have been shown to improve symptoms of hyperemesis in intractable cases.

Ginger and acupressure are alternative evidence-based treatments.

Thiamine

Thiamine (oral 50 mg daily or intravenous 100 mg weekly) should be given to all women with hyperemesis as Wernicke's encephalopathy has been reported from severe vitamin B_1 deficiency as a result of persistent vomiting.

Folic acid

Women with hyperemesis are usually folate-deficient and need to take 5 mg folic acid daily.

Any underlying cause of vomiting, such as UTI, should be treated.

Mallory–Weiss tears occur from prolonged vomiting and may be managed by ranitidine and antacids, though gastrointestinal referral is indicated if there is significant pain or the bleeding does not settle.

Some women are admitted repeatedly with hyperemesis and in these cases a social history may reveal other causes of difficulty coping with the pregnancy.

Heartburn

Delayed gastric emptying, the pressure effect of the gravid abdomen and smooth-muscle relaxation of the gastro-oesophageal sphincter cause a high incidence of gastro-oesophageal reflux in pregnancy. Heartburn is the symptom of retrosternal pain. Up to 70% of pregnant women report heartburn by the third trimester.

Treatment includes diet advice (reduced fat, small frequent meals and remaining upright after eating), posture advice (tilt head of bed up to reduce reflux), antireflux agents (e.g. Gaviscon or magnesium trisilicate) and antacids. Metoclopramide may help by increasing gastric emptying. H_2 antagonists such as ranitidine and proton pump inhibitors such as omeprazole are also effective and are not shown to be harmful in pregnancy, though they are not licensed for this indication.

Constipation

Constipation affects nearly half of pregnant women. The smooth-muscle effect of progesterone, the pressure of the gravid uterus, dietary changes or ferrous sulphate are contributing factors.

Severe constipation may lead to abdominal bloating and pain, nausea, vomiting, haemorrhoids and anal fissures.

Treatment is initially with dietary advice (high fibre, such as bran or wheat supplementation, balanced with appropriate fluid intake). Bulk-forming laxatives (e.g. ispaghula husk), stimulant laxatives (e.g. senna) or osmotic laxatives (e.g. lactulose) can also be used. Stimulant laxatives are more effective than bulk-forming agents but have a higher associated incidence of diarrhoea and abdominal pain.

Haemorrhoids

Haemorrhoids occur in 8% of pregnant women, due to increased intra-abdominal pressure causing decreased venous return, and are exacerbated by constipation. They may present with itching or bleeding. Pain occurs if haemorrhoids become thrombosed. Local preparations containing soothing agents are helpful and any constipation should be treated. Surgical treatment should only be considered very rarely, for unresolving thrombosed haemorrhoids. Haemorrhoids usually disappear spontaneously postpartum.

Urinary frequency

Frequency is normal in pregnancy, exacerbated by the pressure effect of the gravid uterus on the bladder. Infection should be excluded with an MSU sample if the symptoms are severe, suddenly worse or are associated with pain, offensive urine or pyrexia.

UTIs are discussed later in the chapter.

Breathlessness

Most women feel breathless during pregnancy because of increased ventilation, splinting of the diaphragm by the pregnant uterus, anaemia and general tiredness. Consideration should be given to the differential diagnoses if the symptoms are severe, sudden or associated with suspicious features such as pain, cough or wheezing. Other diagnoses include asthma, pulmonary embolism, pneumonia and cardiac causes. All women complaining of breathlessness should have a recent haemoglobin level checked, with iron supplementation as appropriate.

Skin problems

Itching

Many pregnant women experience itching, commonly over the abdomen. It is generally not associated with a rash, except for that due to excoriation, and liver function tests are normal. Suspicious features warranting further investigation are itching on the palms and soles, abnormal liver function or a rash (see obstetric cholestasis, below).

Pigmentation

Linea nigra (midline linear abdominal pigmentation), melasma (facial pigmentation), areolar darkening and striae gravidarum (stretch marks) all occur as features of normal pregnancy. There is no treatment and all fade after pregnancy, though striae never fully resolve.

Spider naevi and palmar erythema both occur in pregnancy, with spontaneous resolution in most cases.

Backache

Backache occurs in 40–60% of pregnant women as a result of progesterone causing relaxation of the ligamentous supports of the back and from the weight of the gravid uterus, with an exaggerated lumbar lordosis. Management, after assessing for neurological and orthopaedic abnormalities, is with reassurance, simple analgesia and physiotherapy for severe cases. Exercise in water, Ozzlo pillows (nest-shaped pillows to help sleep and posture in bed) and acupuncture are also shown to be effective at relieving symptoms.

Symphysis pubis dysfunction

Symphysis pubis dysfunction presents as discomfort or pain in the pelvic area, which may radiate to the upper thighs or perineum. The pain usually occurs initially with walking. It occurs in 3% of pregnant women and it may be severe enough to reduce mobility. On examination, the woman often reports severe pain on pressure over the symphysis pubis or on compression of the pelvis.

Treatment is supportive with crutches, pelvic support braces and analgesia.

Carpal tunnel syndrome

Oedema of the wrist causes compression of the median nerve and pain, numbness or paraesthesia, with possible impaired motor function or muscle wasting. Wrist splints are generally helpful and corticosteroid injections can be considered for intractable symptoms in pregnancy, with limited evidence of benefit. The symptoms usually resolve spontaneously postnatally.

Concentration

Some women report impaired concentration in pregnancy. The cause of this is not clear and it may relate to poor sleep and general tiredness.

Oedema

Dependent oedema occurs in 80% of pregnant women and may be mild or severe and uncomfortable. Simple measures such as elevation of the legs are helpful. Blood pressure and urinalysis are necessary to exclude pre-eclampsia as the cause of the oedema. Oedema often worsens immediately after delivery, with a natural diuresis then occurring within the next 72 hours.

Varicose veins

Varicose veins are common, due to impaired venous return and progesterone effect on valve function and the vein wall. They may be asymptomatic or cause aching or itching. Vulval varicosities are rare, but cause a throbbing discomfort and may bleed excessively at delivery. Varicose veins are generally treated by ligation and stripping, injection or avulsion after the completion of the family. During and after pregnancy, compression stockings may be helpful to relieve symptoms.

Vaginal discharge

Physiological discharge increases in pregnancy. It is white and smooth. Any itching, offensive odour, blood or change in the nature of the discharge should be investigated with swabs for *Candida*, bacterial vaginosis and sexually transmitted infection. It should be noted that endocervical swabs are not recommended in pregnancy.

Candida occurs more commonly in pregnancy due to the state of relative glucose intolerance. Antifungal pessaries and creams are safe in pregnancy, but oral treatments are not recommended. Creams or pessaries are most effective when given for a 1-week course. There is no evidence that the fetus or neonate is affected by maternal vaginal candidiasis.

HYPERTENSIVE DISORDERS OF PREGNANCY

Definitions

Hypertension in pregnancy

There are various definitions in use for the diagnosis of hypertension in pregnancy. Generally accepted criteria for diagnosis are:

- Diastolic blood pressure >90 mmHg on two occasions or >110 mmHg on a single occasion

Or

- An increase in diastolic blood pressure of 20 mmHg or more above booking

Or

- An increase in systolic blood pressure of 30 mmHg or more above booking.
- **Chronic hypertension:** This is hypertension diagnosed before pregnancy or in the first trimester.
- **Essential hypertension:** Essential hypertension is diagnosed before pregnancy or in the first trimester, not secondary to another cause.
- **Pregnancy-induced hypertension:** Pregnancy-induced hypertension is diagnosed after 20 weeks' gestation (most hypertension developing between 12 and 20 weeks will be chronic hypertension, but it may occasionally be due to severe early-onset pre-eclampsia).

Pre-eclampsia

Pre-eclampsia is a pregnancy-specific multisystem disorder with various clinical manifestations. The classic definition involved hypertension, proteinuria and oedema, but now the diagnosis may be made on a combination of possible maternal and fetal features. These include intrauterine growth restriction (IUGR), haematological abnormalities, biochemical abnormalities and clinical symptoms or signs.

Incidence

Ten per cent of women develop high blood pressure or mild pre-eclampsia in pregnancy. Of these, 10% develop severe pre-eclampsia. Women with pre-existing hypertension have double the risk of developing superimposed pre-eclampsia. The incidence of pregnancy-induced hypertension and pre-eclampsia is higher in first pregnancies than in multiparous women.

Aetiology

Chronic hypertension may be due to endocrine disease (e.g. Cushing's and Conn's syndromes) or secondary to renal disease or cardiac disease.

The aetiology of pre-eclampsia is still poorly understood. There is, however, a known genetic component (20% risk of daughters of affected women developing pre-eclampsia).

Prediction

Risk factors for the development of pre-eclampsia are shown in Table 12.1.

Uterine artery Doppler studies at 20–24 weeks can be used to identify women at high risk of pre-eclampsia, in whom a high resistance and 'notched' waveform is seen. This is still a research tool and has not been widely accepted in the general antenatal population

Pathophysiology

The features of pre-eclampsia originate from abnormal placental trophoblast invasion in early pregnancy. The usual low resistance and high flow do not develop in the spiral arteries of the uterus and diffuse maternal vascular endothelial dysfunction results, with vasoconstriction and platelet aggregation.

Table 12.1. Risk factors for pre-eclampsia

Primiparity
Multiple pregnancy
Obesity
Extremes of age
New partner
In vitro fertilization – egg donation
Diabetes
Chronic hypertension
Antiphospholipid syndrome
Renal disease
Molar pregnancy

Clinical features

Hypertension may be the first sign of pre-eclampsia and women with chronic hypertension are likely to develop pre-eclampsia. Differentiation between the two conditions may be difficult clinically.

History

Women with hypertension may report headache or visual disturbance. Pre-eclampsia may also present with epigastric pain, nausea, vomiting and oedema. Oedema is commonly in the face and fingers and women may notice that they cannot take off their rings. Alternatively, their partner may have noticed facial swelling.

Examination

Blood pressure should be measured at 45°, with an appropriate cuff. If the circumference of the arm is more than 80% of the cuff size, a larger cuff should be used to avoid underestimation of the blood pressure.

The first Korotkoff sound (phase I), that is, the beginning of the audible beats, signifies the systolic blood pressure. The diastolic reading is taken at the level of the fifth Korotkoff sound (phase V), that is, when silence occurs. In a minority of women silence does not occur, in which case the phase IV sound (muffling) is used.

The legs, hands and face should be examined for oedema and the reflexes checked for hyperreflexia and clonus (signs of cerebral irritability). Palpation of the abdomen may reveal epigastric tenderness. The symphyseal–fundal height should be measured and a subjective assessment made of liquor volume.

Investigations

The following investigations should be performed for all women with pregnancy-induced hypertension or other features suggestive of possible pre-eclampsia. In established pre-eclampsia the tests should be repeated twice weekly, or more often if the clinical condition deteriorates.

Urinalysis

If +1 proteinuria or more is present, then an MSU sample should be sent to exclude UTI as the cause and a 24-hour urine collection commenced. More than 0.3 gram of protein per 24 hours is diagnostic of pre-eclampsia in the absence of other causes such as infection or chronic renal disease.

Full blood count

Platelets usually fall in pre-eclampsia. Low haemoglobin and very low platelets are suspicious signs as they may signify the syndrome of haemolysis, elevated liver enzymes and low platelet count (HELLP).

Urea and electrolytes

Urea and creatinine may rise in pre-eclampsia. The normal range for creatinine is lower in pregnancy, so creatinine concentration greater than about 80 µmol/l is significant.

Uric acid (urate)

Uric acid is a non-specific marker of pre-eclampsia. As a general rule in singleton pregnancies, the value of the uric acid should be less than the number of weeks' gestation, divided by 100. For example, at 36 weeks, uric acid is normally <0.36. Serial values are more beneficial as a marker of disease progression rather than one level in isolation.

Liver function tests

Alanine and aspartate transaminases rise in pre-eclampsia. If gamma glutamyl transaminase and bilirubin are raised, then HELLP syndrome is the likely diagnosis.

Albumin

Albumin falls in pre-eclampsia as the kidneys lose protein.

Coagulation tests

International normalized ratio (INR) and activated partial thromboplastin time (APTT) only become prolonged in severe pre-eclampsia and do not need to be checked in all cases of suspected pre-eclampsia.

Ultrasound scan

Fetal well-being should be confirmed with growth, liquor volume and umbilical artery Doppler studies.

Management

Delivery of the baby is the only cure for pre-eclampsia. Otherwise, management of hypertensive disorders involves monitoring the disease process, monitoring fetal well-being, treatment of hypertension, diagnosis and treatment of complications, and appropriate timing of the delivery of the baby.

Monitoring of the disease

Confirmed pre-eclampsia should be managed as an inpatient because of the risk of fulminating disease or placental abruption. Bed rest itself does not alter the outcome of pre-eclampsia. Blood pressure should be checked every 4 hours, urinalysis daily and 24-hour protein clearance weekly. Outpatient management may be suitable for well-controlled hypertension without other features, or in mild pre-eclampsia, with frequent assessment as a day case.

All pre-eclamptic women should have twice-weekly FBC, urea and electrolytes and liver function checked, with more frequent tests if clinically indicated.

Monitoring fetal well-being

In established pre-eclampsia, fetal ultrasound scan should be repeated regularly (between twice weekly and every 2 weeks depending on the findings). Fetal movements should be monitored by the mother but the value of regular cardiotocography (CTG) is debated if scans and fetal movements are normal.

Treatment of hypertension

Hypertension should be treated in both pregnancy-induced hypertensive and pre-eclamptic women, to prevent stroke. However, although antihypertensives correct blood pressure, they do not alter the underlying disease process and the risk of worsening pre-eclampsia or eclampsia remains.

The systolic and diastolic values at which antihypertensive treatment should be commenced are debated, but treatment should always be started if the diastolic reading is repeatedly greater than 100 mmHg or systolic greater than 160 mmHg.

Antenatal management

- First-line management: Methyldopa (centrally acting) should be given at a dosage of 250 mg three times a day, increased up to 1 gram three times daily. Methyldopa has the best safety record in pregnancy, but side effects include drowsiness, depression and reduced fetal movements, though these often settle after a few days. Women on other hypertensives prior to pregnancy are usually converted to methyldopa once pregnancy has been confirmed.

- **Second-line management:** Labetalol (beta-blocker and arterial vasodilator) can be given at a dosage of 100 mg twice daily, increased up to 600 mg four times a day. Rare side effects include fetal growth restriction and neonatal bradycardia. Asthma is a contraindication for use.

   Slow-release nifedipine (calcium antagonist) can also be given at a dosage of 10 mg twice daily, increased to 40 mg twice daily. Care is needed, as nifedipine particularly may cause a sudden drop in blood pressure, compromising the uteroplacental circulation.

   Other beta-blockers are rarely used in pregnancy due to concerns over growth restriction and fetal bradycardia.

   Angiotensin-converting enzyme (ACE) inhibitors are contraindicated in pregnancy and diuretics are only used with extreme caution.

Intrapartum management

Severe hypertension developing in labour or in women presenting with severe sudden pre-eclampsia for whom delivery is indicated may need intravenous treatment with hydralazine or labetalol. A bolus of colloid (250–500 ml) should be given prior to this, to avoid a sudden drop in blood pressure as a result of the depleted intravascular volume in pre-eclampsia. The fetus is monitored with continuous CTG, in case of sudden hypotension causing acute uteroplacental insufficiency.

The mean arterial blood pressure (MAP) should be maintained below 125. MAP is calculated as follows:

MAP = diastolic blood pressure + (systolic – diastolic)/3

Hydralazine

Intravenous hydralazine is given at a dosage of 2.5–5 mg over 5 minutes and the dose repeated after 15 minutes if the MAP has not fallen below 125 mmHg. If more than three doses are required, then an infusion is commenced.

Labetalol

Intravenous labetalol is given at a dosage of 20 mg/hour, doubled every 30 minutes, according to the blood pressure, up to a maximum of 160 mg/hour.

Nifedipine

Slow-release nifedipine may be given intrapartum at a dosage of 10 mg, but careful monitoring of the fetus is important, in case of a sudden severe drop in blood pressure.

Postnatal management of hypertension

Methyldopa should be discontinued after delivery, because of the possible side effect of depression. If hypertension has been moderate or severe, then labetalol or atenolol should be commenced. Calcium antagonists and ACE inhibitors are also safe, even with breastfeeding. If hypertension antenatally or during labour was mild, then consideration should be given to stopping all hypertensives and monitoring the blood pressure for 72 hours.

Discharge should only be arranged when the blood pressure is consistently less than 140/90 mmHg. The woman should have regular blood pressure measurement by the community midwife and see her general practitioner in 6 weeks to consider discontinuing treatment.

Timing of delivery

Delivery is the only 'cure' for pre-eclampsia and is indicated by uncontrolled hypertension, severe clinical, biochemical or haematological abnormalities or fetal concerns. Ideally, delivery should be delayed until after 37 weeks to allow for fetal lung maturity, but each case must be assessed individually and delivery may be much earlier. Usual indications for delivery are:

- Severe hypertension not responsive to double or triple therapy
- Symptomatic pre-eclampsia (e.g. epigastric pain, visual symptoms)
- Severe fetal growth restriction with abnormal umbilical artery Doppler flow
- Decreasing platelets
- Increasing creatinine, alanine transaminase (ALT) and aspartate transaminase (AST)
- HELLP syndrome
- Eclampsia
- Placental abruption.

Women with likely premature delivery under 36 weeks should be given a course of steroids to aid fetal lung maturity.

Severe hypertension or pre-eclampsia in labour

A protocol should be adhered to for all women with significant disease. Important considerations in the management are summarized in Figure 12.1 and include:

1. Monitoring:
   a. Blood pressure should be monitored every 15–60 minutes, depending on the severity of disease.
   b. Fluid balance should be calculated with urinary catheter and measurement of all intravenous and oral intake. Low urine output is common and should be managed expectantly unless urine output is less than 80 ml over 4 hours, in which case a central venous pressure line should be inserted to guide fluid management.
   c. Full blood count, coagulation, renal and liver function, and urate should be checked every 6 hours in severe disease.
   d. Clinical signs of hyperreflexia and clonus should be checked.
   e. Fetal well-being should be monitored with continuous CTG.
2. Fluid restriction: fluid input should be restricted to 85 ml/hour, due to the intravascular depletion associated with pre-eclampsia.
3. Treatment of blood pressure: the treatment of blood pressure is outlined above.
4. Delivery: induction of labour or caesarean section (depending on obstetric factors) should be initiated when the maternal haemodynamic condition is stable. Epidural is encouraged as it reduces blood pressure, though platelets should be checked first as there is a risk of epidural haematoma if the platelet count is less than $80 \times 10^9/l$. Syntocinon alone is used for the third stage as ergometrine may precipitate a further rise in blood pressure.
5. Magnesium sulphate: magnesium sulphate decreases the likelihood of an eclamptic fit and should be considered in severe pre-eclampsia. A loading dose of 2 grams (diluted in 20 ml normal saline) over 5 minutes is followed by an infusion of 1–2 g/hour. Side effects are hot flushing sensation, loss of tendon reflexes, respiratory depression and cardiac arrest. The urine output, reflexes, blood pressure, respiratory rate and

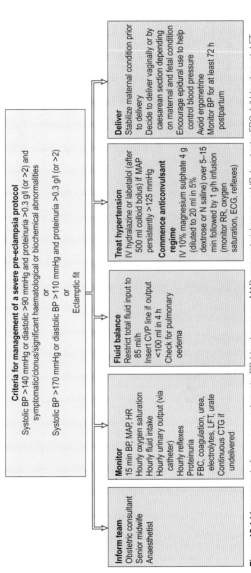

Criteria for management of a severe pre-eclampsia protocol

Systolic BP >140 mmHg or diastolic >90 mmHg and proteinuria >0.3 g/l (or >2) and symptomatic/clonus/significant haematological or biochemical abnormalities

or

Systolic BP >170 mmHg or diastolic BP >110 mmHg and proteinuria >0.3 g/l (or >2)

or

Eclamptic fit

Inform team
Obstetric consultant
Senior midwife
Anaesthetist

Monitor
15 min BP, MAP, HR
Hourly oxygen saturation
Hourly fluid intake
Hourly urinary output (via catheter)
Hourly reflexes
Proteinuria
FBC, coagulation, urea, electrolytes, LFT, urate
Continuous CTG if undelivered

Fluid balance
Restrict total fluid input to 85 ml/h
Insert CVP line if output <100 ml in 4 h
Check for pulmonary oedema

Treat hypertension
IV hydralazine or labetalol (after 500 ml colloid bolus) if MAP persistently >125 mmHg
Commence anticonvulsant regime
IV 10% magnesium sulphate 4 g (diluted to 20 ml in 5% dextrose or N saline) over 5–15 min followed by 1 g/h infusion (monitor RR, oxygen saturation, ECG, reflexes)

Deliver
Stabilize maternal condition prior to delivery
Decide to deliver vaginally or by caesarean section depending on maternal and fetal condition
Encourage epidural use to help control blood pressure
Avoid ergometrine
Monitor BP for at least 72 h postpartum

Figure 12.1 Management of severe pre-eclampsia. BP, blood pressure; MAP, mean arterial pressure; HR, heart rate; FBC, full blood count; LFT, liver function tests; CTG, cardiotocograph; CVP, central venous pressure; IV, intravenous; RR, respiration rate; ECG, electrocardiogram.

oxygen saturation should be monitored closely, with cardiac monitoring. Magnesium sulphate also lowers blood pressure and care is needed with other hypertensives to prevent a sudden drop in blood pressure, which may cause fetal distress. Magnesium sulphate should be continued for 24 hours postpartum.

Postnatal management

Haematology and biochemistry results need to be monitored postnatally until normal. The fluid balance chart should be continued until diuresis occurs, which may be up to 72 hours following delivery. Management of postnatal hypertension is outlined above.

Prognosis

In most women, blood pressure returns to normal within 6 weeks. However, a few women remain hypertensive in the long term.

Pregnancy-induced hypertension commonly recurs in subsequent pregnancies. The risk of recurrence of pre-eclampsia in otherwise healthy women is 10%. However, it is more likely in women with hypertension or other medical risk factors. The severity of the disease tends to reduce with each subsequent pregnancy.

Prevention of pre-eclampsia

Aspirin reduces the incidence of pre-eclampsia in women with a history of previous severe pre-eclampsia necessitating delivery prior to 34 weeks' gestation. Calcium helps to prevent pre-eclampsia in women with inadequate dietary supply or who are vitamin D-deficient, and vitamin C and E supplements may provide benefit in women at high risk of pre-eclampsia.

Complications of pre-eclampsia

Fetal growth restriction

Pre-eclampsia is associated with uteroplacental insufficiency, which causes impaired fetal growth and reduced liquor volume. Eventually fetal blood flow is impaired and reduced, absent and eventually reversed end-diastolic flow occurs in the umbilical artery. Ultrasound monitoring, fetal movement recording and CTG are used to determine timing of delivery. In rare severe cases, fetal growth restriction occurs early, before the fetus has reached a viable weight and intrauterine death occurs.

Haemolysis, elevated liver enzymes and low platelets

HELLP syndrome presents with epigastric pain, nausea, vomiting and right upper quadrant tenderness. Onset is often acute, with patients not necessarily having presented with pre-eclampsia symptoms or signs prior to the development of HELLP.

Management is as for severe pre-eclampsia, with monitoring of haematological and biochemical abnormalities, treatment of hypertension and urgent delivery. Renal failure, liver haematoma or rupture and abruption are all complications.

Pulmonary oedema

Pulmonary oedema occurs as a result of the hypoalbuminaemia and vascular endothelial dysfunction.

Disseminated intravascular coagulation

Disseminated intravascular coagulation (DIC) results from a generalized stimulation of coagulation activity and subsequent depletion in clotting factors and platelets. The clinical presentation is, therefore, of uncontrolled bleeding and the diagnosis is confirmed by increased fibrin degradation products, decreased fibrinogen and platelets, and prolonged TT, APTT and INR. It is most likely after HELLP syndrome or abruption.

Cerebral haemorrhage

Stroke is the result of uncontrolled hypertension and is one of the main causes of death in pre-eclamptic women.

Abruption

Placental abruption is a common complication of pre-eclampsia and cannot be predicted by the clinical severity of the disease. It usually presents with sudden severe abdominal pain, with or without vaginal bleeding. Initial management involves stabilization of the haemodynamic status of the mother by blood transfusion and correction of any coagulopathy. Urgent delivery by caesarean section should be arranged if the fetus is alive, otherwise by induction of labour if intrauterine death has already occurred.

Eclampsia

Eclampsia affects 0.05% of pregnancies (about 1 in 2000). Forty per cent of episodes occur postpartum and eclampsia commonly occurs in women not previously diagnosed with pre-eclampsia. Seizures are generalized and generally self-limiting within 2–3 minutes.

Specific management is covered in Chapter 17.

ANTEPARTUM HAEMORRHAGE

Antepartum haemorrhage (APH) is a significant cause of maternal mortality. Any bleeding should be taken seriously, with a high index of suspicion for placenta praevia or placental abruption. It should always be remembered that hypovolaemic shock can occur rapidly, despite minimal vaginal loss, where a concealed placental abruption has occurred.

Definition

APH is vaginal bleeding occurring once the fetus has reached viability. This is usually defined as more than 24 weeks' gestation.

Incidence

Two to 10% of women report an APH at some stage in pregnancy.

Aetiology

Bleeding may occur from a maternal, fetal or placental site (Table 12.2). Both placental and maternal sites involve loss of maternal blood, whereas in the case of vasa praevia fetal blood is lost.

In many cases the cause of bleeding cannot be identified. It is likely that these small bleeds represent minor abruptions and such women should be carefully monitored as they are at risk of further abruption. If repeated bleeds occur, then fetal growth restriction also may develop. The term 'marginal bleed' is sometimes used to refer to such bleeding.

Non-vaginal causes of bleeding also may occur. Bleeding from haemorrhoids is common in pregnancy, for example, and haematuria may also be mistaken for vaginal blood loss.

Table 12.2. Causes of antepartum haemorrhage

Maternal	Placental	Fetal
Vaginal infection (e.g. *Candida*, *Trichomonas*)	Placenta praevia	Vasa praevia
Cervical ectropion	Placental abruption	
Cervical infection		
Cervical malignancy		
Bloody show		
Uterine rupture		

History

Important features in the history of a woman presenting with suspected APH are:

- The colour, consistency and amount of blood loss. Placenta praevia blood loss tends to be fresh and red whereas blood associated with abruption may be darker. It is useful to attempt to quantify loss by comparing it to the patient's usual menstrual loss or number of pads used.
- The duration of bleeding and any possible triggering factors, such as sexual intercourse.
- Any previous bleeding episodes.
- Abdominal pain – a feeling of uterine 'tightening' or pelvic discomfort are all important features suggesting a possible placental abruption. Bleeding associated with a placenta praevia tends to be painless (80%), unless labour has started.
- Labour – a small amount of blood loss is common with a 'show' and more significant bleeding may occur during precipitate labour. A mucus-like blood loss, rupture of membranes or contractions may, therefore, suggest APH due to labour.
- Fetal movements – bleeding with loss of fetal movements is suspicious of abruption.
- The date and result of the most recent cervical smear and details of any previous sexually transmitted or other genital infections, such as *candida*.
- Placental site, as described in the most recent ultrasound report.
- The Rhesus status of the woman.

Examination

Owing to the increased circulating volume of pregnancy, a woman may lose more than 500 ml of blood before her vital signs are affected. Even where little blood loss is noted vaginally, in cases of placental abruption there may be significant 'concealed' loss within the uterus, resulting in hypovolaemia. Therefore, other indicators of shock should be noted carefully, such as pallor, peripheral vasoconstriction ('cold and clammy'), dizziness or a general feeling of being unwell. Overt signs such as tachycardia, hypotension and a reduced level of consciousness imply life-threatening haemorrhage has occurred.

Abruption is also often associated with pre-eclampsia and hypertension or proteinuria may, therefore, be present.

Abdominal palpation may elicit tenderness, uterine tightenings (spontaneous uterine contractions that may not be felt by the mother) or uterine irritability (uterine contractions in response to palpation of the uterus). Placental abruption may be associated with either high-frequency contractions or with a hard uterus ('woody') due to tonic contraction.

A high fetal head or malpresentation, with a soft uterus, is suggestive of placenta praevia (obstructing the descent of the presenting part into the pelvis).

Speculum examination in women with APH should never be performed until placenta praevia has been excluded by ultrasound scan. Where the placenta is known to be low, speculum examination should usually be avoided as it will be unlikely to add further information and may risk precipitating further bleeding.

If the placenta is not low, speculum examination should be performed and the colour, consistency and volume of any blood or of liquor or other discharge seen should be noted. Bleeding may be seen to come from the endocervical canal or it may be possible to identify the cervix or vagina as the source of bleeding.

The cervix itself should be inspected for dilatation, ectropion, polyps and signs of infection or possible malignant lesions.

Any lesions of the vulva or anus should also be noted if they might be possible alternative sources of blood loss.

Investigations

Women reporting APH should all have the following investigations:

- FBC
- Blood group
- Serum save
- Crossmatch – depending on the estimated blood loss
- Coagulation studies – if a coagulopathy is suspected or blood loss is massive. Low fibrinogen, increased D-dimer, prolonged prothrombin time and APTT, and low platelets suggest DIC, usually following abruption
- Kleihauer test – particularly important for Rhesus-negative women to determine the dose of anti-D required. The result of a Kleihauer test is not immediate enough, however, to help in initial management.
- CTG – commenced as early as possible to ascertain fetal well-being and monitor uterine activity.
- Ultrasound – requested urgently if the placental site is unclear, to look for placenta praevia. Retroplacental blood clot may be visualized on scan after an abruption, but it is often not, and if a large clot is present then the likelihood is that fetal demise has already occurred and the woman is extremely unwell. Abruption is, therefore, essentially a clinical diagnosis, though ultrasound may help to exclude placenta praevia as an alternative cause of the bleeding.
- High vaginal swab – to exclude *Candida* and full vaginal and cervical swabs should be sent if an infective cause of bleeding is suspected.

Management

All women reporting APH should be admitted to hospital. Further management is determined by the severity of the maternal haemorrhage, the fetal condition and gestational age. (The only exception to routine admission may be where bleeding is confirmed to be due to a non-obstetric cause and has ceased, such as a single postcoital bleed associated with an obvious visible cervical ectropion, in a woman with a high placenta and no other risks for placental abruption.)

If estimated blood loss is slight, intravenous access should be obtained and the woman may be observed and discharged 24 hours after the last fresh (red) loss. Rhesus-negative women should be given anti-D.

Women with significant bleeds should have two large-bore intravenous cannulae inserted and aggressive fluid resuscitation and transfusion if necessary. Other blood products, such as platelets and fresh frozen plasma, should be given where indicated. Intensive monitoring and continuous CTG are indicated. Specific management thereafter depends on the cause of the loss.

Both placenta praevia and placental abruption are associated with a high risk of postpartum haemorrhage, and active management of the puerperium with Syntocinon and ergometrine at delivery followed by a Syntocinon infusion is necessary. The management of postpartum haemorrhage is covered in Chapter 17.

Placenta praevia

Placenta praevia is implantation of the placenta in the lower segment of the uterus, occurring in 1% of pregnancies at term. It is classified according to how close the leading edge of the placenta is to the internal cervical os, as shown in Figure 17.1. Bleeding may occur due to the thinning of the cervix and lower segment of the uterus in late pregnancy or in early labour. If bleeding occurs in a woman with placenta praevia, then admission until delivery is normally necessary. The mother should have regular haemoglobin measurement and anaemia treated with iron or blood transfusion, if necessary. Four units of crossmatched blood should be readily available in case of sudden haemorrhage.

The fetus is generally not affected by bleeding from a placenta praevia unless maternal hypovolaemia occurs, but regular CTG is advisable. Delivery by caesarean section at term should be performed unless bleeding is uncontrolled or labour occurs, in which case premature delivery may be necessary. Delivery should be carried out by a senior obstetrician and senior anaesthetist with blood for transfusion immediately available.

In some cases a low placenta may still move from the internal os near term and the clinical finding of a deeply engaged head and accurate determination of the placental site by transvaginal ultrasound may confirm this.

In rare cases where the placenta is suspected to be clear of the os, but some doubt exists, examination under epidural in theatre may confirm the presence of the head and no palpable placenta in the pelvis, and artificial rupture of membranes (ARM) can be carried out. Theatre staff should be ready for immediate caesarean section if bleeding occurs.

Placental abruption (abruptio placentae)

Placental abruption is the premature separation of a part of the placenta from the uterus, before delivery of the baby. Bleeding occurs from the placental bed and a haematoma develops beneath the placenta, shearing it from the uterus. Bleeding may be seen vaginally, or it may be concealed entirely inside the uterus. As a result, the amount of visible or external bleeding may not necessarily correlate with maternal blood loss or grade of abruption.

The fetus is at risk from an abruption due to hypoxia from the sudden reduction in placental gas exchange function. Intrauterine death is, therefore, common.

Abruption is the commonest identifiable cause of intrauterine death and occurs in approximately 0.5–1% of pregnancies, but the reported incidence depends on the diagnostic criteria used. Risk factors for abruption are hypertension, pre-eclampsia, previous abruption (10% recurrence), multiple pregnancy, diabetes, tobacco or cocaine use and trauma (e.g. road traffic accident or assault to the abdomen).

A mild abruption may present with a small amount of pain or bleeding that settles spontaneously with no apparent effect on fetal well-being. Major abruption usually presents with constant lower abdominal or back pain and varying amounts of vaginal blood loss, depending on the degree to which the blood is concealed behind the placenta. A small amount of visible blood loss associated with a woman who is in pain, pale, clammy, tachycardic or hypotensive is classical, and should be treated as a life-threatening emergency.

Management of a suspected abruption includes admission to the labour ward, insertion of two large-bore intravenous cannulae, crossmatching of 4 units of blood and correction of any coagulopathy. If the estimated blood loss is significant, the urinary output should be monitored via a urinary catheter and a central venous line may be inserted to manage fluid balance more accurately. The management of obstetric haemorrhage is covered further in Chapter 17. Continuous CTG is commenced if the fetus is still alive.

Minor abruption, with minimal estimated blood loss and no apparent maternal or fetal compromise, may be managed expectantly, with observation and regular monitoring of CTG, fetal movements and fetal growth by ultrasound.

More commonly, delivery will be indicated. Vaginal delivery in the context of abruption is associated with less blood loss and less risk to the mother than caesarean section. Commonly, abruption stimulates spontaneous labour and delivery is quick. Alternatively, prostaglandin or ARM may be used to induce the labour.

Emergency caesarean section may be indicated if the CTG suggests fetal compromise or the blood loss is uncontrollable. At caesarean, couvelaire uterus may be found, where blood has penetrated the myometrium, resulting in a purplish bruised appearance and inability for the uterus to contract.

In view of the risk of clotting deficiency, epidural or spinal anaesthesia is avoided until clotting studies have been performed.

If pre-eclampsia is present, this must be treated simultaneously.

The dose of anti-D for a Rhesus-negative woman who has had an abruption depends on the size of the fetomaternal haemorrhage. This may be determined by the Kleihauer test.

● **Complications of placental abruption:** The most serious complication to the mother is DIC, with low clotting factors, fibrinogen, platelets and renal failure. This should be anticipated and treated aggressively. Postpartum haemorrhage is also common due to the coagulopathy and to the often poorly contractile uterus.

Table 12.3 summarizes the differences between the typical presentations of placenta praevia and placental abruption, but it should be remembered that many presentations are atypical and that the two conditions may coexist.

Uterine rupture

Uterine rupture is an extremely rare cause of vaginal bleeding, usually occurring in labour in a woman with a history of previous uterine surgery such as caesarean section or myomectomy. The predominant feature

Table 12.3. Summary of the differences between placenta praevia and placental abruption

Placenta praevia	Placental abruption
Painless (80%)	Constant pain or high-frequency contractions
Clinical condition correlates with visible blood loss	Clinical condition suggests more blood loss than visualized
Soft, non-tender uterus	Tender, tense uterus
High presenting part or malpresentation	May be unable to palpate fetal parts due to tense uterus
Ultrasound diagnosis	Clinical diagnosis
Low risk to the fetus	Fetus at high risk
Caesarean section essential	Caesarean only if bleeding uncontrolled or fetal compromise

is pain (though this may be partially masked by an epidural), with sudden cessation of contractions and CTG abnormalities. Haematuria and maternal tachycardia are other clinical signs. Immediate laparotomy should be performed to deliver the baby and control maternal haemorrhage.

Vasa praevia

'Vasa praevia' is the term used where umbilical cord vessels abnormally traverse the membranes and overlie the internal cervical os. It occurs in 1 in 3000 pregnancies and is associated with either a velamentous insertion of the cord into the placenta (from the side) or with a succenturiate (satellite or accessory) lobe of placenta (Fig. 12.2). The vessels are at risk of tearing when they are stretched during cervical dilatation in labour or during ARM.

Fetal mortality from vasa praevia is 35–95% as the fetus exsanguinates unless the condition is quickly diagnosed, immediate caesarean section performed and the neonate transfused.

There is no significant risk to the mother from vasa praevia.

Diagnostic tests for fetal blood from the vagina are available, but are not in general clinical practice and the diagnosis must, therefore, be suspected clinically by a combination of relatively small-volume blood loss (less than 500 ml), no maternal pain and an abnormal CTG, often following ARM.

Occasionally, vasa praevia may be diagnosed antenatally on ultrasound with demonstration of Doppler flow in the vessels beneath the fetus, in which case elective caesarean section should be arranged.

Cervical lesions

Various cervical lesions may account for APH. The commonest is a cervical ectropion, which may be diagnosed on speculum and managed conservatively. Cauterization is avoided in pregnancy and the ectropion often resolves in the puerperium. Infections such as *Trichomonas* may cause cervicitis and bleeding and should be treated accordingly (see Chapter 9).

Cervical polyps are occasionally found in pregnancy and again should be managed expectantly, with consideration of avulsion only if bleeding is uncontrolled, and with great care paid to haemostasis due to the increased cervical vascularity in pregnancy.

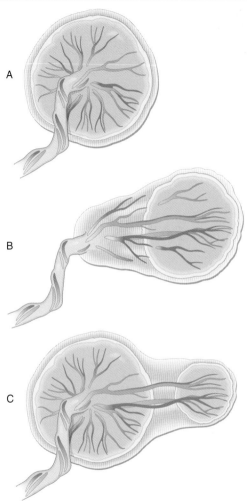

Figure 12.2 Illustration of a normal placenta showing (A) central cord insertion, (B) a velamentous (lateral) cord insertion and (C) a placenta with a succenturiate lobe. B and C both predispose to vasa praevia.

Cervical cancer is rarely suspected or diagnosed in pregnancy. Biopsy should generally be reserved for cases where suspicion is very high, because of the risk of heavy bleeding. If cervical cancer is confirmed, then multidisciplinary team management should determine the optimum time and method of delivery.

INFECTIONS OF PREGNANCY

Urinary tract infection

Asymptomatic bacteriuria, UTI and pyelonephritis are discussed under the maternal systemic disorders section, below.

Chickenpox

Chickenpox, caused by the varicella-zoster virus, occurs in up to 3 in 1000 pregnancies. Spread is by respiratory droplets and incubation is 14–21 days.

Maternal infection

The typical itchy vesicles appear over the trunk, face and limbs following prodromal malaise and fever. The vesicles burst, with scabs developing over the next few days. Sufferers are infectious from 48 hours before the rash until the last vesicles have crusted over. Ninety per cent of women are immune because of childhood infection and this can be confirmed on the booking blood sample.

If infected, pregnant women develop more severe complications, with a 10% risk of pneumonia and up to 1% mortality. Other complications are encephalitis, hepatitis and DIC.

Diagnosis is usually clinical, but if there is doubt an increase in immunoglobulin (IgG) G can be detected over a 2-week period. Non-immune women with definite exposure to chickenpox may benefit from varicella-zoster immunoglobulin given in the first 10 days after exposure to prevent clinical disease.

Women should be seen in the community, avoiding exposure to other pregnant women, with admission for antiviral and supportive therapy if pneumonia is suspected.

Risk to the fetus

Two per cent of fetuses develop fetal varicella syndrome (dermatomal skin scarring, eye defects, limb hypoplasia and neurological defects) if infection occurs prior to 16 weeks. Occasional cases have occurred up to 20 weeks. Urgent assessment in the fetal medicine department should be arranged for ultrasound signs of fetal infection.

Chickenpox developing from 48 hours before to 5 days after delivery carries a >25% chance of varicella infection of the newborn, though it may rarely occur with infection any time in the last 4 weeks of pregnancy. The condition is fatal in 30%. If delivery cannot be delayed until more than 5 days after the onset of the rash, then the baby should be treated with intravenous aciclovir and varicella-zoster immunoglobulin.

Rubella

Rubella (German measles) is very rare, as a result of widespread immunization of teenagers and now infants. Spread is by person-to-person contact and the incubation period is 14–21 days.

Maternal infection

The typical clinical features involve a flu-like illness with associated fine macular rash, particularly over the trunk, though 20–50% of infections are asymptomatic. The disease lasts a few days and no specific maternal management is required. Women are infectious from 1 week before to 1 week after the onset of the rash.

Susceptibility varies with vaccination trends and immigration, but approximately 2% of nulliparous women are susceptible. Infection is thought to occur in 2/1000 of these susceptible (absent or low-level antibody) women.

Diagnosis is confirmed by serological testing for antibody levels.

Risk to the fetus

If the mother develops rubella in the first trimester, there is an 80% chance of the baby becoming infected, compared with a 25% chance at the end of the second trimester. One hundred per cent of infected babies have the characteristic rubella abnormalities, which include cataracts, congenital heart disease, sensorineural deafness, learning difficulties, hepatosplenomegaly and microcephaly. The teratogenic effects are worst for infections at earlier gestations.

Many parents opt for termination of pregnancy if infection occurs, especially in the first trimester.

Adult rubella and congenital rubella syndrome are notifiable diseases.

Toxoplasmosis

Toxoplasma gondii is a parasite and maternal infection may occur by ingestion of cysts or oocytes from raw, cured or poorly cooked meat, unwashed fruit and vegetables, unpasteurized goats' milk, or food contaminated by soil or cat faeces. Lambing is also a risk factor for infection.

Maternal infection

The incidence of toxoplasmosis in pregnancy is about 2 in 1000, in whom about 40% fetal infection occurs (15% in the first trimester and 70% in the third trimester). Thirty per cent of pregnant women in the UK are immune due to previous infection. Incubation is 5–23 days. Clinical features are uncommon, but can include flu-type symptoms and lymphadenopathy, with a rare prolonged glandular fever-type illness.

Diagnosis by serial serological testing in the mother is complex, as seroconversion does not indicate timing of infection, which may have been up to 12 months earlier.

Treatment of the mother with spiramycin may reduce the chance of fetal infection.

Risk to the fetus

Transplacental *Toxoplasma* infection may occur 4–8 weeks after maternal infection and the effects include miscarriage, stillbirth, growth restriction, hydrocephalus, deafness and blindness. Although fetal infection is more likely at later gestations (15, 25 and 65% affected in first, second and third trimesters, respectively), the effect on the fetus is worse at earlier gestations. Amniocentesis or cordocentesis may be used to diagnose fetal infection. Babies infected in the third trimester often appear normal at birth, with blindness developing during childhood.

Prevention of toxoplasmosis involves washing all raw food and vegetables before cooking, ensuring meat is thoroughly cooked before eating, not reheating cooked meals, wearing gloves to garden and avoiding cat litter.

Salmonella

Salmonella is a Gram-negative bacterium that may be contracted by ingestion of contaminated raw or partially cooked eggs, raw meat and chicken. The incubation period is 12–72 hours and gastroenteritis occurs with severe vomiting, dehydration and fever. The infection appears to be more common in pregnancy, but there is no direct effect on the fetus.

Cytomegalovirus

Cytomegalovirus (CMV) infection affects at least 3 in 1000 of all live births. CMV is the leading infective cause of congenital neurological impairment in children.

The virus is transmitted through urine, saliva and other body products.

Maternal infection

CMV has a 3–12-week incubation period and the illness is usually asymptomatic (90%) but may cause a flu-like illness. The virus often continues to be shed after infection. One per cent of women develop either primary or reactivated CMV infection in pregnancy.

Maternal immunity can be detected by IgG in the blood and primary infection can be confirmed with IgM.

Risk to the fetus

If primary infection occurs in pregnancy, then there is a 10–15% risk to the fetus. If the mother is already seropositive and continuing to shed following infection then the risk to the fetus is only 1%.

Fetal infection may occur at any gestation and be diagnosed by identification of the virus on amniocentesis or cordocentesis samples. From 10 to 20% of infected babies may have evidence of infection at birth (e.g. hydrops, IUGR, microcephaly, hydrocephalus, hepatosplenomegaly and thrombocytopenia), but 80–90% develop symptoms later such as mental handicap, visual impairment, progressive hearing loss or psychomotor retardation.

Screening for CMV in pregnancy is not indicated as there is no treatment, women with positive serology can have reactivated disease and it is not possible to predict which babies will be affected and how seriously.

Listeria

Listeria monocytogenes, a Gram-positive coccus, is found in unpasteurized dairy products such as soft cheese and in pâté, soil and animal faeces. Lambing is a specific risk factor for infection.

The incidence in pregnancy is higher than in the normal population (12 versus 0.7 cases per 100 000 women) and the illness may be more severe with fever, headache, malaise, backache, abdominal pain, pharyngitis or conjunctivitis. Severe respiratory complications and meningitis can also occur. The incubation period varies from 3 to 70 days. Diagnosis is made by identification of the organism in blood culture, placenta or neonatal swab culture and treatment is with high-dose penicillin.

Infection in the fetus can result in miscarriage, stillbirth, preterm delivery and neonatal listeriosis (50% mortality).

Parvovirus

Parvovirus B19 infection occurs in fewer than 1% of adults in the UK each year. Transmission occurs via respiratory droplets and the incubation period is about 18 days. Infectiousness occurs from 5 to 15 days after infection. Outbreaks of infection tend to occur in schools (erythema infectiosum, fifth disease, slapped-cheek syndrome). Infection in adults may involve fever, malaise and arthralgia, and is asymptomatic in 20%. Immunity is confirmed by detection of IgG in the serum. Diagnosis of infection is made on serial IgM measurements, 3 weeks apart.

Risk to the fetus

Transplacental infection occurs in up to 30% of pregnant women with parvovirus, with fetal death in 9%. The risk is highest when infection occurs in the second trimester. The commonest finding is non-immune hydrops (from a chronic haemolytic anaemia and myocarditis).

Fetal monitoring with ultrasound to detect hydrops should be performed for up to 12 weeks after maternal infection. Intrauterine transfusion or early delivery may be needed.

Pregnant women exposed to parvovirus, such as staff at a school during an epidemic, should probably be advised to take time off for a few weeks, especially in the second trimester.

HIV

Human immunodeficiency virus (HIV) infection is discussed in Chapter 9. The incidence of HIV infection is up to 1 in 200 pregnant women in some areas of the UK. Transmission occurs by sexual contact (heterosexual or homosexual), infected blood products (e.g. needle sharing) or vertical transmission.

In pregnancy, many women are now diagnosed as a result of inclusion of HIV testing in routine antenatal screening programmes. Some women, however, will be known to be infected prior to pregnancy.

Pregnancy does not have an adverse effect on HIV disease or viral load. The pregnancy may be affected, however, by HIV infection if the mother is very underweight or has another HIV-associated illness.

Infection of the baby may occur by transplacental spread, by infected blood at delivery (through mucous membranes at the mouth, nose, conjunctivae) or through breast milk.

Neonatal HIV infection is more likely in the presence of:
- High viral load
- Low CD4 lymphocyte count
- Preterm labour
- Prolonged rupture of membranes (>4 hours)
- Invasive procedures (fetal blood sampling, instrumental delivery, episiotomy, fetal scalp electrode).

Antenatal management

Management in pregnancy involves careful counselling and support. Antiviral therapy is usually started and viral load, CD4 count and platelet count are monitored.

Confidentiality is paramount, as many women will not have told their partners, friends and family about the infection.

Management around delivery

The following four strategies combined reduce the chance of neonatal HIV infection from about 25% to less than 5%:
1. Caesarean section delivery, ideally maintaining intact membranes until the head has been delivered and avoiding contact between the baby and the maternal blood
2. Delivery within 4 hours if spontaneous rupture of membranes occurs, ideally by caesarean section
3. Zidovudine prophylaxis intravenously to the mother for 4 hours prior to delivery and to the baby orally for 6 weeks postnatally
4. Avoidance of breastfeeding.

The baby can be tested for infection by polymerase chain reaction techniques in the neonatal period, or by antibody test, once the maternal antibody has cleared from the baby's circulation (about 3 months).

Group B streptococcus

Group B streptococcus (GBS) (*Streptococcus agalactiae*) colonization of the vagina occurs in approximately 25% of women at some stage in their pregnancy. It is generally asymptomatic in the mother, but is responsible for early-onset neonatal sepsis in 1 in 2000 births. This disease is fatal in 6% of term infants and 18% of preterm infants, accounting for approximately 1 in 65 of all neonatal deaths.

The risk factors for neonatal group B streptococcus infection are shown in Table 12.4. Women with any of these risk factors should be treated with intrapartum high-dose intravenous penicillin (3 grams stat followed by 1.5 grams every 4 hours) or 8-hourly clindamycin 900 mg (if penicillin-allergic).

Neonatal death has not been shown to be reduced by either routine screening in pregnancy with lower vaginal and rectal swabs or antenatal treatment of colonized women.

Bacterial vaginosis

Bacterial vaginosis is present in 12% of pregnant women in the UK and is asymptomatic in at least 50%. Symptoms are a fishy odour and creamy discharge. Presence of bacterial vaginosis in early pregnancy almost doubles the risk of preterm delivery and late miscarriage. However, although antibiotics such as metronidazole eradicate the infection effectively, they do not reduce the perinatal risks. Therefore, treatment is only indicated for symptomatic women.

Sexually transmitted infections and *Candida* in pregnancy are discussed further in Chapter 9.

MATERNAL SYSTEMIC DISORDERS

Maternal systemic disorders are a common reason for referral of women to the obstetrician-led antenatal clinic. Multidisciplinary team management is important for many such conditions, in particular diabetes, thyroid disease, cardiac, renal and haematological disorders.

Haematological disorders

Anaemia

Anaemia is the commonest medical disorder of pregnancy.

- **Aetiology:** Anaemia may be pregnancy-related, in which case iron deficiency is the commonest cause. Other causes are folate deficiency (e.g. poor diet, thalassaemia), chronic disease (e.g. renal disease), pre-existing anaemia (e.g. from menorrhagia, recent pregnancy) and haemoglobinopathy.

Table 12.4. The maternal risk factors for neonatal group B streptococcus (GBS) infection and indications for antibiotic prophylaxis

Previous GBS-affected baby
Colonization with GBS at any time in the current pregnancy
GBS bacteriuria in the current pregnancy
Preterm labour (<37 weeks)
Prolonged rupture of membranes
Pyrexia in labour

- **Pathophysiology:** In pregnancy, iron absorption increases in response to the increased maternal, placental and fetal demands. The subsequent increase in red cell mass is about 20%. However, plasma volume expands by 40–50% and the haemoglobin concentration therefore falls. This is exacerbated if dietary iron is insufficient. The normal lower limit for haemoglobin concentration at booking is 11 g/dl and drops to 10.5 g/dl after 28 weeks.

- **Clinical features:** Breathlessness, palpitations, tiredness and dizziness are the common symptoms of anaemia, though some women are asymptomatic.

  Pallor, pale nails and pale conjunctivae as well as tachycardia may be noted on examination.

  Low haemoglobin is associated with low birth weight and preterm labour as well as increased risk of transfusion for the mother if haemorrhage occurs at delivery.

- **Investigations:** Routine FBC at booking and at 28 weeks may detect anaemia. Otherwise, FBC should be checked when anaemia is suspected clinically.

  Iron deficiency is diagnosed with a low mean cell volume (MCV), mean cell haemoglobin and mean cell haemoglobin concentration. It may be confirmed if necessary by a low serum iron, total iron-binding capacity and low serum ferritin.

  Folate deficiency presents with a raised mean cell volume and may be confirmed by a low serum and red cell folate concentration.

  Pregnant women may have a mixed folate and iron-deficiency picture.

  Haemoglobinopathy screen should be checked if not done at booking.

- **Treatment:** Many types of iron therapy are available and the ferrous compounds are better absorbed than the ferric compounds. The usual preparation is ferrous sulphate 200 mg three times a day. Liquid preparations, such as ferrous fumarate, may be prescribed for women intolerant of tablets. Side effects of oral iron include nausea, epigastric discomfort and constipation.

  A course of injectable iron is used rarely for women intolerant of any oral preparations, but does not increase iron concentration any faster than oral preparations. The expected increase in haemoglobin from oral or injectable iron is 2 grams in 3–4 weeks.

  Transfusion is rarely used for anaemia in pregnancy.

  Folic acid 5 mg daily should be given for folate deficiency, women taking anticonvulsants and those with haemoglobinopathies. There is no evidence for routine iron or folic acid supplementation for prophylaxis in pregnancy except for women with multiple pregnancies.

Venous thromboembolism

- **Incidence:** VTE remains the leading cause of maternal death. The incidence in non-pregnant women is 5 in 100 000 per year and in pregnant women is 60 in 100 000 per year. VTE occurs at all gestations and is also common postnatally.

- **Risk factors:** Risk factors for VTE are shown in Table 12.5.

- **Pathophysiology:** Virchow's triad describes the pathophysiological factors contributing to thrombus development:

1. Increased blood viscosity (e.g. increased clotting factors in pregnancy, thrombocythaemia, antiphospholipid syndrome (APS))
2. Decreased blood flow (impeded circulation in lower limbs from gravid uterus, reduced mobility)

Table 12.5. Risk factors for venous thromboembolism in pregnancy and the puerperium

Pre-existing risk factors:
Previous venous thromboembolism
Age over 35 years
Smoking
Obesity (body mass index >30 kg/m^2 at booking)
Parity >4
Gross varicose veins
Paraplegia
Congenital thrombophilia
   antithrombin deficiency
   protein C deficiency
   protein S deficiency
   factor V Leiden
Acquired thrombophilia
   antiphospholipid syndrome
Thrombocythaemia
Polycythaemia
Sickle-cell disease
Inflammatory disorders, e.g. inflammatory bowel disease
Other systemic disease, e.g. nephrotic syndrome, cardiac disease

Risk factors developing during pregnancy:
Hyperemesis
Dehydration
Ovarian hyperstimulation syndrome
Long-haul travel
Severe infection, e.g. pyelonephritis
Immobility (>4 days' bed rest antenatally, intrapartum or postnatally)
Surgical procedure in pregnancy or puerperium, e.g. caesarean section, evacuation of retained products of conception, postpartum sterilization
Pre-eclampsia
Excessive blood loss
Prolonged labour
Midcavity instrumental delivery
Immobility after delivery

3. Endothelial damage (e.g. pelvic vein trauma at delivery).

- **Clinical features:** Clinical features are often non-specific and have a poor predictive value in the diagnosis of VTE. VTE may present at any stage in the pregnancy or puerperium.

- **History:** Women may report a swollen and red calf, usually on the left. Symptoms may be vague or acute and severe. Deep-vein thrombosis (DVT) in the ileal or femoral vein may present with a swollen leg, which may be painful and white in extreme cases (phlegmasia alba dolens).

    Pulmonary embolism characteristically causes breathlessness, pleuritic chest pain, cough or haemoptysis. Collapse or sudden death may occur with a large pulmonary embolism. Many small emboli are asymptomatic.

- **Examination:** General examination may reveal a low-grade pyrexia, or tachycardia. A swollen tender red calf or leg may be seen. Iliofemoral DVT is common in pregnancy and may be asymptomatic or show the classical white swollen leg.

A large pulmonary embolism may be associated with hypotension, tachypnoea, raised jugular venous pressure, loud second heart sound or right ventricular heave. Reduced air entry and a pleural rub may also be heard.

Investigations

- **D-dimer:** D-dimer, a fibrin degradation product, is usually raised in pregnancy, but the test has good negative predictive value if normal.
- **Imaging:** Duplex ultrasonography can be used to image the veins, looking for DVT in the lower limb. However, thrombosis below the knee or above the inguinal ligament may be difficult to visualize and ultrasound imaging for DVT is operator-dependent. Further imaging, for example with magnetic resonance venography, should be requested if there is clinical suspicion. Contrast venography, with abdominal shielding, is occasionally still used to diagnose DVT where ultrasound is not available.

  Investigations where pulmonary embolism is suspected include electrocardiogram (sinus tachycardia, right axis deviation, right bundle branch block or occasionally the classical 'S1Q3T3'), oxygen saturation, arterial blood gas and chest X-ray (hypoperfusion, infarction, effusion). Spiral computed tomography (CT) or V/Q scan causes minimal radiation to the fetus and may be needed to confirm the diagnosis. Angiography and magnetic resonance imaging are alternative investigations.

- **Treatment:** Women should be treated on clinical suspicion of VTE until the diagnosis has been confirmed or refuted. The commonest treatment now is a therapeutic dose of low-molecular-weight heparin (LMWH), calculated according to maternal weight. This is safe and effective in pregnancy, but intravenous unfractionated heparin is an alternative, with monitoring of APTT.

Graduated elastic compression stockings should be worn and the affected leg should be elevated initially, with mobilization after a few days.

Pulmonary embolism should be managed in liaison with the physicians. Treatment is essentially anticoagulation and supportive measures such as oxygen and monitoring of pulse, blood pressure, oxygen saturation and electrocardiogram.

Thrombolysis or embolectomy should be considered where a thrombus is large or the symptoms do not improve on anticoagulation treatment.

Long-term heparin in pregnancy is associated with some loss of bone mass, but osteoporosis is rare. The platelet count may also drop and women should have platelets checked at 3 days and after 1 month of treatment.

The rest of the pregnancy should be managed in liaison with a haematologist, with a decision made whether to commence warfarin or continue heparin. The woman should remain on prophylactic anticoagulation until at least 6 weeks after delivery. Warfarin, though usually avoided in pregnancy, is safe in the puerperium and with breastfeeding.

VTE prophylaxis during pregnancy, delivery and postpartum

Women with a past history of VTE should be offered LMWH prophylaxis for 6 weeks postpartum. If there is a persisting risk factor, history of recurrent VTE, a positive family history or the thrombophilia screen is positive, then LMWH should also be prescribed antenatally.

All women should be encouraged to mobilize early after delivery and keep well hydrated.

Additional measures such as thromboembolic stockings and prophylactic heparin should be considered after delivery for women with other significant risk factors. Generally, all women with three or more existing risk factors from Table 12.5 should be given LMWH prophylaxis for 3–5 days following delivery. However, age over 35 and obesity are particularly significant risks and prophylaxis should be considered for women who have both risk factors.

Postpartum LMWH should be given as early as possible, though if an epidural or spinal anaesthetic has been given, it should be delayed until 4 hours after the spinal or insertion or removal of the epidural catheter.

Pneumatic boots are another method of reducing VTE risk associated with caesarean section.

Thrombophilia

Women with a history of previous DVT or a strong family history of VTE should be tested for thrombophilia. If positive, depending on the history, consideration should be given to prophylactic heparin either throughout pregnancy or at high-risk times, such as admission to hospital and postpartum. Care should be taken in interpreting results in pregnancy as, for example, protein S concentration falls in pregnancy.

- Inherited thrombophilias:
- Protein C and S deficiency
- Antithrombin III deficiency
- Activated protein C resistance.
- Acquired thrombophilias:
- APS
- Lupus.

Antiphospholipid syndrome

APS, an acquired thrombophilia, causes arterial and venous thrombosis, recurrent miscarriage, and increased risk of pre-eclampsia, fetal growth restriction and placental abruption. Antiphospholipid antibodies (anticardiolipin antibody and lupus anticoagulant) are found in 2% of the general population, but it is unclear what proportion of these women has the syndrome. APS may be primary, or secondary to lupus disease.

Diagnosis of APS depends on:
- Three first-trimester miscarriages

or
- One midtrimester miscarriage

or
- Severe pre-eclampsia, IUGR or abruption, necessitating delivery prior to 37 weeks

and the presence (on two samples, at least 6 weeks apart) of:
- Anticardiolipin antibodies

or
- Lupus anticoagulant.
- **Treatment:** The management of APS depends on the presenting features. Recurrent miscarriage and pregnancy complications such as pre-eclampsia, growth restriction and abruption are discussed in the relevant sections of this book.

In subsequent pregnancies, women with APS and a previous poor obstetric history should be given aspirin prophylaxis (75 mg daily), which is safe and effective at prolonging pregnancy and improving outcome. Daily prophylactic dose LMWH is also indicated in some women to reduce the chance of VTE, IUGR and pre-eclampsia.

All women with APS should have regular blood pressure and fetal growth monitoring.

Women with APS are also at increased risk of thrombosis during and after pregnancy and a low threshold for thromboprophylaxis should be used for prolonged immobilization or operative delivery. Women with previous thrombosis need thromboprophylaxis throughout pregnancy and the puerperium.

A multidisciplinary approach with a haematologist is recommended.

Thrombocytopenia

Up to 10% of women have a low platelet count in pregnancy, most commonly due to gestational thrombocytopenia. The causes of thrombocytopenia are shown in Table 12.6.

- **Clinical features:** Most women are found to have an incidental low platelet count on routine antenatal testing, or in labour. Haemorrhage or easy bruising occurs when the platelet count is less than $50 \times 10^9/l$.
- **Investigation:** Initial low platelet results should be repeated to exclude clumping of platelets as a cause. It may also be necessary to confirm the low platelet count on a blood film or citrate sample. Where the cause of thrombocytopenia is not immediately clear, platelet autoantibodies and HIV status should be checked and blood pressure and urinalysis should be checked to exclude pre-eclampsia.

Gestational thrombocytopenia

The platelet count decreases for most women throughout pregnancy. If it falls below $150 \times 10^9/l$, it is termed gestational thrombocytopenia.

Once diagnosed, the platelet count should be monitored every 2 weeks antenatally and checked again in labour. It is rare for the platelets to fall below $100 \times 10^9/l$. Epidural is usually contraindicated with platelets less than $80 \times 10^9/l$.

There is no effect on the baby.

Autoimmune idiopathic thrombocytopenia

Autoimmune idiopathic thrombocytopenia is caused by antiplatelet antibodies resulting in maternal platelet destruction and thrombocytopenia. It is not pregnancy-specific, but is commonly diagnosed in and exacerbated by pregnancy. Diagnosis is normally made after exclusion of other causes, or by detection of the antibodies.

Management involves monitoring the platelet count every 2 weeks. High-dose corticosteroids are indicated when the platelet count falls below

Table 12.6. Causes of thrombocytopenia in pregnancy

Common causes:
Gestational thrombocytopenia
Autoimmune idiopathic thrombocytopenia

Uncommon causes:
Thrombotic thrombocytopenic purpura
Antiphospholipid syndrome
Human immunodeficiency virus (HIV)-related
Drug-induced thrombocytopenia
Pre-eclampsia
Haemolysis, elevated liver enzymes and low platelets (HELLP) syndrome
Disseminated intravascular coagulation

$50 \times 10^9/l$. Intravenous gammaglobulin can also be used to increase the platelet count rapidly, with an effect lasting for about 2 weeks.

Platelet transfusions are only rarely given for autoimmune thrombocytopenia, for example if regional anaesthesia or operative delivery is anticipated, with no opportunity for IgG or steroids to work.

The fetus is affected in approximately 5% of cases of idiopathic thrombocytopenia where IgG antibodies cross the placenta and cause neonatal thrombocytopenia. The clinical features include neonatal or antepartum cerebral haemorrhage. Babies of affected mothers should therefore have regular platelet checks for the first 4 days.

Alloimmune thrombocytopenia

Alloimmune thrombocytopenia is fetal thrombocytopenia as a result of maternal antiplatelet antibodies directed against fetal platelets. The maternal platelet count is normal.

It occurs in 1 in 2000 births and is usually diagnosed after a first affected pregnancy where the baby shows signs of thrombocytopenia and haemorrhage. Thereafter, all pregnancies are at high risk and are managed in a fetal medicine department with serial fetal platelet counts (by cordocentesis) and intrauterine platelet transfusions as necessary. Instrumental deliveries, fetal blood sampling and fetal scalp electrode are all contraindicated at delivery and caesarean section is usually considered to minimize risk of haemorrhage for the baby.

ENDOCRINE DISORDERS

Insulin-dependent diabetes mellitus

Incidence

Insulin-dependent diabetes mellitus (IDDM) affects 4 in 1000 pregnant women.

Pregnancy is a state of insulin resistance and glucose intolerance, due to the anti-insulin effects of human placental lactogen, cortisol and glucagon from the placenta. Insulin requirements in diabetic women, therefore, increase in pregnancy.

The fetus in a diabetic pregnancy becomes hyperinsulinaemic because of the high maternal glucose level. Neonatal hypoglycaemia then occurs due to the sudden loss of maternal glucose.

Diabetes is associated with a variety of pregnancy complications, as listed below, but good glycaemic control prior to and during pregnancy reduces these, and all diabetics must be strongly advised to see their diabetic team before becoming pregnant, for comprehensive counselling. For the fetus, the risks of maternal IDDM are miscarriage, fetal abnormality (5–25%), IUGR, macrosomia, polyhydramnios, sudden intrauterine death and increased neonatal mortality. Specific congenital abnormalities include cardiac disease, neural tube defects and sacral agenesis. For the mother, pre-eclampsia (especially if she has pre-existing hypertension or nephropathy), infections and difficult glycaemic control with more hypoglycaemic attacks, as well as increasing insulin requirements, are likely. Diabetic nephropathy and renal disease are likely to worsen, and should preferably be screened for and treated before pregnancy.

The risks of maternal IDDM are summarized in Table 12.7.

Clinical features

Insulin requirements usually double during pregnancy and the increase is most marked as the fetus grows most rapidly between 28 and 32 weeks. Hypoglycaemic episodes are also more common in pregnancy and women

Table 12.7. The risks of diabetic pregnancies

Maternal risks:
Difficult glycaemic control and increased hypoglycaemic episodes
Occasional diabetic ketoacidosis (e.g. with undercurrent infection, hyperemesis, steroids or tocolytics)
Worsening of diabetic retinopathy
Worsening of diabetic nephropathy
Increased risk of pre-eclampsia (especially with pre-existing hypertension or nephropathy)
Increased risk of infections

Fetal risks:
Congenital abnormality (5–25%)
Miscarriage
Infection (*Candida*, urinary tract infection, wound infection, endometritis)
Preterm delivery (20% risk)
Intrauterine growth restriction
Macrosomia
Polyhydramnios
Shoulder dystocia
Cord prolapse
Sudden intrauterine death

Neonatal risks:
Neonatal hypoglycaemia
Neonatal respiratory distress syndrome
Jaundice
Polycythaemia
Increased neonatal mortality

may be less aware of these in pregnancy. However, hypoglycaemia does not affect the fetus as long as the mother is given appropriate oral carbohydrate or glucagon.

Management

- **Prepregnancy:** Prepregnancy consultation, as discussed in Chapter 11, is crucial for diabetic women as tight glycaemic control prior to pregnancy reduces the risk of fetal congenital abnormality and miscarriage. The number of insulin injections may be increased and a different combination of short- and longer-acting insulins used to maintain the blood glucose between 4 and 5 mmol/l. Non-insulin-dependent diabetics are usually converted from oral hypoglycaemic agents to insulin.
- **Antenatal:** Hyperemesis may need to be managed as an inpatient if the blood glucose control is poor. Antenatal management should then be based in a specialist antenatal diabetic clinic, with visits generally every 2 weeks initially and then weekly from 34 weeks.

A detailed scan is needed in the first and second trimesters in view of the increased risk of fetal abnormality and a fetal cardiac scan should also be arranged for the second trimester. Serum screening for Down's syndrome must be used with an appropriate reference group as oestriol, βhCG and alpha-fetoprotein are all reduced in diabetic women. Nuchal translucency may, therefore, be a better screening test in diabetic women.

Retinopathy should be screened for, as there is a risk of significant deterioration in pregnancy. Nephropathy should be assessed initially with urinalysis testing for proteinuria and if present, with a 24-hour urinary protein collection and urea, creatinine and electrolytes.

Blood glucose measurements should be recorded before and after meals at least 3 days per week, with confirmation of these results with glycosylated haemoglobin and random glucose measurements in clinic. Ideal measurements are <5.0 mmol/l fasting and <7.5 mmol/l postprandial. To achieve this, most women have their insulin regime altered in pregnancy, if not prepregnancy, to improve glucose control, for example with a greater number of injections (three short-acting and one intermediate/long-acting at night). Polyhydramnios occurs when maternal glucose levels are high.

Ultrasound scans are arranged every 4 weeks until 32 weeks, then every 2 weeks to detect macrosomia and polyhydramnios.

If steroids are to be administered, or tocolytics such as ritodrine are indicated, insulin-dependent women need admission for intravenous sliding-scale insulin.

- **In labour:** The risk of sudden stillbirth in babies of diabetic mothers is the indication for early delivery. Most diabetic women should be delivered between 38 and 39 weeks.

The mode of delivery depends on previous obstetric history, estimated fetal weight and predicted risk of shoulder dystocia. Overall, 60% of diabetic women are delivered by caesarean section.

A sliding scale of insulin and dextrose should be commenced in labour (or prior to caesarean section) as stress and abnormal eating patterns in labour disrupt the mother's normal insulin regime and also because good predelivery maternal glucose control reduces the chance and severity of neonatal hypoglycaemia.

The baby should have early regular blood glucose measurement and feeds.

- **Postnatal:** The insulin dose is reduced immediately after delivery to the prepregnancy regime, as insulin requirements return to the nonpregnant state within 24 hours. In practice this is done when the woman first eats after delivery. In breastfeeding women, the insulin should be reduced to only two-thirds of the normal dose due to the risk of hypoglycaemia.

All diabetics should have a 6-week endocrinological review.

Gestational diabetes mellitus

Gestational diabetes mellitus (GDM) is defined as carbohydrate intolerance of varying severity with onset or first recognition during pregnancy. The incidence is up to 3%, depending on the diagnostic criteria used and the ethnic background of the relevant pregnant women.

Diagnostic criteria

The diagnostic criteria for GDM are controversial, but the most commonly quoted are World Health Organization definitions after a 75-gram glucose load:

- 2-hour venous glucose <7.8 mmol/l: normal
- 2-hour venous glucose 7.8–11 mmol/l: impaired glucose tolerance
- 2-hour venous glucose >11 mmol/l: gestational diabetes.

These definitions may overdiagnose GDM because they are based on a non-pregnant population and there is a slowed glucose response in normal pregnancy.

A glucose tolerance test for all pregnant women is not recommended, but screening tests are recommended for women with higher risk factors:

- Glycosuria
- Macrosomia or polyhydramnios
- Previous GDM
- Previous macrosomic baby or stillbirth
- Body mass index greater than 30
- Strong family history of diabetes.

As glucose tolerance worsens with advancing gestation, GDM is best diagnosed in the second trimester.

Clinical features

Most women have no clinical features, but are diagnosed after screening because of high-risk features as outlined above. GDM is associated with an increased risk of macrosomia and pre-eclampsia, but not of congenital abnormality.

Management

Initial management is dietary, involving reduced fat and carbohydrate and increased fibre in the diet. Postprandial blood glucose level above 7.5 mmol/l or fasting blood glucose above 5.5 mmol/l is an indication for insulin in addition to diet restriction.

Ultrasound scan at 28, 32 and 36 weeks will detect macrosomia and polyhydramnios, which help the decision regarding timing and mode of delivery.

Screening for pre-eclampsia involves vigilant monitoring of blood pressure and urinalysis. Postnatally, women should have a glucose tolerance test at 6 weeks to exclude diabetes.

Prognosis

Women with a history of GDM have a 50% risk of developing type 2 diabetes within 15 years and should be advised about weight control, exercise and regular blood glucose monitoring. Most women have GDM again in subsequent pregnancies.

Thyroid disease

Hyperthyroidism

The rate of hyperthyroidism in pregnancy is 0.2%. Ninety-five per cent of these have Graves' disease, in which increased circulating T_4 levels are the result of TSH receptor-stimulating antibodies. Hyperthyroidism may improve or deteriorate in pregnancy.

Clinical features

Most women are on antithyroid treatment prior to pregnancy, but features of thyrotoxicosis may be present if the dose is insufficient or the diagnosis has not been made. Symptoms include heat intolerance, weight loss, insomnia, palpitations and vomiting and clinical signs are tachycardia, lid lag and exopthalmos.

Investigations

In untreated hyperthyroidism TSH is low and free T_3 and T_4 are raised.

Management

Carbimazole and propylthiouracil both cross the placenta, but are relatively safe in normal doses, though carbimazole can occasionally cause scalp defects in the fetus. Beta-blockers may rarely be needed for severe thyrotoxicosis in pregnancy. Radioiodine is contraindicated in pregnancy and for 4 months before conception because of the risk of fetal thyroid destruction.

Women with hyperthyroidism should be seen monthly and T_4 maintained at the high end of the normal range.

Effect on the baby

Babies may be hypothyroid due to transplacental passage of antithyroid drugs, or hyperthyroid due to passage of thyroid-stimulating antibodies, especially if the thyrotoxicosis is of recent onset or poorly controlled. At delivery the baby should have thyroid function checked from cord blood and repeated in the neonatal period if breastfed. The baby should also be monitored for clinical signs of abnormal thyroid function for the first few weeks until maternal antibodies and medications have cleared.

Breastfeeding is safe on antithyroid medication in normal doses, but breastfed babies may need more prolonged monitoring for abnormal thyroid function.

Hypothyroidism

One per cent of pregnant women are hypothyroid. The most common causes are Hashimoto's thyroiditis and atrophic thyroiditis, both microsomal autoantibody disorders.

Clinical features, if T_4 dose is insufficient or if the condition has not yet been diagnosed, are weight gain, lethargy, depression and constipation. Bradycardia or goitre may be present on examination.

- **Investigations:** T_4 is low and TSH is raised. Thyroid autoantibody measurement has limited value, as antibodies may be present in many women who do not have clinical features of disease.
- **Management:** Women on long-term T_4 replacement should have T_4 and TSH checked at booking and again in the second and third trimesters if normal. Some women require an increased dose of T_4 in pregnancy but this may represent previous underreplacement prior to pregnancy.
- **Effect on the fetus:** If untreated, hypothyroidism is associated with miscarriage and later fetal loss and low birth weight. If treated, then fetal complications are rare.

  T_4 crosses the placenta in very small amounts and, therefore, neonatal thyrotoxicosis is rare. The autoantibodies also cross, but neonatal hypothyroidism is also extremely uncommon.

ASTHMA

Asthma occurs in 3% of pregnant women. The disease may deteriorate, improve or be unaffected by pregnancy. The pregnancy is not affected by asthma unless the mother is chronically severely hypoxic, which is rare.

Clinical features

Women present with wheeze, cough or shortness of breath, which may be exacerbated by pollen or upper respiratory tract infection.

Examination should look firstly at general appearance. Inability to complete sentences, tachycardia and increased respiratory rate are signs of severe disease. Wheeze should be audible on chest examination and peak expiratory flow rate should be compared with the patient's normal best value.

Management of asthma is as for the non-pregnant woman and advice should be given about good compliance with medication. Reassurance that there is no evidence of harm to the fetus from bronchodilators or inhaled corticosteroids is important.

RENAL DISORDERS

Asymptomatic bacteriuria

Asymptomatic bacteriuria is persistent bacterial colonization of the urinary tract (>100 000 organisms/ml) without symptoms. The prevalence is up to 15% in pregnant women.

The risk to the mother is pyelonephritis (1.8–28%) and to the fetus is preterm birth (2.1–12.8%).

Diagnosis of asymptomatic bacteriuria is made on MSU culture. Screening by reagent strip for nitrites, leukocytes, blood or protein detects only 50% of cases. Treatment with a 7-day course of antibiotics effectively eliminates bacteriuria and reduces pyelonephritis (relative risk 0.24) and preterm birth (odds ratio 0.6).

Urinary tract infection

The incidence of UTI in pregnancy is 1%. The factors predisposing to infection are the short female urethra, smooth-muscle relaxation effect of progesterone, the pressure of the gravid uterus and constipation.

Clinical features

Symptoms may include suprapubic pain, fever, increased frequency, dysuria or offensive urine. Examination may reveal pyrexia, tachycardia and suprapubic tenderness.

Diagnosis

Diagnosis is confirmed on MSU culture and the usual causative organism is *Escherichia coli*.

Treatment

Treatment is indicated for both confirmed infections and for suspected infection on the basis of symptoms and more than a trace of proteinuria or positive nitrite or leukocytes on reagent strip testing. Amoxicillin and cefadroxil are effective and safe in pregnancy. Treatment should be continued for 7 days, with repeat MSU culture after completion of treatment. Women should be advised to increase oral fluids, wipe from front to back and pass urine after sexual intercourse to help prevent recurrences. Recurrent UTI indicates further investigation with renal tract ultrasound and prophylactic antibiotics should be considered, such as 500 mg cefadroxil each night.

Pyelonephritis

Pyelonephritis is common in pregnancy due to the dilatation of the ureters and collecting system increasing the chance of ascending infection. Severe UTI with bacteraemia is associated with a risk of miscarriage and preterm labour and should be treated aggressively.

Clinical features

Most women with pyelonephritis are very unwell with fever, rigors, anorexia, nausea and vomiting. Abdominal pain, loin pain, dysuria and frequency may be absent. Women may report uterine tightenings.

General examination findings include pyrexia, signs of dehydration, tachycardia and hypotension. Abdominal tenderness and uterine tenderness or irritability may be present on palpation. Renal angle tenderness is usually present.

Investigations

MSU culture, blood culture, FBC, renal function and C-reactive protein should all be checked. Renal ultrasound is necessary to exclude obstruction (e.g. renal calculi) and congenital abnormality (e.g. duplex ureter).

Treatment

Intravenous antibiotics (amoxicillin, ampicillin or cephalosporins first-line) should be given until the woman has been apyrexial for at least 24 hours and is tolerating oral fluids and antibiotics. Severe pyelonephritis may need additional gentamicin, which must be carefully monitored to avoid potentially ototoxic levels for mother and fetus. Other management includes hydration, analgesia, paracetamol and rest.

Most women improve within 48 hours, though loin pain and malaise often continue for 2–3 weeks. A total antibiotic course of 2 weeks is necessary, with a repeat urine culture after completion.

Chronic renal disease

Chronic renal disease (e.g. glomerulonephritis, reflux nephropathy and diabetic nephropathy) carries risks to the pregnancy and the mother.

Risks to the mother are:
- Deterioration in renal function
- Proteinuria
- Pre-eclampsia.

Risks to the fetus are:
- Miscarriage
- Intrauterine death
- Preterm delivery
- IUGR.

Poor renal function, hypertension or proteinuria predicts poor outcome. If the prepregnancy creatinine is greater than 250 µmol/l, then 50% of women will experience long-term worsening of renal function and at least 50% of babies will have IUGR and prematurity.

Management

The mother should have a baseline 24-hour urinary protein measurement, urea and creatinine measurement and creatinine clearance. These are repeated at intervals depending on the severity of disease. Close monitoring and treatment of hypertension are also essential. Pre-eclampsia may be difficult to diagnose in a woman with pre-existing proteinuria. Fetal growth should be monitored with regular ultrasound scans.

Renal transplant patients generally do well in pregnancy if renal function is normal prior to conception and immunosuppressive therapy is continued throughout pregnancy. Women should be advised to avoid pregnancy for 2 years after transplant as good renal function at that stage predicts very good long-term survival.

Pre-eclampsia, IUGR and premature delivery are all more likely, especially if proteinuria or hypertension is present before pregnancy. MSU should be sent at each visit, as infection is more likely and also likely to damage the transplanted kidney. Renal and liver function as well as haemoglobin should all be closely monitored.

Delivery should be managed according to obstetric indications, with the addition of antibiotic and steroid cover.

NEUROLOGICAL DISORDERS

Epilepsy

The incidence of epilepsy in pregnancy is about 1 in 200. Seizures may be generalized tonic–clonic, petit mal (absences) or temporal lobe (complex partial seizures).

Risks to the mother
Some women have an increased number of fits in pregnancy and this may relate to poor compliance with medication, increased plasma volume, hyperemesis or excessive tiredness.

Risks to the pregnancy
Anticonvulsant medication is associated with an increased risk of fetal abnormality (7%), which increases further with the number of different medications taken. Typical abnormalities are neural tube defects, orofacial clefts, cardiac defects and dysmorphic features. The fetus does not seem to be adversely affected by maternal fits, if self-limiting, despite transient fetal bradycardias being observed.

Management
Preconceptual management is outlined in Chapter 11. Folic acid 5 mg daily should be continued throughout the pregnancy because of the risk of folate deficiency in the mother as well as neural tube defects in the fetus.

First-trimester ultrasound identifies gross neural tube defects such as anencephaly. Cardiac scan should be arranged at about 18 weeks and detailed anomaly scan at 20 weeks.

Anticonvulsant medication should be continued throughout the pregnancy and emphasis placed on the risk to the mother of persistent fits. If the incidence of fits increases, the dose of anticonvulsants should be increased after checking drug levels.

Vitamin K 10 mg should be taken daily from 36 weeks as anticonvulsants inhibit production of clotting factors and, therefore, increase the risk of cerebral haemorrhage in the fetus and neonate. Babies should also be given intramuscular vitamin K at birth.

Breastfeeding is not contraindicated with anticonvulsants.

Pregnant epileptics should try to shower rather than bath and if bathing have another person present, due to the risk of drowning if a fit occurs.

Differential diagnosis of fits in pregnancy
A fit in the second half of pregnancy should always be assumed to be eclampsia until proven otherwise, by assessment of blood pressure, urinalysis, FBC, urea, creatinine, urate and liver function. Other causes of fits are hypoglycaemia, cerebrovascular accident, pseudoepilepsy and drug or alcohol withdrawal.

Once eclampsia has been excluded, a first fit in pregnancy should warrant further investigation with blood glucose, calcium and magnesium, CT or magnetic resonance imaging and electroencephalogram.

Multiple sclerosis

Multiple sclerosis is a demyelinating condition of the brain and spinal cord affecting about 1 in 1000–2000 people in the UK. It results in a variable clinical picture of neurological symptoms and signs including optic neuritis and limb weakness.

The condition commonly improves in pregnancy, though the relapse rate is 40% after delivery. No specific management is indicated antenatally or for delivery.

Bell's palsy

Bell's palsy is a unilateral lower motor neurone disorder affecting the seventh cranial nerve (facial nerve). It causes facial muscle weakness, loss of taste on the anterior two-thirds of the tongue and pain around the ear.

It occurs in 4 in 10 000 pregnancies and is 10 times more common in pregnancy than in the non-pregnant population.

The diagnosis is made on examination. Ramsay Hunt syndrome (varicella-zoster infection of the facial nerve) is the important differential diagnosis, which can be excluded by checking that no vesicles are present in the ear.

Recovery from Bell's palsy over a few weeks is spontaneous in 90%, but prednisolone 40 mg/day for 1 week speeds recovery if given within the first day of symptoms.

LIVER DISORDERS

Obstetric cholestasis

Obstetric cholestasis is a pregnancy-specific condition of impaired bile acid excretion. It has little serious effect on the mother, but is associated with poor fetal outcome. The aetiology is unknown, but it appears to relate to the oestrogen concentration during pregnancy.

Clinical features
Women present with severe itching, especially on the limbs, trunk, palms and soles.

No rash is present unless it is due to excoriation.

Investigations
Liver function tests are deranged in some women (elevated ALT and AST, alkaline phosphatase and gamma glutamyl transaminase). Bile acids are markedly increased and may be the only abnormality on which to confirm the diagnosis, but results can take up to 2 weeks to obtain. Coagulation tests should only be monitored when liver function is abnormal.

If abdominal pain or other features are present, then ultrasound and hepatitis serology should be arranged to exclude other causes of itching and abnormal liver function.

Maternal risks
Vitamin K deficiency and subsequent risk of postpartum haemorrhage have very rarely been reported with obstetric cholestasis.

Effect on the fetus
The main concern with obstetric cholestasis is the risk of sudden intrauterine death, but fetal distress in labour, spontaneous preterm delivery and intracranial haemorrhage can also occur. The fetal outcome cannot be predicted by severity of symptoms in the mother.

Management
- **Management of pruritus:** Antihistamines such as chlorphenamine are safe and effective for mild symptoms of itch. For severe symptoms, ursodeoxycholic acid reduces serum bile acids and relieves itching at a dose of 8–12 mg/kg per day, in divided doses.

- **Clotting factors:** Vitamin K 10 mg/day given to the mother should reduce the risk of maternal and fetal haemorrhage.
- **Fetal well-being:** Fetal growth, liquor volume and umbilical artery Doppler should be monitored, though these may not help to predict sudden intrauterine death. CTG in labour is also recommended. Delivery is aimed at 37–38 weeks to minimize the risk of intrauterine death without disproportionately increasing the risks of prematurity.

Prognosis

Obstetric cholestasis recurs in about 50% of pregnancies and symptoms may also occur with use of the combined oral contraceptive pill.

Acute fatty liver of pregnancy

Acute fatty liver of pregnancy is a rare condition (1 in 10 000 births) with a maternal mortality of up to 20%. The aetiology is unknown.

Clinical features

Anorexia, malaise, diarrhoea, vomiting and abdominal pain are common presenting features, generally in the third trimester. Signs include jaundice, mild hypertension or proteinuria or signs of fulminant hepatic failure.

Investigations

Investigations reveal markedly deranged AST, ALT and alkaline phosphatase, with renal and clotting abnormalities in severe cases. Hypoglycaemia and very high uric acid help to differentiate acute fatty liver from HELLP syndrome.

The diagnosis is usually made on clinical findings and CT or magnetic resonance imaging of the liver, but may be confirmed on liver biopsy if necessary, with its associated risks.

Management

Management involves urgent delivery after correction of blood glucose, clotting factors and hypertension if present. Renal failure and DIC should be treated if they occur. Transfer to a liver unit is usually indicated, or to an intensive care unit if that is not possible. Liver transplant is sometimes performed in severely ill women.

CARDIAC DISEASE

The overall incidence of heart disease in pregnancy is about 1%. It is a major cause of indirect maternal death. The commonest problems are atrioseptal defect, ventriculoseptal defect and rheumatic mitral disease (stenosis or incompetence). Pregnancies in these women are generally well tolerated, especially if the defects have been corrected. Cyanotic heart diseases such as Eisenmenger's syndrome are significantly more difficult to manage in pregnancy, with 30% maternal complication rate, 50% fetal loss rate and significant maternal mortality.

Pathophysiology

The changes in maternal physiology that affect cardiac disease in pregnancy are:

- Increased plasma volume
- Increased cardiac output
- Catecholamine release from pain and anxiety at delivery
- Sudden increase in blood volume at delivery (about 500 ml) as the uterus contracts

● Sudden decompression of the vena cava at delivery.

Heart disease in pregnancy may be practically classified as high-, moderate- or low-risk, according to the severity of the effect on the mother in terms of:

● The degree of cyanosis
● The presence of pulmonary hypertension
● The New York Heart Association functional class (degree of breathlessness/exercise tolerance).

Table 12.8 gives a classification of cardiac disease in pregnancy according to maternal risk.

Assessment

Antenatal clinical assessment of heart disease is often difficult due to the overlap between pregnancy symptoms and cardiac symptoms. For example, oedema, breathlessness and palpitations are all normal pregnancy symptoms. However, chest pain, breathlessness at rest or at night and haemoptysis are all suspicious features.

On examination, normal pregnancy features can include bounding pulse, ejection systolic murmur, sinus tachycardia and third heart sound. However, pansystolic or diastolic murmurs are abnormal, as are features of cyanosis.

Management

Multidisciplinary team

Women with serious cardiac disease should be managed within a multidisciplinary setting with cardiologist, obstetrician, anaesthetist and, occasionally, cardiothoracic surgeon.

Table 12.8. Cardiac disease according to maternal risk in pregnancy

High-risk (mortality up to 50%):
Eisenmenger's syndrome
Tetralogy of Fallot
Transposition of the great vessels
Pulmonary hypertension (primary or secondary)
Ischaemic heart disease
Hypertrophic obstructive cardiomyopathy
Severe aortic stenosis

Moderate-risk (mortality up to 15%):
Valve stenosis
Coarctation of the aorta
History of myocardial infarction
Marfan's syndrome
Mechanical prosthetic valve

Low-risk (mortality around 1%):
Valve regurgitation
Mitral valve prolapse
Uncomplicated ventriculoseptal defect/atrioseptal defect/patent ductus arteriosus
Porcine valve replacement

Prepregnancy counselling

This is discussed in Chapter 11. Women should be assessed for the nature and severity of the lesion and the risk to mother and fetus during a potential pregnancy should be discussed.

Termination of pregnancy

The maternal mortality is so high that termination is recommended for women with Eisenmenger's syndrome, other pulmonary hypertension, Marfan's syndrome with aortic root diameter more than 4 cm or previous peripartum cardiomyopathy.

Medication

Most medication, except diuretics and ACE inhibitors, can be continued in pregnancy after consideration of risks and benefits to the mother.

Fetal abnormality

The risk of fetal cardiac abnormality is considerably raised in women with cardiac disease (2–5%) and detailed fetal echocardiography should be performed in the second trimester to assess for this and plan appropriate management. Fetal echocardiography detects about 80% of structural problems.

Fetal growth and well-being

Regular growth scans should be performed from 28 weeks due to the increased risk of growth restriction in utero, related to poor cardiac output or hypoxia.

Cardiac failure

Anaemia, infections, hypertension and arrhythmias all contribute to cardiac failure and should be screened for and treated aggressively if diagnosed.

Delivery

Most women with cardiac disease will deliver vaginally, unless there are specific obstetric indications for caesarean section. There is no overall benefit to mother or baby from caesarean section. However, effective pain relief and an instrumental delivery help to minimize the impact of the second stage. Epidural may be contraindicated if there is poor cardiac reserve and oxytocin infusion (without ergometrine) is generally used for the third stage to avoid sudden vasodilatation and tachycardia (both avoided in heart failure). Fluid balance must be managed carefully to avoid overload and a wedge to maintain left lateral tilt should be used to avoid the supine position.

Antibiotics

Endocarditis prophylaxis is essential for women with artificial heart valves and generally recommended for those with other structural problems such as congenital abnormality, rheumatic valve disease, cardiomyopathy and valve prolapse.

The current recommendation is 1 gram intravenous amoxicillin (1 gram vancomycin if penicillin-allergic) and 120 mg intravenous gentamicin at the onset of labour, anaesthesia or rupture of membranes and a second dose of oral amoxicillin 500 mg 6 hours later.

Thromboprophylaxis

Many cardiac diseases predispose to thrombosis. Heparin (or warfarin) prophylaxis should be continued throughout pregnancy for women with mechanical heart valves and considered in other clinical situations such as prolonged immobilization or cardiomyopathy.

Specific cardiac diseases

Coarctation of the aorta

Coarctation of the aorta is well tolerated if corrected. If uncorrected, blood pressure must be well controlled and angina, hypertension and pulmonary oedema are risks.

Marfan's syndrome

Marfan's syndrome is an autosomal-dominant condition characterized by increased height, large arm span, high arched palate, depressed sternum, aortic dilatation and dissection.

Aortic root imaging should be performed before conception and elective aortic root replacement planned if the root is dilated because of risk of dissection or rupture in pregnancy.

Fallot's tetralogy

Fallot's tetralogy is characterized by a large ventriculoseptal defect, right ventricular outflow obstruction, overriding aorta and right ventricular hypertrophy.

If pulmonary hypertension occurs, these women have a very high risk of morbidity and mortality in pregnancy, as cardiac output cannot be increased due to fixed pulmonary vascular resistance. There is also a risk of paradoxical embolus causing cerebrovascular accident or arterial embolism in the mother.

Cyanosis itself causes a high risk of IUGR and prematurity for the fetus.

Eisenmenger's syndrome

Eisenmenger's syndrome is another cyanotic condition whereby an original left-to-right shunt is reversed due to the development of pulmonary hypertension causing the pulmonary pressure to exceed the systemic pressure. Symptoms of fatigue, breathlessness, palpitations, syncope and chest pain develop in adult life. It is an important cause of maternal mortality.

Mitral stenosis

Mitral stenosis is caused by rheumatic fever and is the commonest acquired heart disease.

The disease usually presents in childhood and results in residual valve disease. The diagnosis is often made in pregnancy in women from high-risk countries with no previous medical input.

In pregnancy, the clinical condition may deteriorate with increased breathlessness and pulmonary oedema. Treatments include beta-blockers to prevent tachycardia and allow adequate diastolic left ventricular filling, diuretics for pulmonary oedema, balloon valvotomy and valve replacement prior to or after pregnancy.

Artificial heart valves

Women with mechanical heart valves need full anticoagulation throughout the pregnancy because of the high risk of thrombosis. Warfarin is, therefore, usually continued throughout pregnancy, in consultation with the haematologists, with intravenous heparin around the time of delivery.

Women with artificial valves also need antibiotic prophylaxis around the time of delivery to cover the risk of endocarditis.

Puerperal cardiomyopathy

Puerperal cardiomyopathy can occur from 36 weeks' gestation to 6 months postpartum. The incidence is 1 in 3000–15 000. Clinical features are shortness of breath, palpitations, oedema and possible cerebrovascular accident. Signs of pulmonary oedema or dysrhythmia may be present.

The diagnosis is made on echocardiogram, showing dilated atria and ventricles and poor left ventricular function.

Treatment is with diuretics or ACE inhibitors for left ventricular failure and, in extreme cases, heart transplantation. Thromboprophylaxis is essential because of the risk of emboli from the dilated heart. Delivery should be expedited if the woman has not yet delivered. Recurrence is common and mortality high, so further pregnancies should be avoided.

PSYCHIATRIC DISORDERS

The Confidential Enquiry into Maternal Deaths has identified mental illness as a major cause of indirect maternal death, both during and after pregnancy. Women with a history of previous psychiatric or mental health problems are at higher risk of psychiatric morbidity during and after pregnancy.

Women should be asked about a history of psychiatric problems at booking and any ongoing problems should be referred to a psychiatric team. Most psychiatric units have a pregnancy liaison team. A delivery and postnatal plan should be made that may involve the psychiatric, obstetric, midwifery, neonatal and social services teams. Some women will need treatment, support and observation in a mother and baby unit after delivery.

Depression

Depression in early pregnancy is not uncommon and may be pre-existing or relate to feelings about an unwanted pregnancy, relationship issues or be secondary to severe hyperemesis.

It is estimated that up to 13% of women have symptoms suggestive of depression by 32 weeks' gestation. At this stage, fear of labour or anxiety about parenthood may be contributing factors.

Although unlicensed in pregnancy, there is little evidence of adverse fetal effects from antidepressant medication, except tricyclic drugs which may cause transient neonatal tachycardia and irritability.

Postnatal depression is discussed in Chapter 15.

Schizophrenia

Women with psychotic disorders need to continue treatment throughout the pregnancy and should be reassured that the importance of treatment outweighs any potential harm to the baby. There are no clear teratogenic effects of antipsychotics, though occasional extrapyramidal effects in neonates are observed. Benzodiazepines cause neonatal respiratory depression and dependency and these babies need neonatal monitoring.

Hypomanic disorder

Lithium causes congenital defects, including cardiac abnormalities. It is, therefore, not recommended in pregnancy. However, owing to the nature of the condition, the benefit often outweighs the risk. The dose of lithium increases with gestation, but the requirement then falls abruptly at delivery.

Domestic violence

Domestic violence accounts for a significant number of indirect maternal deaths. Violence in pregnancy may cause direct morbidity such as placental abruption or preterm birth, but can also cause depression and anxiety in the antenatal period or prevent access to proper antenatal care. Women should be asked at booking about any history of violence or abuse and referred for appropriate counselling, psychiatric and social services support.

SUMMARY

- Half of pregnant women experience nausea or vomiting, but hyperemesis gravidarum, with excessive symptoms, occurs in only 1%.
- Thiamine replacement should always be included with fluids and antiemetics in the management of hyperemesis, to avoid the risk of Wernicke's encephalopathy.
- Hypertension diagnosed prior to 20 weeks' gestation is generally due to pre-existing chronic hypertension, rather than pregnancy-induced hypertension.
- Ten per cent of pregnant women develop hypertension or mild pre-eclampsia and 10% of these develop severe pre-eclampsia.
- Pre-eclampsia may be diagnosed by a combination of fetal and maternal features, including IUGR, haematological or biochemical abnormalities, as well as clinical symptoms and signs.
- Treatment of hypertension in pregnancy is important to reduce the risk of cerebrovascular accident, but does not alter the development of, and may mask, underlying pre-eclampsia.
- Women with confirmed pre-eclampsia should be managed as inpatients, because of the risk of fulminating disease or placental abruption.
- Vertical transmission of HIV can be reduced to less than 5% by zidovudine prophylaxis to the mother and baby, elective caesarean section and the avoidance of breastfeeding.
- Maternal group B streptococcal infection is an important cause of neonatal morbidity and mortality, and prophylaxis protocols should be adhered to.
- VTE is still the leading cause of maternal mortality.
- Some cardiac diseases, such as Eisenmenger's syndrome, carry a very high maternal mortality risk, and termination of pregnancy should be seriously considered in such cases.

CHAPTER CONTENTS

MALPRESENTATIONS

Breech

The presentation of the fetus refers to the part of the fetus that occupies the lower uterine segment, which in this case is the fetal buttocks. This is the commonest malpresentation, occurring in 3–4% of singleton pregnancies at term, but in up to 25% in preterm labour. There are three types of breech presentation (Fig. 13.1):

1. Frank breech – buttocks presenting with the legs extended.
2. Complete breech – legs flexed so that feet present beside the buttocks.
3. Footling breech – one or both feet presenting below the buttocks.

Aetiology

In most cases of breech presentation, no cause is found, but there are situations that predispose to this presentation.

- Maternal causes:
- Grand multiparity results in uterine laxity so that the fetus has an increased likelihood of changing position
- Uterine abnormalities, e.g. bicornuate or septate
- Pelvic tumours or bony abnormalities that prevent engagement of the head
- Full bladder in labour.
- Placental causes:
- Placenta praevia
- Oligo- or polyhydramnios.
- Fetal causes:
- Multiple pregnancy
- Fetal abnormality
- Prematurity.

Investigations

Clinical examination is known to pick up only 50% of breeches at term but it may detect the presenting part as wider than normal and the harder head will be felt in the fundus of the uterus, which will be ballotable. An extended leg breech has the head in the midline compared to the flexed breech, where the head is more lateral. An ultrasound scan will confirm the diagnosis and determine the type of breech, the liquor volume, the placental site, the estimated fetal weight and the presence of a fetal abnormality. Despite this, approximately one-third are undiscovered until during labour.

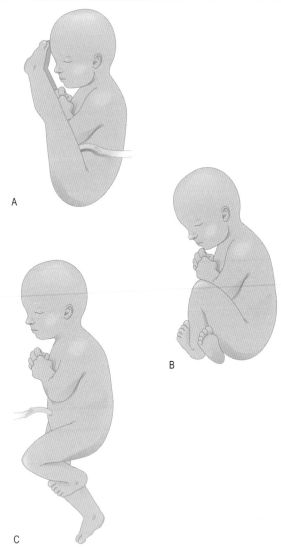

A

B

C

Figure 13.1 Breech presentations. (A) Extended (frank); (B) flexed (complete); (C) footling. (Redrawn with permission from Rymer J, Davis G, Rodin A et al. 2003 Preparation and Revision for the DRCOG, 3rd edn. Edinburgh: Churchill Livingstone, p. 235.)

Management

If a breech presentation is diagnosed antenatally women can be offered external cephalic version which has a 1% risk of cord accident or abruption. This is a method to manipulate the lie of the fetus into a cephalic presentation with the aid of tocolysis to relax the uterus. The procedure is successful in 40% of primiparous and 60% of multiparous patients if performed after 37 weeks. If the breech presentation persists, then a decision must be made about the mode of delivery, which remains controversial. Most obstetricians would now advocate an elective caesarean section for all persistent breech presentations at term. However, the multiparous patient with a breech may be offered the option of a vaginal delivery in the presence of a normal pelvis and an estimated fetal weight of 2500–3500 g.

Breech delivery is becoming less common, but is a skill that all obstetricians should be familiar with, as unexpected breech deliveries will always occur.

Vaginal delivery of the breech

Most practitioners would not induce a woman with a breech presentation, as the best chance for a successful vaginal delivery is spontaneous labour and, likewise, few would advocate augmentation for slow progress in labour. The fetus should be monitored continuously, often with the scalp electrode attached to the buttock, and epidural anaesthesia is advised.

Once full dilatation is reached, the breech must be allowed to descend to the perineum before an episiotomy is performed. As the breech is delivering, the sacrum is guided gently to the anterior position with the operator's fingers and thumbs over the iliac crests and lumbar spine of the fetus, respectively, and the breech, legs and abdomen allowed to deliver spontaneously. The legs may need to be flexed to assist delivery (Pinard's manoeuvre). Pushing is encouraged until the scapulae are visible and at this stage Lovset's manoeuvre (rotation of the trunk) can be used to assist delivery of the shoulders and arms. Delivery of the head should be controlled manually (Mauriceau–Smellie–Veit manoeuvre) or by using forceps.

Regardless of the mode of delivery, breech presentation is associated with an increased perinatal morbidity and mortality, and, therefore, must be considered a high-risk pregnancy.

Transverse (and oblique) lie

The lie of the fetus is the relationship of the fetus to the long axis of the uterus. The lie is oblique if the head or buttocks are found in one or other iliac fossa, and the lie is transverse if they are found in the patient's flanks. Unless these positions convert during pregnancy, vaginal delivery will not be possible and a caesarean section must be performed.

The aetiologies of both these presentations are similar to those outlined for breech presentation and also an ultrasound assessment should be performed for the same reasons (Fig. 13.2).

Management

Both transverse and oblique lie are uncommon at term and, if this is the case, the woman should be admitted for the remainder of her pregnancy for observation, as she is at high risk for cord prolapse if the membranes rupture from 37 to 38 weeks. If an identifying cause can be found on ultrasound scan, e.g. placenta praevia, then an elective caesarean section should be arranged. If no cause can be found, then the patient is observed until the lie stabilizes to cephalic for at least 48 hours, at which stage the labour can be induced.

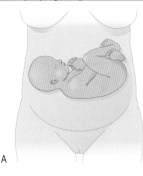

Figure 13.2 Fetal lie describes the relationship of the long axis of the fetus to the long axis of the uterus. (A) Transverse; (B) oblique; (C) longitudinal. (Redrawn with permission from Symonds E M, Symonds I M 2003 Essential Obstetrics and Gynaecology, 4th edn. Edinburgh: Churchill Livingstone, p. 80.)

A

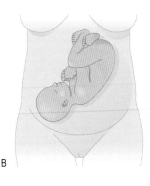

B

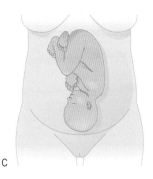

C

A caesarean section for transverse lie can be technically difficult and should only be performed by an experienced obstetrician, especially if the fetal back is presenting and particularly so if there is oligohydramnios. This is because it is more difficult to access a fetal foot in order to perform a breech extraction. In this situation a general anaesthetic may be preferred (to allow more uterine relaxation). The other potential problem with a transverse lie is that the lower uterine segment is poorly developed and a vertical uterine incision may be required.

Cord prolapse

If the membranes rupture in the presence of a transverse or oblique lie then cord prolapse is likely and an immediate vaginal examination should be performed to exclude or confirm the prolapse. If the cord is found in the vagina then the woman should be placed in a knee–chest position or on all fours (with her buttocks higher than her head) to allow gravity to assist in avoiding cord compression against the pelvic cavity by the presenting part. The examiner's hand should remain in the vagina, which will also assist in preventing cord compression until caesarean section can be performed. The examiner's hand should not be withdrawn from the vagina until the surgeon has opened the uterus. An alternative strategy is to catheterize and fill the bladder to 500 ml, which may prevent the presenting part compressing the cord until caesarean section can be performed.

MULTIPLE PREGNANCY

The incidence of twin pregnancy is approximately 1 in 100 and that of triplets is 1 in 1000, although the incidence of all multiple pregnancies is increasing because of increasing use of assisted conception techniques.

Aetiology of twin pregnancy

Twinning can be either mono- or dizygotic, referring to the number of maternal eggs used in fertilization.

Dizygotic twins are the commonest (60%) and result from the fertilization of two separate ova by separate sperm and are, therefore, no more genetically similar than siblings in the same family and may be of different sex. Monozygotic twins result from mitotic division of a single fertilized ova (zygote) into identical twins.

Therefore, dizygotic twins are always dichorionic and diamniotic, whereas monozygotic twins can share the same amnion and chorion depending on the stage at which the mitotic division occurred.

Predisposing factors include:

- Increasing maternal age and parity
- Family history
- Race
- Assisted conception (approximately 20% of all in vitro fertilization pregnancies).

Management

1. Diagnosis – women will often have exaggerated symptoms of pregnancy, including hyperemesis gravidarum. On examination the uterus feels larger than would be expected for her dates. Ultrasound assessment is usually performed in all pregnancies and should reveal the diagnosis.
2. Multiple pregnancy is not a normal pregnancy and should be closely monitored.
3. Both congenital abnormality and intrauterine growth restriction (IUGR) are more common in multiple pregnancy and so regular ultrasound assessment is important at 28, 32 and 36 weeks or more frequently if necessary.
4. An early ultrasound scan should determine chorionicity at 12 weeks or less.

Complications of multiple pregnancy

Maternal
- Hyperemesis often requiring admission for rehydration
- Miscarriage
- Pregnancy-induced hypertension and pre-eclampsia, which often presents earlier and is more aggressive than in singleton pregnancies
- Gestational diabetes
- Anaemia
- Antepartum and postpartum haemorrhage
- Placenta praevia
- Maternal discomfort.

Fetal
- Perinatal mortality is increased fourfold
- Congenital abnormality, especially in monozygotic twins
- Preterm labour occurs in 40% of twin pregnancies. More than 50% of babies from multiple pregnancies are less than 2500 grams compared with 6% of babies from singleton pregnancies
- Placental insufficiency or IUGR, especially in monochorionic twins
- Twin–twin transfusion in monochorionic twins, due to anastomosis of vessels within the single placental mass of a monochorionic twin pregnancy. In this condition one twin gains at the expense of the other, i.e. one twin becomes anaemic and the other polycythaemic
- Malpresentation of the first twin occurs in 20% of cases.

A twin delivery is high-risk, especially for the second twin. There may be added complications of preterm labour, malpresentation and postpartum haemorrhage. A plan for labour and delivery should be discussed antenatally with the consultant. A trial of vaginal delivery will generally be recommended if the first twin is cephalic and there are no added complications.

Delivery

The decision on mode of delivery depends on the presentation of the leading twin and on the presence of maternal or fetal complications. There is no evidence to suggest that caesarean section is advantageous if the first twin is cephalic, regardless of the presentation of the second twin. However, 50% of twins at term in spontaneous or induced labour will need caesarean delivery, usually because of fetal distress in the second twin. Caesarean section is indicated for all the usual reasons of a singleton pregnancy or if the first twin is breech or a transverse lie.

It is usual to induce labour for twins between 38 and 40 weeks and continuous monitoring of both twins throughout labour is essential as the fetuses, particularly the second twin, are at increased risk of hypoxia.

An epidural is recommended, as the second twin may need to be delivered by breech extraction. Labour is closely monitored and the first twin is delivered in the usual manner and the cord clamped and cut. The lie of the second twin is determined and presentation can be confirmed by ultrasound if necessary. If the lie is not longitudinal then external cephalic version can be used. Once the head or breech enters the pelvis the membranes are ruptured (often with fundal pressure) and pushing begins again. If contractions diminish, then an oxytocin drip is commenced. The second twin is then delivered in the usual manner, but breech extraction may be required if the second twin is not cephalic. The cord is double-clamped and cut, and the placenta is delivered. It is recommended that an oxytocin infusion is commenced as there is an increased risk of postpartum haemorrhage.

Complications
- Inefficient uterine action, especially after delivery of the leading twin
- Fetal distress, especially of the second twin
- Cord prolapse when rupturing membranes of second twin
- Locking is rare but can occur if leading twin is breech and the second twin is cephalic
- Postpartum haemorrhage
- Postpartum thrombosis.

SUMMARY

- All women with a malpresentation should deliver in hospital.
- Breech presentation is associated with an increased perinatal mortality rate and, therefore, is considered a high-risk pregnancy.
- Transverse and oblique lie at term are uncommon and women should be admitted after 37 weeks as cord prolapse is more common in these situations and is an obstetric emergency.
- Multiple pregnancies have significantly increased fetal and maternal morbidity and mortality and, therefore, require regular specialist monitoring.

Labour 14

CHAPTER CONTENTS

LABOUR

Definition

Labour is defined as the process whereby the fetus and the placenta are expelled by the uterus at term, i.e. between 37 and 42 completed weeks of pregnancy.

Features of labour

The diagnosis of labour is crucial as this will determine the duration of labour. Labour is diagnosed by regular painful uterine contractions accompanied by dilatation and effacement of the cervix, often with the passage of a mucous plug or 'show' (the operculum). There are three stages of labour:

1. First stage: from the diagnosis of labour to full dilatation of the cervix
2. Second stage: from full dilatation of the cervix to delivery of the fetus
3. Third stage: the interval from delivery of the fetus to delivery of the placenta.

Cervical ripening or change is characterized by softening, effacement (when the normally tubular cervix is drawn up into the lower uterine segment) and then dilatation. This cervical change is caused by the onset of regular uterine contractions.

Mechanical features of labour

There are three mechanical features of labour commonly described:

1. The powers: this is the uterine force of contractions that will expel the fetus. In labour an efficient uterus will contract regularly for 40–60 seconds every 2–3 minutes. These contractions will cause descent of the presenting fetal part, allowing effacement and subsequent dilatation of the cervix. By definition, the nulliparous uterus is inefficient, in that the uterus often contracts irregularly, as opposed to the multiparous uterus.

2. The passage: the bony pelvic canal has to be traversed by the fetus in labour and, therefore, the diameters of the pelvis need consideration (Figs 14.1 and 14.2). The pelvic inlet has two diameters:
   a. The transverse diameter is usually approximately 13 cm.
   b. The anteroposterior diameter is approximately 11 cm.
      The pelvic outlet is the opposite, with a transverse diameter of 11 cm and an anteroposterior diameter of 13 cm. The ischial spines can be palpated vaginally and are used as the landmarks to define the descent or station (in centimetres above or below) of the fetal presenting part.

3. The passenger is the fetus and the fetal head diameters (Fig. 14.3) are important to allow ease of descent:
   a. The attitude of the fetal head in labour is the degree of flexion, and the smallest diameter of the fetal head to allow ease of passage through the pelvis is at maximum flexion when the diameter is approximately 9.5 cm. A lesser degree of flexion (deflexed) will increase the diameter of the vertex or fetal head, with increasing deflexion resulting in a brow or face presentation.
   b. Position of the fetal head describes the relationship of its sagittal suture to the pelvis and is described by the position of the fetal occiput. Usually, the fetal head enters the pelvis in a left occipital transverse (LOT) position and then rotates as it passes through the pelvis by 90° clockwise to an occiput anterior (OA) position. However, failure

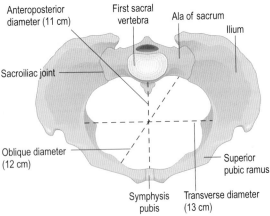

Figure 14.1 Diameters of the pelvis, the pelvic brim. (Redrawn with permission from Rymer J, Davis G, Rodin A et al. 2003 Preparation and Revision for the DRCOG, 3rd edn. Edinburgh: Churchill Livingstone, p. 382.)

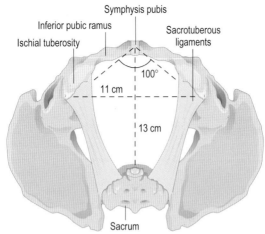

Figure 14.2 Diameters of the pelvis, the pelvic outlet. The boundary of the outlet from the symphysis pubis, down the inferior rami of the pubic bones to the ischial tuberosities, and then obliquely upwards and posterior along the sacrotuberous ligaments to the tip of the fifth sacral vertebra. Anteroposterior: 13 cm; transverse: 11 cm; oblique diameter 12 cm. (Redrawn with permission from Rymer J, Davis G, Rodin A et al. 2003 Preparation and Revision for the DRCOG, 3rd edn. Edinburgh: Churchill Livingstone, p. 383.)

of the fetal head to rotate results in a persistent occiput transverse (OT) position and in fewer than 5% of cases the opposite is the case, where the occiput faces posteriorly (OP); both situations that result in a difficult spontaneous delivery without assistance.

c. The size of a normally formed fetal head will rarely cause obstruction. The fetal head is highly malleable and will mould as it passes through the pelvis, resulting in palpable overlapping suture lines on vaginal assessment. Cervical pressure on the fetal scalp during labour may result in scalp swelling or oedema, which is called caput. Both caput and the degree of moulding will be an indication of possible obstruction.

Mechanical features of the vertex in labour

The mechanics of labour described above cause changes in the attitude of the fetal head during descent into the pelvis (Fig. 14.4) and are summarized in stages as:

1. Descent: the fetal head often descends during the last few weeks of pregnancy in the nulliparous patient, but this descent may not occur until just before the onset of labour in multiparous patients or also in Afro-Caribbean women because of the shape of their pelvises.

2. Engagement: this occurs when the maximum diameter of the fetal head has passed through the pelvic inlet. It is usually described in fifths of the fetal head that can be palpated abdominally, with engagement being defined as less than or equal to two-fifths of the fetal head palpable above the pelvic brim.

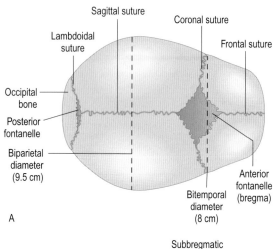

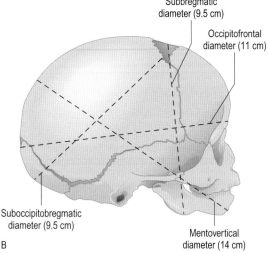

Figure 14.3 The fetal skull diameters. (Redrawn with permission from Rymer J, Davis G, Rodin A et al. 2003 Preparation and Revision for the DRCOG, 3rd edn. Edinburgh: Churchill Livingstone, p. 381.)

3. Flexion: the fetal head flexes as it descends through the pelvis in order to allow its smallest diameter to traverse the pelvis. With maximum flexion the posterior fontanelle can be easily palpated vaginally.
4. Internal rotation: as the fetal head descends it rotates from a LOT position to OA, as described above (Fig. 14.5).

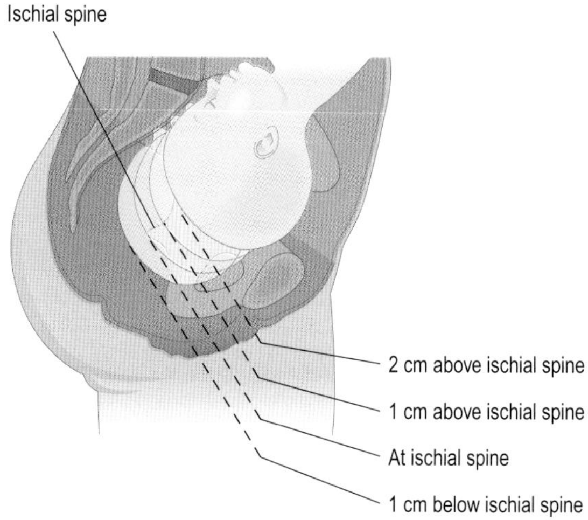

Ischial spine

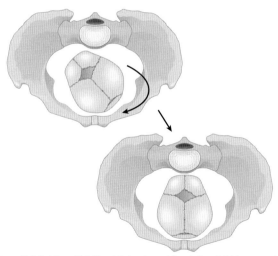

2 cm above ischial spine

1 cm above ischial spine

At ischial spine

1 cm below ischial spine

Figure 14.4 Descent of fetal head vaginally described in relation to the ischial spine.

Figure 14.5 Rotation of fetal head during descent from left occipital transverse to occiput anterior.

5. Extension: the fetal head remains flexed until it reaches the perineum and then begins to extend as the head crowns as it is about to be delivered.
6. External rotation (restitution): as the fetal head is delivered it reverts to the transverse position (OT).

7. Lateral flexion: when the head is delivering the anterior shoulder appears, followed by the posterior shoulder with the trunk delivering by lateral flexion.

Assessment of labour

The prompt and accurate diagnosis of labour is crucial in the management and assessment of the progress of labour.

1. History: the history on admission should include specific questioning on the following:
   a. The time of onset, frequency and duration of contractions
   b. The presence of a show and whether the membranes are ruptured (and if so, the colour of the liquor).
2. Examination:
   a. General assessment of maternal well-being, including vital signs
   b. Abdominal palpation to assess symphyseal–fundal height, lie and position of the fetus, presentation and descent of the presenting part in the pelvis
   c. Vaginal examination with a sterile speculum to confirm drainage of liquor if this is in doubt. Digital examination to assess cervical dilatation and station of the presenting part.
3. Fetal well-being:
   a. Ask about fetal movements
   b. Cardiotocograph (CTG)
   c. Presence of meconium in the liquor.

Management

Once the diagnosis of labour has been made then the membranes can be ruptured to assess the liquor for the presence of meconium, which will provide information on fetal well-being. A partogram is a visual record of labour progress and records a variable amount of information depending on each individual obstetric unit. The following is a list of usual information recorded in a partogram (Fig. 14.6):

1. Patient details
2. The date and time of admission
3. Maternal vital signs
4. A progressive representation of cervical dilatation (descent of the head). The partogram may include an action line denoting a minimum acceptable rate of cervical dilatation (usually 1 cm/h for a primigravid patient). If progress falls below the action line, then medical intervention may be considered
5. Details on the contractions should include frequency (usually described as the number occurring in 10 minutes), duration and strength
6. The fetal heart rate by intermittent auscultation or continuous fetal monitoring
7. Colour of liquor and time of rupture of membranes
8. Drugs given, including oxytocin and analgesics
9. Maternal urine production and urinalysis for ketones and/or protein.

Progress of labour

The fundamental process of labour is progressive dilatation of the cervix and descent of the presenting part.

Primiparous and multiparous patients are very different in their labour progress. A primiparous labour is often slow, but a slow multiparous labour is always of concern.

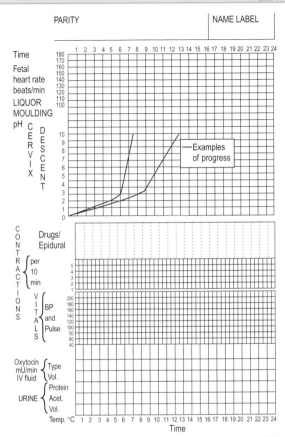

Figure 14.6 Typical partogram illustrating graphically essential information of labour progress. BP, blood pressure.

Primiparous labour

Labour should proceed at a rate of at least 1 cm cervical dilatation per hour in a primiparous patient. The first stage should, therefore, last for 10 hours with 2 hours for the second stage. Labour that lasts for longer than 12 hours is said to be prolonged. However, the primiparous uterus is notoriously inefficient as it has not experienced labour before, so that even if the contractions feel strong and frequent they may be having little effect on cervical dilatation. This is correctable if diagnosed early by performing an amniotomy if the membranes are still intact and by commencing an oxytocin infusion to augment labour. Careful clinical monitoring is required to ensure that contractions do not exceed one every 2 minutes or hypertonia results, with fetal hypoxia caused by restriction of the maternal placental blood flow. Oxytocin is, therefore, administered by titrating the infusion against the uterine contractions to achieve efficient uterine action and each obstetric unit will have protocols for concentration and infusion rates (Fig. 14.6). If full dilatation is not foreseeable within 12 hours, then caesarean section may need to be considered as the woman will become exhausted and there will be increasing risk of fetal hypoxia. The partogram is a crucial guide to labour progression. An individual decision is taken by each woman on the recommendation of the obstetrician and midwife.

Cephalopelvic disproportion is diagnosed when a woman has been unable to deliver a fetus despite adequate uterine activity and in the absence of malposition of the fetus. This disparity between the size of the fetus and the maternal pelvis is uncommon in the UK in the absence of pelvic abnormality.

Multiparous labour

The multiparous uterus is not inefficient as it has laboured previously. However, it should be noted that a multiparous patient may not have laboured before (i.e. caesarean section) and in this case the uterus will behave in the same way as that of a primiparous woman. Therefore, slow progress is a cause for concern and is usually the result of a larger baby in this pregnancy or because of malposition. The multiparous uterus is prone to rupture and so the use of oxytocin should only be considered after careful evaluation.

Fetal surveillance in labour

The aim of fetal monitoring in labour is to detect fetal hypoxia. Each fetus will behave differently during the stresses of labour depending on its individual reserve and in particular a fetus that is compromised antenatally is more vulnerable during labour.

Methods

1. Amniotic fluid and liquor: the absence of liquor is associated with intrauterine growth retardation. Meconium is the passage of stool by the fetus in utero and is caused by vagal stimulation of the gut as a result of an episode of hypoxia. Some units will grade the meconium during labour from 1 to 3. Grade 1 meconium is lightly stained fluid (meconium that is very diluted by adequate liquor), grade 2 is moderately stained and grade 3 is a heavy, thick liquid associated with the fresh passage of meconium in the presence of reduced liquor, which is of particular concern, indicating fetal hypoxia.
2. Intermittent auscultation with either a Pinard's stethoscope or a Sonicaid. This is sometimes the method of choice in monitoring a low-risk labour and should be performed for 1 minute after a contraction and every 15 minutes to detect accelerations or decelerations of the fetal heart rate.
3. Continuous fetal monitoring using either an abdominal transducer (as part of the CTG) or a fetal scalp electrode. This will give a continuous real-time record of the fetal heart rate response to labour. The CTG should always be interpreted as part of the whole clinical picture, including stage of labour, maternal analgesia and status of the uterine contractions.
4. Fetal blood sampling is performed when the CTG suggests fetal compromise in labour and is interpreted on the basis of the fetal blood pH. A pH of greater than 7.25 is considered normal; a pH of between 7.20 and 7.25 is a borderline result that will need to be repeated within 1 hour; and a pH of less than 7.20 is abnormal, indicating immediate delivery.

Fetal heart rate patterns

There are three features of the fetal heart rate that should be noted – the baseline, beat-to-beat variability and the presence of accelerations or decelerations (see Fig. 14.7 for examples of CTG traces):

- Normal: the normal baseline should be between 110 and 160 beats per minute (bpm). Baseline beat-to-beat variability should be 5–25 bpm. Accelerations from baseline of 10–15 bpm will indicate a healthy fetus.
- Baseline tachycardia: a baseline fetal heart rate of greater than 160 bpm can be associated with prematurity, hypoxia, maternal pyrexia or drugs and fetal distress if also in the presence of any other abnormality.
- Baseline bradycardia: a baseline fetal heart rate of less than 110 bpm may be associated with postmaturity, hypoxia or heart block. A baseline of less than 90 bpm is usually indicative of impending fetal demise.
- Baseline variability: variability is the presence of irregular accelerations from baseline, and loss of beat-to-beat variability can indicate a sleep pattern if it lasts for less than 40 minutes. If it is prolonged beyond this it indicates hypoxia. Increase in variability may also indicate acute hypoxia.
- Early decelerations: these occur with the onset of a contraction and the fetal heart rate returns to baseline by the end of the contraction. These are usually caused by fetal head compression during descent and are benign.
- Late decelerations: these occur when the fetal heart rate drops after the peak of the contraction, with slow recovery to baseline after the contraction. Late decelerations are associated with fetal hypoxia.
- Variable decelerations: these decelerations, as the name suggests, occur at variable times during labour, often with no association to the contraction, and usually indicate cord compression.

Third stage of labour

The third stage of labour is the period between delivery of the fetus and delivery of the placenta. In a normal physiological third stage, the uterus continues to contract, which in combination with the reduced surface area of the uterus causes the placenta to separate from the uterine wall. During this phase there is usually a small gush of blood indicating that separation has occurred. The normal haemostatic processes that occur during this stage will be interfered with in the following situations:

- Morbid adherence of the placenta
- A prolonged labour
- When the uterus has been overdistended as a result of a multiple pregnancy
- As a result of halothane anaesthesia.

Physiological management

Inform the woman of the benefits of active management and document her choice in her notes. Physiological management is contraindicated where there has been any intervention (e.g. induction of labour), previous postpartum haemorrhage or cause for current obstetric concern (i.e. antepartum haemorrhage, postpartum haemorrhage or preterm labour).

Following delivery of baby, wait until cord pulsation has stopped, unless the baby requires resuscitation, is ill or requires observation, in which case active management should be undertaken. The baby can be handed to the mother, but kept at the same level as the uterus until the cord has

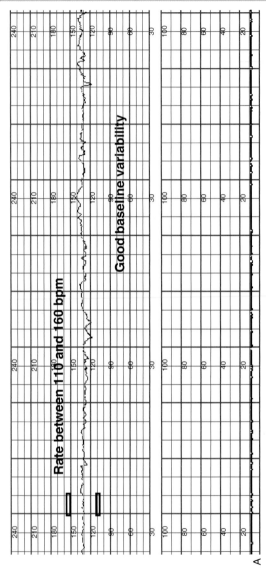

Figure 14.7 (A) Normal baseline (between 110 and 160 beats per minute (bpm)) is indicated by the fetal heart rate when stable (note: accelerations and decelerations are absent in this trace section).

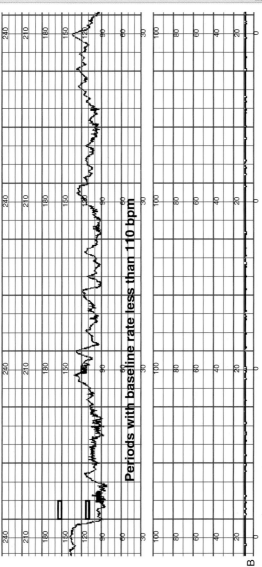

Periods with baseline rate less than 110 bpm

Figure 14.7—cont'd (B) Bradycardia is defined as a baseline heart rate of <110 bpm.

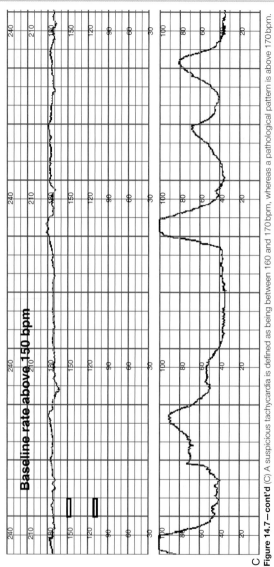

Baseline rate above 150 bpm

Figure 14.7—cont'd (C) A suspicious tachycardia is defined as being between 160 and 170 bpm, whereas a pathological pattern is above 170 bpm.

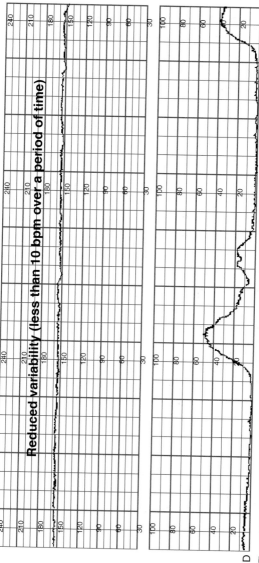

Reduced variability (less than 10 bpm over a period of time)

Figure 14.7—cont'd (D) Reduced variability (a flat trace).

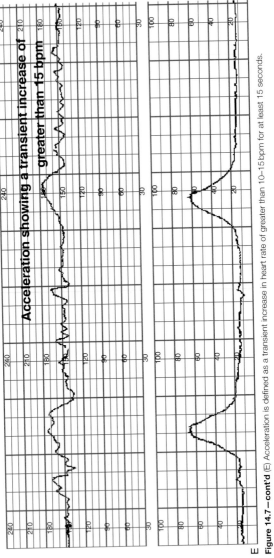

E

Figure 14.7 – cont'd (E) Acceleration is defined as a transient increase in heart rate of greater than 10–15 bpm for at least 15 seconds.

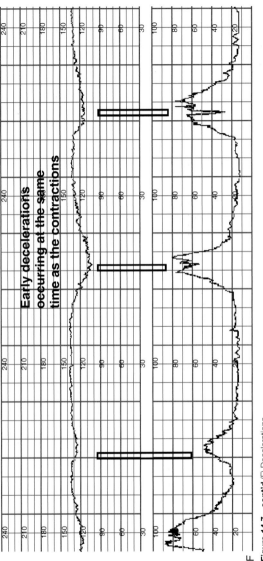

Early decelerations occurring at the same time as the contractions

Figure 14.7 – cont'd (F) Decelerations.

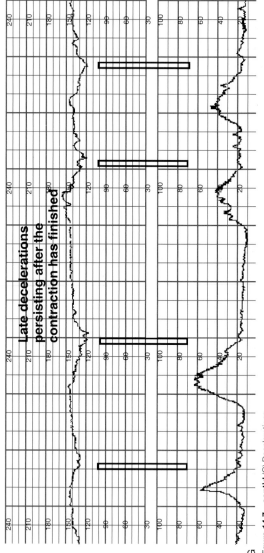

Figure 14.7—cont'd (G) Decelerations.

Late decelerations persisting after the contraction has finished

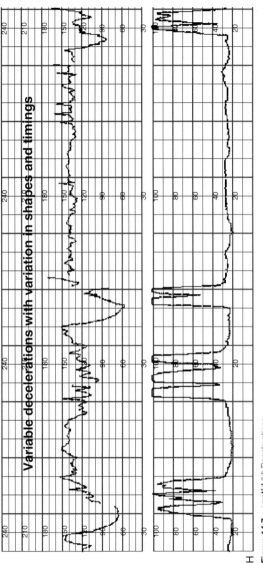

Variable decelerations with variation in shapes and timings

Figure 14.7 —cont'd (H) Decelerations.

been clamped and cut. When the cord pulsation has stopped, the cord is then clamped and cut and the mother should be encouraged to breast-feed. Release the clamp on the placental cord and allow cord blood to drain. Measure blood loss and observe the mother's colour, pulse rate and respirations.

Active management

In order to reduce the risk of postpartum haemorrhage because of retained placenta many units have a policy of active management of the third stage unless the woman requests physiological management.

The active management of the third stage of labour is carried out with the use of drugs, early clamping and cutting of the umbilical cord and controlled cord traction for the delivery of the placenta. Controlled cord traction is performed using the Brandt–Andrews technique, which involves downward traction on the cord with the other hand placed suprapubically to lift the uterus upwards.

The oxytocic drug of choice is Syntometrine 1 ml (a combination of oxytocin and ergometrine), given intramuscularly as the anterior shoulder of the baby is delivered. Women who are anaemic or who have a history of postpartum haemorrhage should be given ergometrine 250 µg intravenously instead or in addition.

Contraindications to the use of Syntometrine/ergometrine include:

- Hypertension
- Cardiac conditions
- Asthma
- History of cholecystitis
- Women who have received betamimetics.

In these cases, give 10 units of oxytocin intramuscularly/intravenously and await signs of placental separation (a gush of blood, lengthening of the cord, contracted uterine fundus), which should occur within 10–15 minutes. The placenta may become visible at the vulva or the mother may feel a heavy sensation or an urge to push. If the signs of separation have occurred, but the placenta has not delivered, vaginal examination will confirm whether the placenta is in the vagina. If the placenta is undelivered by 30–60 minutes, then manual removal of the placenta under anaesthesia (epidural will suffice, if in place, otherwise a spinal or general) may need to be considered.

Once the placenta has delivered it should be carefully inspected to ensure completeness and the genital tract should be inspected for any lacerations that may need to be repaired.

CEPHALIC MALPOSITIONS

1. OP: this is the commonest malposition and is caused by a posterior rotation of the fetal head during descent and results in deflexion of the fetal head and thus a larger head diameter traversing the pelvis so that obstruction is caused. It is associated with inefficient uterine action, pelvic shape variants and epidurals. This malposition may be corrected as labour progresses spontaneously or with an oxytocin infusion if the contractions are poor. The earlier slow progress is diagnosed as being caused by an OP presentation, the better the chance there is of rotation to OA. However, the fetus may be delivered in that position (face to pubis) spontaneously if the pelvic diameters are adequate, but an instrumental delivery may be required to rotate the fetal head to OA or to deliver face to pubis.

2. OT: again this is caused by incomplete rotation of the fetal head during labour. If this position persists in the second stage, then delivery will not occur unless rotated to OA manually or with Kielland forceps or the ventouse. Both OP and OT instrumental deliveries are increasingly being performed in theatre, with early recourse to caesarean section if required.

3. Brow presentation: this is caused by hyperextension of the fetal neck in labour and is generally incompatible with a vaginal delivery (may deliver if fetus is preterm) as the presenting diameter is too large (mento-vertex diameter is usually 13 cm), and a caesarean delivery is indicated unless flexion occurs during the course of labour.

4. Face presentation: this is the result of complete extension of the fetal neck. The facial features can be felt on vaginal examination and vaginal delivery may be possible if the chin is anterior (mento-anterior) as it will catch on the pubic bone during descent in the pelvis, causing the fetal neck to flex and, therefore, allow for further rotation. If the chin is posterior (mento-posterior), flexion is impossible and caesarean section is indicated.

INDUCTION OF LABOUR

Labour is induced when external methods are used to start labour artificially. This is different to augmentation, which is use of external methods to enhance uterine contractions after labour has begun spontaneously. After induction of labour has commenced, the risk of operative vaginal delivery is increased 1.5-fold and that of caesarean section is increased 1.8-fold.

Indication

This is a decision made between the obstetrician, midwife and patient. There are few definite indications for induction and the decision is usually a carefully weighted one to ensure the delivery of a healthy baby from a healthy mother, weighing up the risk/benefit ratio of the fetus remaining in utero versus delivery. In all these decisions two factors must always be considered:

1. The risk to mother and fetus if the pregnancy were allowed to continue
2. The risk to the mother of complications of induction and to the fetus of prematurity.

Common reasons for induction include:

- Postmaturity: when pregnancy extends beyond the due date, as studies have demonstrated an increase in perinatal mortality with increasing postmaturity as a result of decreased placental function. The time frame for this varies between units, but is usually at 41–42 weeks (despite the definition of term being until 42 weeks)
- Intrauterine growth retardation or antepartum haemorrhage
- Maternal hypertension
- Diabetes
- Poor obstetric history
- Maternal request.

Contraindications are defined as the following:

- Absolute: acute fetal compromise, unstable lie (if the lie stabilizes to cephalic, then controlled artificial rupture of the membranes (ARM) may be performed), placenta praevia and pelvic obstruction.
- Relative: previous caesarean section (although there are differing opinions in this situation), breech presentation and prematurity.

Method

The method of induction will usually depend on the cervical assessment, which will normally be undertaken at the time of the decision to induce (Table 14.1):

- Medical: insertion of prostaglandin gel or pessaries into the posterior vaginal fornix. Particular care should be exercised when using prostaglandins in a multiparous woman or a woman with a uterine scar, because of the risk of overstimulation. All prostaglandin administrations should be followed by a CTG for a minimum recording of 1 hour. Usually, following the second dose of prostaglandin, labour will start spontaneously. Alternatively, the cervix will have ripened sufficiently to allow surgical induction to proceed.
- Surgical induction of labour (ARM): if the cervix is favourable (Bishop's score of >7) (Table 14.1), or the hindwaters are ruptured, there is no advantage in further use of prostaglandin. A vaginal examination should reveal the presence of fetal membranes in advance of the fetal head, and ARM can be performed using an amnihook.
- Following ARM multiparae may go into labour spontaneously as prostaglandins are released as the membranes rupture. To reduce unnecessary venous cannulation they may be left to mobilize for 2–4 hours to allow spontaneous contractions to begin. This will rarely be effective in primiparae and, therefore, an oxytocin infusion should be commenced immediately. The oxytocin regime for induction of labour is the same as that used for augmentation.

Complications

- Uterine hypertonia with possible rupture
- Fetal distress
- Precipitate delivery
- Operative delivery
- Iatrogenic prematurity
- Amniotic fluid embolus
- Systemic effects of prostaglandins, including vomiting and diarrhoea.

OPERATIVE DELIVERY

Instrumental delivery allows the use of traction, usually combined with maternal effort, to expedite delivery of the fetus in the second stage of labour. The shape of the maternal pelvis will only allow the fetal head

Table 14.1. Bishop's score used to assess suitability for induction

	Score			
	0	1	2	3
Cervical length (cm)	>2	1 or 2	<1	Fully taken up
Cervical dilatation (cm)	Closed	1–2	3–4	>4
Cervical consistency	Firm	Medium	Soft	NA
Position of cervix	Posterior	Central	Anterior	NA
Station of presenting part (cm above ischial spines)	3	2	1 or 0	Below ischial spines

to deliver if it is in the OA or, occasionally, if the pelvis is adequate, the OP position. Therefore, rotation to these positions may be required either manually or with the use of a ventouse or rotational forceps.

Indications

- Fetal distress in the second stage
- Delivery of the aftercoming head in a breech delivery
- Prolonged second stage (usually after 1 hour of active pushing) or maternal distress
- Maternal disease where active pushing would be harmful, e.g. cardiac disease
- Dural tap.

Criteria for operative vaginal delivery

If an operative vaginal delivery is deemed appropriate, the operator must be confident that delivery will be easily achieved. If there is any doubt, then the procedure should be performed in the operating theatre (trial of instrumental delivery) with a full team present (obstetrician, midwife, anaesthetist and paediatrician) and ready to proceed immediately to caesarean section.

The following criteria must be met before proceeding to operative vaginal delivery, as both forceps and ventouse are potentially dangerous instruments:

- Patient understands and accepts the need for intervention.
- There is a valid indication for expediting delivery.
- Fetus must be in a cephalic presentation and the head not palpable above the pelvic brim (the exception being the use of forceps to aid delivery of the aftercoming head in vaginal breech delivery). On vaginal examination the head must be at or below the level of the ischial spines.
- Cervix must be fully dilated and the membranes ruptured.
- Maternal bladder should be empty.
- There should be no excessive moulding or caput, and the operator must be certain of the position of the fetal head.
- There must be adequate analgesia.

Forceps

The two blades of an obstetric forceps fit around the sides of the fetal head and should easily come together when correctly applied. Non-rotational forceps (e.g. Neville–Barnes, Simpson's or Wrigley's) have a cephalic curve for the head and a pelvic curve to follow the contours of the sacral hollow. Rotational forceps (e.g. Kielland's) do not have a pelvic curve to minimize soft-tissue trauma during rotation to the OA position before traction is applied (Figs 14.8 and 14.9).

Vacuum extractor (ventouse)

This instrument has either a metal or soft cap connected to a handle and then to a suction device that can be controlled either by a hand or foot release device. The cup must be carefully applied to an optimal point on the fetal head and the position checked before the vacuum is commenced. Traction is applied in the correct direction in combination with maternal effort and rotation can occur to the OA position as the head follows the curve of the pelvis during descent. The soft cup is more popular, but metal cups can be used for more difficult deliveries (Fig. 14.10).

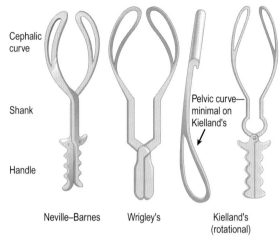

Cephalic
curve

Shank

Handle

Neville–Barnes   Wrigley's   Kielland's
(rotational)

Pelvic curve—
minimal on
Kielland's

Figure 14.8 Types of forceps.

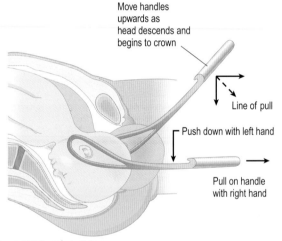

Move handles
upwards as
head descends and
begins to crown

Line of pull

Push down with left hand

Pull on handle
with right hand

Figure 14.9 Forceps technique.

Type of instrumental delivery

The type of instrumental delivery and the choice of instrument depend on the position and descent of the head:

- Low cavity: the head is well below the ischial spines and is usually in the OA position.
- Mid cavity: the head is not palpable abdominally and is at or just below the level of the ischial spines. The head may be in the OA position, but

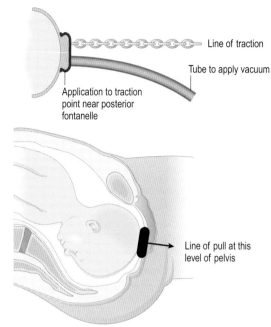

Line of traction

Tube to apply vacuum

Application to traction
point near posterior
fontanelle

Line of pull at this
level of pelvis

Figure 14.10 Ventouse technique.

is more commonly malpositioned in an OT or OP position, which will require rotation. Often these deliveries should be undertaken in theatre, with early recourse to caesarean section if progressive descent is not immediate.

Complications
- Failure to achieve delivery
- Soft-tissue trauma: vaginal lacerations and, in particular, third-degree tears are more common following instrumental delivery (by a factor of eight)
- Fetal trauma: facial bruising or abrasions.

Analgesia
Ideally, the patient should have a functioning epidural or spinal anaesthetic. If a formal block is not available or there is no time because of fetal distress, then local infiltration of the perineum or a pudendal block may be sufficient.

Procedure
The procedure should be performed with the patient in the lithotomy position. Once the operator is satisfied that the criteria have been met then the chosen instrument should be applied to the fetal head using the standard method for that instrument.

Traction should only take place during uterine contractions. The force used should be the minimum required to sustain the advancement of the

Essentials of Obstetrics and Gynaecology

fetal head. Excessive force must not be used under any circumstances. An episiotomy may be required as the perineum is becoming distended to aid with delivery.

A maximum of three uterine contractions should be enough for delivery to be completed, or at the very least imminent with the next contraction. If this is not the case, the procedure should be abandoned and caesarean section performed.

If one instrument fails, another should not be used, the exception being the use of forceps at the end of the procedure following descent and rotation of the head with the aid of the ventouse (Fig. 14.11).

Caesarean section

Caesarean section rates are continuing to rise throughout the world and this is a cause for concern for many, including the World Health Organization. In the developed world, rates of 15–25% are common. The procedure is described later, but is usually performed through a Pfannenstiel incision and an incision through the lower uterine segment. A classical caesarean section is one performed through a vertical upper uterine segment incision.

Indications
- Emergency:
- Fetal distress in the first stage of labour
- Failure to progress in the first stage

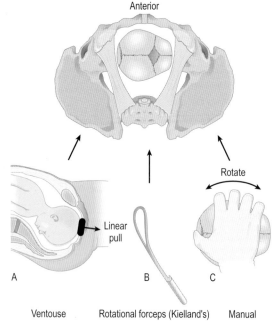

Figure 14.11 Methods of rotation from right occipitotransverse position.

- Either of the above in the second stage if an instrumental delivery is not possible
- Cord prolapse.
- Elective:
- Placenta praevia
- Abnormal lie or malpresentation at term
- Antenatal fetal compromise
- Previous classical caesarean section
- Multiple pregnancy if the presenting fetus is not cephalic
- Relative indications include breech, preterm delivery, various maternal medical disorders, poor obstetric history and, increasingly, maternal request.

Complications
- Haemorrhage
- Infection: although this is less of a problem when prophylactic antibiotics are used
- Thrombosis: less common if anticoagulants are used appropriately in at-risk patients
- Ileus.

Labour following caesarean section
The indication for repeat caesarean section depends on the reason for the first caesarean section and a clear history of that labour is essential in this decision-making. There is little clear evidence on the appropriate choice of delivery for women who have had one previous caesarean section, although most would advise a woman with two previous sections to have caesareans for any future pregnancy. Some obstetricians would advocate the adage 'once a caesarean, always a caesarean'; however, approximately 70% of women with one previous caesarean will achieve a vaginal delivery. Rupture of the uterine scar can occur in up to 0.5% of these women and so a 'trial of labour' must be carefully managed.

Management
- Caution regarding induction of labour. If the cervix is favourable, an ARM may be performed with cautious use of oxytocin, but few would consider administering prostaglandins to ripen the cervix.
- Continuous fetal monitoring should be carried out.
- Epidurals are appropriate.
- Avoid prolonged labours: failure to progress should alert the obstetrician to consider caesarean section. Women with a previous caesarean section who present in spontaneous labour should not have augmentation for slow progress.

Complications
The major complication of 'trial of labour' (or 'trial of scar') is that of scar rupture. This is an obstetric emergency and can be recognized by:
- Evidence of fetal distress
- Scar pain and tenderness
- Vaginal bleeding (and occasionally haematuria)
- Diminished contractions
- Maternal collapse.

In this situation or if there is even suspicion of scar rupture, the woman must be resuscitated (see Chapter 17, unconscious patient) and immediate arrangements made for laparotomy and caesarean section.

PRELABOUR RUPTURE OF MEMBRANES

At term, this occurs in 10% of women and the cause is often unknown. A clear history can be taken from the woman, who characteristically will describe a 'gush' of fluid followed by a continuous trickle. The diagnosis is crucial as many women at term may experience urinary incontinence. Diagnosis can only be made by direct visualization of amniotic fluid draining through the cervix by speculum examination. Ultrasound and the use of nitrazine sticks are of limited benefit.

If rupture of the membranes is suspected, digital examination should be avoided and the diagnosis made using a sterile speculum. A vaginal swab is taken and maternal observations recorded to ensure there is no evidence of infection. Similarly, the fetal heart rate is monitored to assess fetal well-being. The majority of women (80%) will labour within 24–48 hours, and if this is not the case then augmentation of labour is recommended. If there is any evidence of compromise – maternal infection, fetal distress on CTG or meconium – then labour should be augmented immediately.

Preterm prelabour rupture of membranes (PPROM) is defined as rupture of the membranes before labour at less than 37 weeks' gestation. The cause is often unknown, but it occurs in approximately 40% of all preterm labours. The clinical features are similar to the above and similarly the diagnosis is vital, but the management is very different. In PPROM the risks of maternal and fetal infection must be balanced against the risks of prematurity. At gestations of greater than 34 weeks there is little to be gained by waiting and the labour should be induced. However, at gestations before this the management is conservative and the patient is usually admitted for regular monitoring of both herself and the fetus, and steroids administered. The use of prophylactic antibiotics is now accepted in improving perinatal outcome. Management should involve the following:

- Admit patient for observation
- Four-hourly maternal temperature and pulse
- Daily CTG
- Twice-weekly blood tests for white cell count and C-reactive protein
- Weekly or 2-weekly fetal ultrasound assessment
- Can consider allowing patient home to self-monitor with instruction to return if there are any concerns.

Signs of impending infection or chorioamnionitis include:

- Maternal pyrexia
- Maternal leukocytosis or raised C-reactive protein
- Uterine tenderness
- Fetal tachycardia
- Meconium or foul-smelling liquor.

PRETERM LABOUR

This is defined as the delivery of a fetus between 24 and 37 completed weeks of pregnancy.

Low-birth-weight infants are those weighing less than 2500 grams and very-low-birth-weight infants are those weighing less than 1500 grams at delivery.

Incidence

Preterm labour occurs in 5–10% of cases, but a further 5% of labours are complicated by 'threatened' preterm labours that continue on to deliver at term. Although preterm labour accounts for the main cause of perinatal mortality and morbidity, survival rates are improving as neonatal intensive care advances. However, long-term morbidities, like cerebral palsy, blindness and lung disease, are common in this group of infants.

Aetiology

The pathophysiological processes involved in preterm labour are still unknown, although much research is ongoing and various factors, described below, have been shown to have an association.

Maternal

- Infection (e.g. urinary tract)
- Chorioamnionitis
- Antepartum haemorrhage
- Pre-eclampsia
- Polyhydramnios
- Uterine abnormalities like cervical incompetence.

Fetal

- Intrauterine growth retardation
- Congenital abnormality
- Intrauterine death
- Multiple pregnancy.

Other risk factors include maternal age <20 years, maternal smoking and low socioeconomic group. However, the greatest risk factor for preterm labour is a previous preterm labour.

Maternal genital tract infection has been linked to preterm labour, in particular with the organisms *Trichomonas vaginalis* and *Chlamydia trachomatis*, or infection with bacterial vaginosis. Recent trials have shown benefit in the use of prophylactic antibiotics in women with bacterial vaginosis demonstrated on a high vaginal swab.

Assessment

A correct diagnosis of labour is just as important in preterm patients:

- History and examination will include precipitating factors and cervical assessment.
- Ensure accurate dating information regarding gestation.
- CTG to assess fetal well-being and uterine activity.
- Ultrasound assessment to confirm fetal well-being, exclude fetal abnormality, estimate fetal weight and confirm presentation.

Management

1. Steroids to promote fetal lung maturity: glucocorticoids administered by injection to the mother 24 hours before delivery have been shown to reduce perinatal mortality and morbidity by promoting lung maturity in babies born between 24 and 34 weeks. There is at present no evidence to suggest that repeated doses are of any benefit.
2. Tocolysis: tocolytics act by inhibiting uterine smooth-muscle contractility. The most common agents used are the beta-sympathomimetics like ritodrine and salbutamol given as an infusion intravenously. This delays rather than stops preterm labour, to allow administered steroids to have an effect or if the mother needs to be transferred due to inadequate neonatal facilities being available. Tocolysis is contraindicated in cases with ruptured membranes or following an antepartum haemorrhage and should be used with caution with careful maternal monitoring as these infusions have significant side effects, including tremor, anxiety, tachycardia and pulmonary oedema.

3. Delivery: adequate neonatal care facilities must be available to ensure optimum outcome, otherwise an in-utero transfer should be arranged. Vaginal delivery is usually recommended for preterm delivery, especially if there is a cephalic presentation. Mode of delivery of a breech presentation is controversial, but again can be safely carried out vaginally in the care of an experienced obstetrician. Instrumental delivery is conducted for the usual reasons, but the ventouse is contraindicated in fetuses of less than 34 weeks' gestation, because of possible risk of injury to the immature fetal head and intracranial haemorrhage.

PAIN RELIEF IN LABOUR

Labour is painful, although each woman's response to labour is different, as is each individual woman's experience with her own previous labours.

A woman's expectation of pain can be greatly diminished by carefully addressing her fears and giving precise, accurate and relevant information on the options for pain relief in labour.

Causes of labour pain

- Stretching of the cervix during dilatation
- Ischaemia of the uterine muscular wall during labour
- Stretching of the vagina and perineum during the second stage.

Self-help and natural sources (non-pharmacological methods)

Increasing numbers of women use non-pharmacological methods to maintain control of their labour. An important feature of any labour is the removal of anxiety and the support of a trusted companion and this can be emphasized in the antenatal class:

- Relaxation: being aware of physical tension and being able to relax consciously both during and between contractions helps to reduce pain.
- Changing position and moving: many women find pelvic rocking and other rhythmic movements help with pain.
- Massage can be a great aid to localized pain in the lower back, hips and thighs.
- Music: this can be both relaxing and a distraction from the pain of contractions.
- Warm baths or showers: many women find warm water very soothing, especially in early labour, and some professionals may advocate the options of a water birth in low-risk pregnancies.
- Natural therapies include acupuncture, aromatherapy, herbal remedies, homeopathy and hypnotherapy and many women find these helpful during labour. A properly qualified practitioner must be consulted.
- Transcutaneous electrical nerve stimulation (TENS) consists of a machine which sends small electrical impulses between four electrodes taped to the woman's back. The woman controls the strength of the impulses by turning a small dial. It reduces pain by interfering with the pain messages to the brain and also by increasing the production of the woman's endorphins (natural painkillers). Women are advised to start using TENS in early labour as the pain-relieving effect is built up over time.

Pharmacological methods of pain relief

Entonox is a premixed 50% oxygen/50% nitrous oxide gas that is self-administered and is available in all delivery suites. Entonox has a short half-life, but is safe for both mother and fetus. It is important to educate the woman beforehand as to the correct use of Entonox. Ideally, she should take deep inspirations of the gas at the onset of the contraction and not at the peak of the contraction pain to allow adequate analgesia.

Pethidine is usually administered as an intramuscular injection of between 50 and 150 mg. It generally works within 20 minutes, but many women become nauseous so it is often given in conjunction with an anti-emetic like metoclopramide 10 mg. It may be administered 4–6-hourly, but it is rare that more than two doses are required. It does cross the placenta, causing reduced variability in the fetal heart rate, and, if given within 4 hours of delivery will cause significant respiratory depression in the neonate. If this occurs, then the narcotic antagonist naloxone should be given to the neonate.

Epidural analgesia provides the most effective form of pain relief in labour and is becoming a more popular choice with most women. The epidural space is the potential space lying outside the dura mater. Injection of local anaesthetic into this space will produce analgesia in the spinal nerve roots (Fig. 14.12). The nerve roots T10–L1 need to be targeted to give adequate analgesia during the first stage of labour and

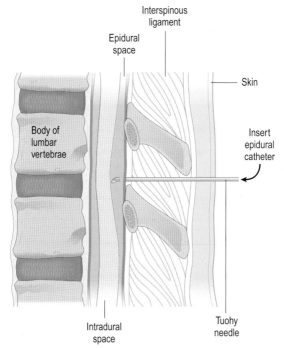

Figure 14.12 Insertion of epidural needle.

the sacral nerve roots for the second stage. A more extensive block to T8 will be required for caesarean sections. To administer an epidural, an indwelling plastic catheter is introduced into the epidural space (usually at L2–3 or L3–4) through a needle with a curved tip (Tuohy needle). The local anaesthetic usually administered is bupivacaine, but this causes motor blockade so that more often it is given in combination with the opioid fentanyl, to good effect. This mixture is becoming more popular as it can allow the woman limited mobility with effective analgesia. After an initial test dose, the analgesia can be topped up periodically as required or an infusion pump can be commenced. Contraindications to epidurals include:

- Coagulopathy: this may cause haemorrhage into the epidural space. This may be a particular problem in pre-eclampsia
- Recent antepartum haemorrhage: epidural analgesia may be associated with a profound hypotensive episode, especially in the presence of haemorrhage
- Sepsis at the potential site for epidural
- Spinal abnormalities
- Active neurological disease
- Allergy to local anaesthetic.

Complications of epidurals include the following:

- Dural tap is the inadvertent puncture of the dura and occurs in less than 1% of cases, but will cause a severe postural headache. It can be eased by application of a blood patch where a small sample of autologous blood is injected into the epidural space, which clots and forms a patch to prevent further leakage of cerebrospinal fluid.
- Hypotensive episodes can cause maternal and fetal distress. If this occurs, an infusion of 1l Hartmann's or saline over 20 minutes will generally correct the hypotension.
- Total spinal block can occur if the local anaesthetic is injected into the intrathecal space. It results in marked hypotension, bradycardia and respiratory distress that may lead to apnoea. It must be quickly recognized and the patient may need to be ventilated.

Spinal analgesia is becoming increasingly common for caesarean section, for instrumental delivery or manual removal of the placenta. The local anaesthetic is administered into the cerebrospinal fluid with rapid onset of action and effective analgesia for about 2 hours. The injection is administered with the patient in the sitting position to minimize cephalad spread of the anaesthetic.

Lidocaine (nerve block) can be injected locally for perineal infiltration prior to episiotomy or instrumental delivery. Alternatively, lidocaine can be used for pudendal block by injecting it at the site where the pudendal nerve passes around the ischial spine (Fig. 14.13).

General anaesthesia is still used for 'crash' caesarean sections and in other cases where regional block is not available. However, regional anaesthesia is eight times safer because of the risk of airway problems and aspiration associated with general anaesthesia. To reduce the risk of aspiration most units would advocate the administration of H_2-receptor blocking drugs every 6 hours in labour in case a general anaesthetic is required.

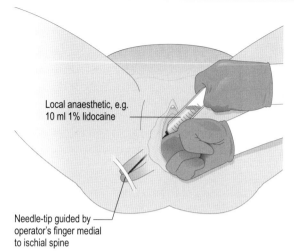

Local anaesthetic, e.g.
10 ml 1% lidocaine

Needle-tip guided by
operator's finger medial
to ischial spine

Figure 14.13 Pudendal block.

SUMMARY

- Primiparous and multiparous labours are very different clinical entities.
- Partograms are important in the assessment of the progress of labour.
- Every labour has a different level of risk and the extent of fetal monitoring should be tailored around this, although many units rely on continuous monitoring for all patients.
- Current methods of intrapartum fetal monitoring are still unreliable and should be used in conjunction with fetal blood sampling.
- The decision to induce labour must be carefully weighted against the risk to both mother and fetus of prolonging the pregnancy.
- Induced labour has a higher incidence of operative delivery compared with spontaneous labours.
- Instrumental deliveries should only be performed for appropriate reasons, using the appropriate instrument and by a skilled practitioner.
- Preterm labour is a major cause of perinatal mortality and morbidity.

The puerperium **15**

CHAPTER CONTENTS

DEFINITION

The puerperium is the time during which physiology and anatomy return to normal after pregnancy. It is usually quoted as starting at delivery of the placenta and ending after 6 weeks, but puerperal problems may in fact present up to 6 months after the birth.

Physiological and anatomical changes in the puerperium include:
- Reduction in cardiac output
- Lowering of respiratory rate
- Loss of the hypercoagulable state
- Return of hormone levels to the normal range
- Involution of the uterus, cervix and vagina
- Lactation.

NORMAL POSTNATAL EVENTS

Lochia

Lochia is the bloody discharge lost from the uterus after delivery, which gradually becomes serosanguineous. It may continue for up to 6 weeks. Any offensive smell or fresh blood loss after the first few days should be investigated for possible infection (endometritis) or retained products of conception (RPOC).

Uterine involution

The uterus is usually at the level of the umbilicus after delivery. It is no longer palpable in the abdomen at 2 weeks and has returned to the prepregnancy size within 6 weeks of delivery.

Sexual intercourse

There is no evidence about when sexual intercourse may be resumed after delivery, but endometritis may be more common from sexual intercourse soon after delivery and it is generally recommended to avoid intercourse for 3 weeks or so.

Many couples do not resume sexual intercourse for weeks or months after delivery. Factors inhibiting intercourse include tiredness, pain from perineal or caesarean section wounds, vaginal bleeding and fear after childbirth.

Breastfeeding

Physiology

In pregnancy, progesterone stimulates proliferation of the alveoli and breast enlargement. Oestrogen causes darkening of the areola and an increase in the number of lactiferous ducts. At delivery, prolactin acts on the alveoli to initiate lactation and sucking further stimulates this. Colostrum, a high-protein, low-volume fluid is released initially and at day 2–3 milk ejection occurs in response to oxytocin.

The advantages of breastfeeding for the baby are:

- Reduced diarrhoea
- Reduced respiratory infection
- Reduced otitis media
- Reduced necrotizing enterocolitis
- Mildly increased IQ
- Half the risk of eczema
- Half the risk of juvenile-onset diabetes mellitus.

The advantages for the mother are:

- Reduced incidence of osteoporosis
- Reduced breast cancer
- Reduced ovarian cancer
- Bonding with the baby.

It is important to encourage breastfeeding as the ideal, although one third of women do not breastfeed at all. This is particularly common if the woman was not breastfed herself, or if her partner does not actively support her breastfeeding.

A small number of women are unable to breastfeed for the following reasons:

- Inverted nipples (2% incidence), which do not evert with attempts at breastfeeding
- Medications that are transmitted into breast milk and harmful to the baby
- Maternal human immunodeficiency virus (HIV) infection
- Inability to establish breastfeeding
- Some types of breast surgery
- Neonatal problems, such as cleft palate.

These women may feel stigmatized by their inability to give their baby 'the best' type of feeding.

Inability to establish feeding

Many women have difficulty breastfeeding. This may have various causes, such as an irritable and hungry baby, tired mother, dehydration, pain or anaemia. Some women find breastfeeding embarrassing, physically repellent or have anxiety about their ability to produce milk. The mother should be assessed for exacerbating factors and the baby reviewed if it is crying excessively or sleepy. Otherwise, management involves consideration of positioning of the baby, reassurance and emotional support, ideally with a specialist breastfeeding counsellor. When the baby is properly attached it should have the whole areola in the mouth (not just the nipple) and the jaw should be seen moving as the baby sucks. Women also need an adequate fluid and calorie intake and rest.

Postnatal visits

Community midwives visit women at home until at least 10 days postpartum. If there are no specific obstetric problems then care is handed over to the health visitor and general practitioner (GP). If there are ongoing obstetric issues, the midwife may continue to visit for up to 1 month following delivery.

Postnatal check

The postnatal check at 6 weeks is usually carried out by a GP. Obstetric input is needed in circumstances such as severe pre-eclampsia, third-degree tear or traumatic delivery.

A history should be taken to establish:

- General well-being
- Whether the lochia has stopped
- Whether there are any breastfeeding difficulties
- If the woman has any urinary or bowel symptoms, specifically incontinence
- The mental state of the woman. Is there anxiety or depression? How is her relationship with the baby?
- If sexual intercourse has resumed, what contraception is being used? Are there any sexual difficulties?
- If a cervical smear is due.

Examination is only carried out if indicated by the history. For example, the perineum may need to be inspected if there is continued pain from a tear or episiotomy.

Contraception

All postnatal women should be given appropriate contraception advice within the first few postnatal days. Factors to consider are previous contraceptive history, wishes for further fertility, age, smoking, weight, breastfeeding and medical problems. Ovulation can occur within 3 weeks of delivery so contraception is essential, especially in non-breastfeeding women:

- The progesterone-only pill is safe with breastfeeding and can be started immediately.
- The combined oral contraceptive pill reduces the quality and quantity of breast milk and is, therefore, contraindicated in lactating women. It should also be avoided for 6 weeks after delivery in non-lactating women due to the increased risk of thrombosis.
- Intrauterine contraceptive devices and the levonorgestrel-releasing intrauterine system can be fitted at 6 weeks postpartum, after uterine involution.

Essentials of Obstetrics and Gynaecology

- Injectable progestogens are safe with breastfeeding, but should be delayed until 6 weeks postpartum, because of risks of erratic bleeding.
- Full breastfeeding is effective contraception for at least 6 months, as long as no formula supplements are given and the woman remains amenorrhoeic.
- Condoms can be used at any time after delivery.

Further information on contraception options is given in Chapter 9.

PROBLEMS IN THE PUERPERIUM

Breast engorgement

The breasts become full and tense on the third to fourth days, resulting in pain, discomfort and mild pyrexia. The management is a tight-fitting bra, paracetamol and continuation of feeding.

Cracked nipples

These are extremely painful and may bleed. Correction of the baby's position, oral analgesia and camomile cream should be tried.

Mastitis and breast abscess

Mastitis is an infection of the lactiferous ducts and occurs in 5% of lactating women. It may be secondary to cracked nipples or to a blocked duct. The common organisms are *Staphylococcus aureus*, *S. epidermidis* and streptococci. The symptoms are pain, fever and malaise or anorexia and signs of redness, swelling and tenderness may be present. Breast milk can be cultured for identity and sensitivity of the organism. Treatment is with fluids, analgesia and antibiotics (flucloxacillin or erythromycin) with continuation of feeding.

Mastitis can develop into an abscess with increased pain and a localized fluctuant swelling. Treatment is repeat aspiration, ideally under ultrasound guidance, and antibiotics. Incision and drainage are rarely indicated. Breastfeeding from that breast should be avoided until resolution, but the woman should continue to express and discard milk to maintain lactation during recovery.

Headache

Headache is commonly caused by:

- Tiredness
- Hypertension
- Anaemia
- Stress.

Intracranial pathology, for example from cerebrovascular accident or meningitis, is very rare. However, a severe headache may occur from cerebrospinal fluid leakage during epidural insertion.

A full examination should include temperature, pulse and blood pressure; meningism and gross neurological signs should be excluded. Blood pressure and full blood count should always be checked.

Treatment of the cause may include iron for anaemia or treatment of hypertension. Where possible, tiredness should be managed with support in caring for the baby.

Constipation

Constipation may occur from the pregnancy hormone effect, dehydration, altered diet, breastfeeding, the progesterone-only pill or due to pain from a tear or sutures. Management involves high-fibre diet, fluids and laxatives.

Hair loss

Women commonly lose hair between 4 and 20 weeks postpartum. This is caused by an increased proportion of hairs entering the telogen (resting) phase in pregnancy. Recovery usually occurs within 6 months.

Postpartum pyrexia

Aetiology
- Labour
- Breast engorgement
- Mastitis
- Breast abscess
- Urinary tract infection
- Endometritis
- Wound infection
- Respiratory tract infection
- Haematoma (pelvic or vulval)
- Venous thromboembolism.

Assessment

The history may reveal the likely source of pyrexia, such as heavy bleeding with endometritis or cough with infection.

A full examination includes checking the lungs for evidence of infection, the breasts for engorgement or mastitis, the abdomen for a tender boggy uterus, the perineum for haematoma or infection and the legs for calf tenderness.

Full blood count, blood culture, vaginal swabs and midstream urine should always be sent. A chest X-ray should also be requested in the presence of chest signs or symptoms.

Treatment

Treatment of the pyrexia depends on the cause. Mild pyrexia in labour is common, especially after prostaglandin induction, and should be investigated only if persistent for more than a few hours after delivery or if the temperature exceeds 37.5°C.

Perineal wound problems

Twenty-three per cent of women report discomfort 10 days after normal vaginal delivery and 66% 10 days after instrumental delivery.

Women with perineal tears or sutures should be advised:

- To take analgesia (paracetamol and non-steroidal anti-inflammatories) as needed, for up to 2 weeks
- To keep the area clean by regular bathing or showering, without soap
- To dry the area with a clean towel or cool hairdryer
- To observe for signs of infection (increased swelling or pain, offensive discharge)
- That the sutures dissolve spontaneously over a few weeks and stitch debris may be seen during this time.

Examination prior to discharge should check for signs of wound dehiscence, haematoma or infection. Occasionally, women feel one or two sutures are particularly 'tight'. In such circumstances individual sutures can be divided 1 week after delivery without compromising healing.

Perineal wound dehiscence is rare and should generally be treated conservatively with wound hygiene and antibiotics if there are signs of infection. Revision of the perineum can be arranged after 6–8 weeks if necessary for perineal deficiency. Haematomas are also managed conservatively with antibiotics and analgesia. Surgical drainage is indicated only where an abscess has developed or the haematoma is increasing in size. Infected perineal wounds should be swabbed and treated with a broad-spectrum antibiotic with anaerobic cover.

Postpartum haemorrhage (PPH)

Definitions

Primary PPH is the loss of more than 500 ml blood in the first 24 hours after delivery. Secondary PPH is the loss of more than 500 ml blood more than 24 hours after delivery. PPH occurs in around 5% of deliveries.

Aetiology

Primary PPH may occur because of uterine atony, vaginal or cervical trauma, retained placental tissue, sepsis or clotting abnormality (e.g. disseminated intravascular coagulation).

Secondary PPH is almost always due to sepsis, RPOC, or both.

Risk factors for PPH include high parity, antepartum haemorrhage in this pregnancy, PPH in a previous pregnancy, placental abruption, placenta praevia and uterine fibroids.

The incidence of PPH may be reduced by routine administration of oxytocin and ergometrine at the delivery of the baby, and by delivery of the placenta by controlled cord traction ('active management of the third stage').

Assessment

Women may show signs of hypovolaemic shock with reduced level of consciousness when profuse haemorrhage occurs. Less severe bleeding may still be associated with signs of anaemia or tachycardia. Speculum and bimanual examination may reveal retained products in the os, an open cervical os or a large, boggy uterus. An assessment should also be made for cervical or vaginal sources of bleeding, under epidural, spinal or general anaesthetic if necessary.

Women should all have full blood count and either serum save or blood crossmatch, depending on the amount of blood loss.

Management

PPH is an emergency and management is covered in Chapter 17.

Endometritis

Postpartum endometritis is still a potential cause of serious morbidity and mortality. Common organisms are *Streptococcus* and anaerobic bacteria. Endometritis is more common after caesarean section than vaginal delivery.

Assessment

Presentation may be with bleeding, offensive discharge, abdominal pain, fever, general malaise or anorexia. Clinical signs are fever, excessive vaginal bleeding, abdominal tenderness, bimanual uterine tenderness and a poorly contracted, soft uterus. High vaginal and endocervical swabs and blood cultures should be sent urgently, with full blood count and C-reactive protein.

Treatment with oral antibiotics should be commenced until the culture results are available. Severe infections should be treated with intravenous antibiotics (for example, clindamycin and gentamicin), fluids and careful haemodynamic monitoring. 'Puerperal sepsis' is a historically important cause of maternal death. Aggressive treatment and monitoring are essential to prevent such severe infection.

Retained products of conception

RPOC may consist of small placental fragments or a whole placental lobe. RPOC may not necessarily be suspected when the placenta is inspected after delivery, especially if the retained lobe is a succenturiate lobe, that is, an accessory or 'satellite' lobe, separate from the main body of the placenta.

Clinical features

Women present with bleeding either as continued fresh loss or as a sudden PPH up to 2 weeks after delivery. Bleeding may be very heavy with haemodynamic compromise. RPOC also predisposes to secondary infection, which may be subclinical or be evident as overt sepsis.

Pyrexia, tachycardia, hypotension and anaemia may be found on general examination. Speculum may reveal an open cervical os and bimanual examination may reveal a soft, bulky uterus.

Investigation

Full blood count, C-reactive protein and vaginal swabs should be taken. Transvaginal ultrasound scan should be performed to confirm the diagnosis of RPOC. Interpretation of the findings may be difficult in the first 5 days postpartum as RPOC may be difficult to differentiate from blood clot.

Management

Antibiotics should be commenced immediately and blood or fluid replacement given as indicated. Evacuation of retained products should normally be delayed until antibiotics have been administered for at least 24 hours. This reduces the risk of haemorrhage at operation.

Urinary retention

Acute urinary retention may occur after delivery where there has been:

- Failure to catheterize a woman with a dense epidural
- Failure to check for bladder emptying within 8 hours of delivery
- Lack of sensation to pass urine after spinal or epidural for caesarean section or other obstetric surgical procedure
- Urinary tract infection
- Inhibition of voiding due to a painful perineum.

Assessment

Symptoms of suprapubic discomfort and the need to pass urine may be present, but some women are unaware of a full bladder and are falsely reassured by passing frequent very small volumes of urine. The full bladder is usually palpable on examination, though tenderness postpartum and the large uterus make examination difficult.

Management

A Foley urethral catheter should be inserted and residual volume checked. If the residual is moderate (<1000 ml), then a trial without catheter can be performed after 24 hours. For severe retention (residual >1000 ml) the catheter should be left for 3–5 days to allow full recovery. Failure to pass good urinary volumes after a trial without catheter necessitates a suprapubic catheter for 10 days and urogynaecological review.

Midstream urine should be sent for culture to exclude infection.

Stress urinary incontinence

Stress incontinence symptoms (the involuntary loss of urine with increases in intra-abdominal pressure) occur in up to 40% of women after delivery. From 3% to 12% of women still report symptoms 6 months after delivery.

The mechanism is a combination of mechanical injury, denervation and ischaemic damage. It is more common after vaginal delivery, but can still occur with caesarean section (8%). Other risk factors are pre-existing incontinence, prolonged second stage, assisted vaginal delivery, episiotomy, high birth weight and multiparity.

Assessment

Examination may be normal or reveal uterovaginal prolapse. Midstream urine sample should be sent to exclude infection.

Management

Pelvic floor exercises, taught by a physiotherapist, are effective if performed both antenatally and postnatally, but the benefit of weighted vaginal cones and electrical biofeedback is unclear. A proportion of women will remain incontinent and may need surgical treatment, usually after completion of their family.

Faecal incontinence

Vaginal delivery is the primary cause of faecal incontinence in women. Symptoms include flatus incontinence, faecal urgency and stool incontinence. The incidence of incontinence varies from 11% to 35% after the first delivery, and from 3% to 12% after subsequent deliveries. Recognized third-degree tears only occur in 3% of deliveries, but occult injury can be seen on endoanal ultrasound in up to 36% of women. Of women with occult injury on ultrasound, only a third have symptoms of incontinence.

Risk factors for faecal incontinence are recognized third-degree perineal tear, high birth weight, forceps delivery, prolonged second stage and persistent occipitoposterior position.

Initial management is conservative with pelvic floor exercises. Referral to a colorectal surgeon should be made if symptoms persist, for consideration of secondary repair of the anal sphincter.

Postpartum thyroiditis

Postpartum thyroiditis occurs in 5% of women, usually 3–4 months postpartum. Antithyroid antibodies cause destruction of the gland, with an initial increase in release of thyroxine followed by a decrease. Hypothyroidism, hyperthyroidism or both may occur, with typical symptoms. However, some women are asymptomatic and symptoms in others may be dismissed as related to the pregnancy and puerperium.

Investigations may reveal increased or decreased thyroid hormones.

Most cases (97%) resolve spontaneously but symptomatic treatment may be needed with beta-blockers or thyroxine, depending on the presentation.

Puerperal cardiomyopathy

Puerperal cardiomyopathy is a dilated cardiomyopathy with presentation from 1 month before to 6 months after delivery. The severity of disease is variable, but some women have severe sudden onset of symptoms, with a high mortality. Other women have a slower, less serious course of disease.

Diagnosis is made on a combination of clinical findings and echocardiography. Treatment is supportive with diuretics and occasionally inotropes. In most women recovery is spontaneous, but this may take a few months. Some women continue to have impaired cardiac function.

Recurrence is common and women are generally advised to avoid future pregnancies.

PSYCHOLOGICAL, EMOTIONAL AND PSYCHOSEXUAL PROBLEMS IN THE PUERPERIUM

Many women find the emotional experience difficult during the puerperium. Contributing factors are:

- Sleep disturbance and tiredness
- Physical pain or discomfort from perineal or caesarean wounds
- Lack of control over the baby's sleep or crying
- Dependence of the baby and lack of freedom
- Change in self-image from partner or lover to mother
- Fear of sexual intercourse due to perineal pain or memory of delivery
- Concerns about body image, lax perineum or weight changes
- Relationship difficulties.

Management involves a careful investigation of the underlying feelings and contributing factors. Counselling and reassurance are generally effective, but women with persistent symptoms should be referred for formal psychosexual or psychological counselling, after addressing the physical factors such as sleep problems.

Postpartum psychiatric illness

Postpartum blues

'Postpartum blues' is a normal feature in about half of postnatal women, commonly occurring from the third postpartum day. Features include tearfulness, anxiety, fatigue, irritability, feeling unable to cope and concern about the baby's well-being. Symptoms may be exacerbated by a difficult delivery, tiredness, difficulty caring for the baby, for example because of pain, and fear about going home with the baby. Symptoms resolve spontaneously within a few days.

Postpartum depression

Postpartum depression occurs in 10% of women. Features are persistent low mood and crying, anxiety about their own or their baby's health, guilt or feeling unable to cope with caring for the baby. Panic attacks, excessive tiredness, poor appetite and poor concentration may also occur. Onset may be from a few days to 6 months after delivery, with the commonest presentation at about 3 months.

Management

Risk of self-harm, suicide or harm to the baby must be assessed urgently. Thereafter, management is with the health visitor, GP, community psychiatric team and psychologist. Family and social support is important. Counselling and antidepressants are the main treatments. Progesterone and oestrogen treatments have not been shown to be effective. Antidepressants are not licensed for breastfeeding, but do not appear to cause harm and breastfeeding is usually continued unless there are signs of drowsiness or irritability in the baby.

Postpartum psychosis

Postpartum psychosis occurs in 1 in 500 women. Clinical features are delusions, hallucinations and impaired perception of reality, with onset within 6 weeks of delivery, usually within the first few days. Some women report delusional ideas relating to their baby, such as their baby is evil or that the baby will be harmed by themselves or someone else. Some women are manic with rapid speech, pressure of speech and feelings of power. Sleep may be minimal. Predisposing factors are a family history of psychotic illness (in 30%), a previous personal history of mental illness, absence of social or partner support, traumatic delivery and age over 30 years.

Management

Psychiatric referral and assessment of the safety of the baby are needed immediately. The baby may be at risk from direct harm or from neglect due to the illness. Treatment with antidepressants or antipsychotics is usually indicated. Severe cases may need sedation, for example with haloperidol or chlorpromazine. Electroconvulsive therapy is used occasionally where the woman is in a psychotic stupor and not eating or drinking.

Prognosis

Recovery usually takes 4–8 weeks, with 15% recurrence in the next pregnancy. There is also a 30% incidence of a repeat psychotic episode outside pregnancy.

SUMMARY

- Lochia may continue for up to 6 weeks but any offensive smell or fresh bleeding after the first few days should be investigated.
- Breastfeeding confers significant advantages to the mother and baby but care should be taken to avoid stigmatization of women who are unable to breastfeed.
- Contraception advice should be given prior to hospital discharge and at the 6-week postnatal check.
- Postnatal depression occurs in 10% of women and is distinct from 'postpartum blues', which only lasts a few days.
- Puerperal sepsis is still associated with serious maternal morbidity and mortality and should always be investigated and treated aggressively.
- Voiding after delivery, after removal of a urinary catheter and after an epidural or spinal anaesthetic should be ensured to minimize the risk of urinary retention and its consequences.

Neonatal medicine 16

CHAPTER CONTENTS

ATTENDANCE OF PAEDIATRICIAN AT DELIVERY

Approximately 70% of babies requiring resuscitation are born following a complicated pregnancy or labour. Attendance of a paediatrician should be anticipated in the following situations:

- Preterm delivery (<37 weeks' gestation)
- Malpresentations (e.g. breech)
- Fetal distress or in the presence of meconium
- Instrumental delivery or caesarean section
- Multiple pregnancy
- Antenatal fetal abnormality
- Rhesus incompatibility
- Maternal narcotic analgesia.

CARE OF THE NORMAL BABY FOLLOWING DELIVERY

Umbilical cord

The umbilical cord should be clamped once the baby has been delivered by replacing the forceps that may have been used at delivery with a sterile clamp.

Temperature control

The newborn infant is at significant risk of hypothermia because of its impaired ability to increase metabolic rate after delivery. There is a natural heat loss, which is exacerbated by a baby's high surface area to volume ratio. Hypothermia will also worsen hypoxia and acidosis and induce respiratory distress.

Vitamin K

Vitamin K is essential for the coagulation pathways so a deficiency, as may occur in breastfed babies, may result in haemorrhagic disease of the newborn. Vitamin K deficiency may also occur in premature infants, small babies or babies who are unable to feed sufficiently. Maternal liver disease, drug abuse, or mothers on anticonvulsant or antituberculous medication are more likely to lead to babies with this problem.

Vitamin K as a single intramuscular administration at birth will prevent this disease.

CARE ON THE POSTNATAL WARD

General care takes place on the postnatal ward. The cord stump should be cleaned daily with soap and water. Vernix, dried blood and meconium can be cleaned soon after birth, but the first bath can be delayed until the following day. Routine observations on the postnatal ward include temperature, heart rate, respiratory rate, bladder and bowel activity, and weight.

Temperature and heart rate

Abnormal temperature (>38 °C or <35.5 °C) or a tachycardia (>160 bpm) that lasts longer than 1 hour is cause for concern and could indicate sepsis.

Respiratory rate

A normal rate is ≤60 breaths per minute. Other than sepsis, the common cause of tachypnoea is transient tachypnoea of the newborn. This is attributed to a build-up of fetal lung fluid, particularly following caesarean section in the absence of labour, and has characteristic chest X-ray appearances. It is diagnosed only after other causes of respiratory distress have been excluded, especially infection. The common causes of respiratory distress in the term baby include:

- Infection – this commonly includes group B β-haemolytic streptococcus, *Escherichia coli, Staphylococcus aureus, Listeria monocytogenes, Klebsiella, Enterobacter* and *Streptococcus pneumoniae*
- Meconium aspiration
- Spontaneous pneumothorax
- Severe anaemia
- Central nervous system depression, especially after birth asphyxia
- Cardiac failure
- Metabolic disease with acidosis
- Transient tachypnoea of the newborn
- Congenital anomalies, including causes of upper airway obstruction like goitre, tracheo-oesophageal fistula, diaphragmatic hernia and pulmonary agenesis.

Respiratory distress should be treated as neonatal sepsis until proven otherwise – usually group B streptococcal infection.

Other signs of respiratory distress include grunting; central cyanosis; subcostal, intercostal and sternal recession.

Blood sugar levels

Small and premature babies have different nutritional needs from larger babies and are more prone to hypoglycaemia. If feeding poorly, 3-hourly assessment of blood glucose (before a feed) should be performed. Signs of impending hypoglycaemia include lethargy, irritability, apnoea and fitting. Healthy term babies do not routinely need blood glucose assessment.

Bladder and bowel activity

Failure to pass urine is rare and is associated with palpable kidneys or bladder. Poor stream or dribbling in male infants may be associated with posterior urethral valves.

Meconium is the green/black stool passed in the first 2–3 days after delivery. This changes colour depending on the type of feeding: yellow/mustard and soft with breastfeeding and a firmer yellow/brown stool with bottle-feeding. A delay in passing meconium may indicate intestinal obstruction or Hirschsprung's disease. Pale stools in a jaundiced baby may indicate obstructive jaundice and extrahepatic biliary atresia should be excluded.

Weight

Babies can lose up to 10% of their birth weight in the first few days of life. As feeding becomes established, birth weight should be reached within the first week and thereafter the baby should gain 20–30 grams a day until 6 months of age.

Feeding

Breastfeeding is becoming more popular and is advised as it has been shown to reduce the risk of gastrointestinal and respiratory infections in term babies as well as necrotizing enterocolitis in premature babies. Human milk has the following advantages:

- It contains the maternal factors that reduce infection in babies:
  - plasma immunoglobulins
  - lysozyme (a bactericidal enzyme)
  - lactoferrin, which competes with bacteria for iron in the gut, thereby inhibiting growth of bacteria, e.g. *E. coli*
  - antiviral agents, like interferon
  - antibacterial agents, such as macrophages, lymphocytes, neutrophils, cytokines, complement.
- The water, fat and protein mix varies throughout a feed to give a balanced diet.
- It lessens the risk of cows' milk intolerance.
- It is associated with a lower risk of sudden infant death syndrome.
- It is cheap and convenient.

In spite of these advantages, breastfeeding is contraindicated in severe maternal systemic disease, maternal human immunodeficiency virus (HIV) infection, or if the mother is taking drugs that may be secreted in the milk (always check in the drug formulary):

- Anticoagulants
- Antibiotics, e.g. chloramphenicol, metronidazole, isoniazid, tetracyclines, trimethoprim
- Antiarrhythmics, e.g. atenolol, amiodarone
- Anti-inflammatories, e.g. indometacin
- Antidepressants, e.g. lithium, doxepin
- Antimalarials, e.g. dapsone preparations
- Antimigraine, e.g. ergotamine
- Immunosuppressives.

Breastfeeding babies will feed on demand and will self-regulate their intake.

Examination of the newborn

All babies should be thoroughly examined at delivery and also before discharge from hospital. Initial complete inspection of the infant in a cot will provide much information, such as colour (cyanosis or pallor), posture (complete movement and tone), abnormal morphological features and evidence of respiratory distress.

Skin abnormalities

- Milia: These are tiny sebaceous retention cysts that look like small white spots and are mainly found over the nose.
- Erythema toxicum (neonatorum): This very common diffuse erythematous rash often occurs in the first week of life, is harmless and is of uncertain cause.
- Vascular naevi: These include capillary haemangiomata, which produce pale pink patches on the neck, forehead and eyelids (often referred to as 'stork marks') and gradually fade away. In contrast, port-wine stains are larger and darker.

Jaundice

Physiological jaundice often occurs within the first 5 days, occurring 24–48 hours after delivery, peaking at day 4, and is due to:

- Shortened lifespan of fetal erythrocytes, resulting in increased breakdown as well as liver enzyme immaturity
- Hepatic immaturity.

However, jaundice is abnormal if it occurs in the first 24 hours after birth or lasts beyond 14 days. The most common causes for onset within 24 hours of birth include: erythrocyte haemolysis due to incompatibility, e.g. Rhesus, ABO or other blood group; infection; and excessive erythrocyte breakdown because of bleeding, e.g. cephalohaematoma or infection.

This excess haemolysis results in an unconjugated hyperbilirubinaemia in the baby with the potential for kernicterus. Guidelines are available to determine management options depending on level of unconjugated bilirubin, gestational age of baby and weight. Kernicterus has serious implications, including cerebral palsy, deafness and death. Unconjugated hyperbilirubinaemia usually after haemolysis can be treated with either phototherapy or, in more extreme cases, with intravenous immunoglobulin or exchange transfusion.

Routine investigations include:

- Full blood count, reticulocyte count and blood film
- Maternal and baby blood group
- Coombs' test
- Urine for culture
- Full infection screen, depending on status of the baby, may be considered, including blood and cerebrospinal fluid for culture.

If baby fails to respond, then investigate further for rarer causes.

The most common cause for prolonged jaundice in the newborn (> 14 days) is breastfeeding. However, other more serious causes like biliary atresia must be excluded. Breast milk jaundice is characterized by a raised unconjugated hyperbilirubinaemia, whereas in biliary atresia the conjugated bilirubin levels are raised. Biliary atresia can be corrected with surgery to the biliary obstruction to prevent chronic liver damage. Other causes of prolonged jaundice include:

- Hypothyroidism
- Galactosaemia

- Viral hepatitis
- Glucose-6-phosphate dehydrogenase deficiency.

Head and neck

The head shape can be distorted by birth, and this will resolve within a few days. Caput succedaneum is the oedematous thickening of the scalp caused by prolonged labour or ventouse delivery, which quickly resolves, but must be distinguished from a cephalohaematoma, a more serious condition caused by a collection of blood between the periosteum and the skull bones.

There are usually two fontanelles: the posterior closes within 3–4 months, but the anterior takes up to 18 months to close.

Observe for typical facial appearances that may be syndromic, paying particular attention to eyes, ears, mouth and tongue.

Chest

Carefully inspect the chest for respiratory rate, symmetry and movement. Auscultation will reveal abnormal breath sounds and confirm heart rate and normal heart sounds and exclude murmurs.

Abdomen

Major defects of the abdominal wall, e.g. gastroschisis or omphalocele, will be evident at birth. The liver, spleen and kidneys are often palpable in normal infants, but any unusually large masses should be further investigated. The anus should be inspected for patency and position. The genitalia should be carefully inspected and in particular it is often quite normal for female infants to have some bloody vaginal discharge. Any ambiguity of the genitalia should be investigated further and chromosome analysis performed as a matter of urgency before confirming the sex of the infant with the parents. Ambiguous genitalia is now referred to as a disorder of sexual differentiation and requires specialist assessment.

Vertebral column

The spine should be continuous and smooth to palpation. Any defects, swelling, birthmarks or hair patches should be investigated with ultrasound as they may indicate an underlying spinal abnormality.

Limbs

The limbs should move freely and have normal posture and tone when still. Birth injuries to the limbs may occur and include fractured humerus or clavicle, brachial plexus injury with the characteristic Erb's palsy and wrist drop as a result of radial nerve injury with fractured humerus. Hands, feet and digits should be carefully inspected. Developmental dysplasia or congenital dislocation of the hips more commonly occurs in female infants, in a breech delivery or in the presence of a family history. It is important that this is discovered early, as intervention at this stage will prevent problems later in life.

Reflexes

A term baby should be able to support its head with minimal lag as the baby is pulled gently to the sitting position. With the baby suspended in the ventral position, again the head should come into line with the axis of the body. The Moro reflex is a useful primitive reflex in the neurological assessment.

Group B streptococcus

This pathogen is the most common cause of serious bacterial infection in the newborn. It can be either early (the first week of life) or late (up to 3 months) in onset and is manifested as pneumonia, septicaemia or meningitis. Early-onset infection is usually acquired from the mother during delivery, and should be suspected if detected in maternal vaginal swabs antenatally, or in cases of maternal pyrexia in labour, prolonged prelabour ruptured membranes and in the premature infant.

Neonatal disease can be prevented by administering antibiotics to the mother in labour, or to the neonate postpartum.

The small baby

Small-for-gestational-age babies are defined as those weighing less than the 10th centile at birth for that gestation. Alternatively, low-birth-weight babies are those weighing less than 2.5 kg at birth. These babies need to be carefully observed in the neonatal period, as they are more prone to hypothermia, hypoglycaemia and hypocalcaemia.

Prematurity is defined as delivery before 37 completed weeks of pregnancy, regardless of the baby's birth weight. Premature infants are susceptible to all the problems of the small baby outlined above, including feeding difficulties, temperature regulatory difficulties, infection and jaundice. Specific problems encountered by premature infants are outlined below.

Respiratory distress syndrome

This is also known as hyaline membrane disease and is caused by a deficiency of surfactant in premature lungs. Surfactant lowers the surface tension within the alveolar sacs, preventing their collapse during normal expiration.

Intraventricular haemorrhage

This is a common condition of prematurity with complicated aetiology, including vascular friability and clotting dysfunction. The haemorrhage can vary from a minimal cerebral bleed to an extensive haemorrhage with severe neurological sequelae.

Retinopathy of prematurity

Excessive oxygenation during ventilation has been associated with this type of retinopathy, which may cause retinal detachment and blindness.

Neonatal resuscitation

Most babies are born in good condition and do not require any special stimulation or resuscitation. Immediately following delivery, the baby should be gently dried and rapidly assessed. Mucus is only removed from the mouth and then nose if necessary or if meconium is present at delivery. The Apgar score is a system developed for the initial assessment of the newborn at 1 and 5 minutes, and thereafter if indicated. It consists of a score from 0 to 2 for each of five variables, giving a score out of 10 (Table 16.1).

Table 16.1. Apgar score

	0	1	2
Heart rate	Absent	<100/min	>100/min
Respiratory effort	Absent	Gasp/shallow breaths	Normal/crying
Muscle tone	Limp	Some flexion	Flexion
Reflex	None	Grimace	Cough/cry
Colour	Pale/blue	Blue extremities	Pink

The umbilical cord should be kept long in infants likely to need special care (for cannulation) and cord blood taken for blood gas analysis and pH.

If the baby is vigorous and pink, then the baby can be wrapped to keep warm and passed immediately to the mother. If a baby fails to breathe by 1 minute despite drying off and stimulation of the feet, then immediate paediatric assistance should be called. If the baby is considered 'flat' or limp at delivery – impaired breathing or heart rate below 100 bpm – then resuscitate immediately following the guidelines outlined in Figures 16.1 and 16.2.

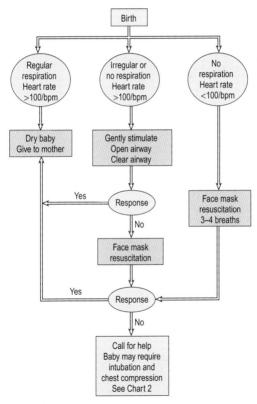

NOTE: If there is particulate meconium and the baby is unresponsive, proceed at once to Chart 2.

Figure 16.1 Neonatal resuscitation, chart 1. (Reproduced with permission from Working party of the Royal College of Paediatricians and Child Health and the Royal College of Obstetricians and Gynaecologists 1997 Resuscitation of Babies at Birth. London: BMJ, pp. 57 and 58.)

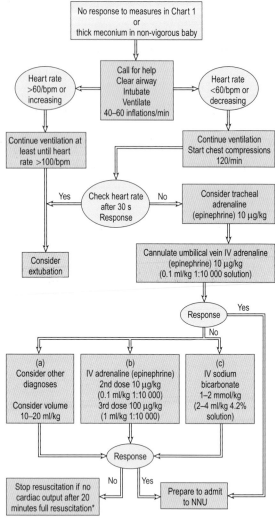

Figure 16.2 Neonatal resuscitation, chart 2. NNU, neonatal unit. (Reproduced with permission from Working party of the Royal College of Paediatricians and Child Health and the Royal College of Obstetricians and Gynaecologists 1997 Resuscitation of Babies at Birth. London: BMJ, pp. 57 and 58.)

Section 4

Emergencies and practical procedures

Emergencies and procedures 17

CHAPTER CONTENTS

OBSTETRIC EMERGENCIES AND PROCEDURES

Antepartum haemorrhage

Antepartum haemorrhage (APH) can be life-threatening to both mother and fetus, and so assessment must be immediate and accurate.

A vaginal examination should not be performed until the source of bleeding has been determined and a diagnosis made in case of placenta praevia.

Severe antepartum haemorrhage

The main causes of severe APH are placenta praevia (Fig. 17.1) and placental abruption. If the patient is collapsed and shocked, then a careful and efficient management protocol must be followed:

● Alert senior medical and midwifery staff.
● Estimate vaginal blood loss from history of pad usage, pooling and other subjective information; assess for signs of hypovolaemic shock, i.e. blood pressure, pulse, respiration rate, temperature.
● Calculate gestation.
● Auscultate fetal heart and commence continuous monitoring if fetal heart is present.
● Observe for signs of labour.
● Administer oxygen by facial mask.
● Insert intravenous (IV) line using large-bore cannula (may need two lines of access) and commence infusion of colloid (e.g. Gelofusine) ± crystalloid (e.g. Hartmann's).
● Take blood samples for urgent full blood count, clotting screen, and crossmatch for 6 units of blood.
● Insert indwelling catheter for urinary output measurement.
● Alert anaesthetic registrar, theatre staff and paediatric registrar, and special care baby unit if the fetal heart is present.
● Arrange transfer to labour ward or theatre if necessary.

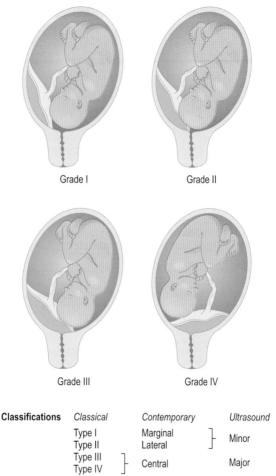

Figure 17.1 Grades of placenta praevia.

If bleeding settles and the fetal heart tracing is normal, the patient may be transferred to the antenatal ward when stable. If bleeding continues and/or fetal distress develops, the situation must be discussed with a senior medical colleague. In cases of severe bleeding the possibility of caesarean hysterectomy should be brought to the mother's attention before consent to the caesarean section.

Labour ward emergencies and procedures

In all obstetric emergencies, it should be remembered that there are two patients – the mother and the fetus. As with any emergency, the basic principles of airway, breathing and circulation are paramount and when resuscitating the mother it is important to bear in mind that the fetus is very susceptible to maternal hypoxia.

Unconscious patient

The main causes include:

- Supine hypotension
- Epilepsy
- Eclampsia.

Additional causes are:

- Cardiovascular, including hypovolaemia (haemorrhage), myocardial infarction, thromboembolus and hypertensive encephalopathy
- Respiratory, including amniotic fluid embolus
- Endocrine, including hyper/hypoglycaemia
- Neurological, including subarachnoid haemorrhage or total spinal anaesthesia
- Other, e.g. septicaemia or drugs.

Management

- Basic first aid: left lateral position, maintain airway, oxygen administration via bag and mask if not breathing.
- Assessment of situation and patient, including pulse, respiratory rate, blood pressure and fetal heart rate.
- Commence cardiopulmonary resuscitation if there is no cardiac output.
- Establish IV access, obtain blood for full blood count, renal function and electrolytes, serum glucose, liver function, coagulation screen and blood group (crossmatch if suspect haemorrhage).
- Intubate if necessary.
- Monitor mother and fetus: electrocardiograph and vital signs, cardiotocograph to assess fetal well-being.
- Establish and treat cause of collapse.
- If there is no cardiac output within 10 minutes, consider an immediate caesarean section.

Uterine rupture

This is an uncommon event that should be considered in the collapsed woman with a previous uterine scar undergoing oxytocin augmentation. Be aware of predisposing situations in which the risk of uterine rupture is increased.

The diagnosis should also be suspected in any woman with a previous scar in labour with pain or scar tenderness between contractions.

Presentation

- Pain or scar tenderness between contractions
- Cessation of contractions
- Evidence of hypovolaemia – tachycardia and/or hypotension
- Haematuria
- Vaginal bleeding
- Fetal heart rate abnormalities.

Management

- General resuscitation
- If oxytocin infusion is in progress, discontinue immediately

- If suspected, alert senior medical staff and arrange immediate delivery by caesarean section
- Postpartum haemorrhage (PPH) in a patient with a previous uterine scar could be due to uterine rupture. The patient should be managed according to the major obstetric haemorrhage guidelines and may require an exploration of the uterine cavity in theatre, with preparation for a laparotomy and caesarean hysterectomy if necessary.

Amniotic fluid embolus

This is an acute and extremely unexpected condition with a high rate of maternal mortality (60%). It can occur in 1–4 per 100 000 deliveries. It presents with respiratory distress and sudden circulatory collapse, and if the patient survives the first hour, there is a 40% chance of developing a coagulopathy.

It is caused by amniotic fluid or debris appearing in the maternal circulation. This quickly deposits in the lung, with a resulting anaphylactic-type reaction resulting in pulmonary vasoconstriction, severe hypoxia, acute left-sided heart failure and often disseminated intravascular coagulopathy. It is a condition that can often only be confirmed at postmortem examination and, therefore, should always be considered in sudden maternal collapse.

- Risk factors:
- Precipitate labour
- Caesarean section
- Polyhydramnios
- Hypertonic uterine action.
- Management:
- As outlined in management of unconscious patient (p. 277)
- Immediate delivery of fetus if alive
- Reversal of bronchospasm and hypoxia
- Administration of clotting factors, including fresh frozen plasma, fibrinogen and platelets
- Inotropic support to reverse vasodilatation.

Uterine inversion

This is inversion of the uterine fundus through the vagina.

- Risk factors:
- Previous inversion
- Uterine atony
- Cord contraction before placental separation
- Fundal placenta.
- Presentation:
- Pain and bleeding with signs and symptoms of cardiovascular and vasovagal shock
- Lump in the vagina following delivery of the placenta, although the placenta may be morbidly adherent.
- Management:
- Resuscitate
- Take blood (including crossmatch for 4 units) and establish IV access
- If the placenta is adherent, do not attempt to separate, but manually replace within the vagina
- Stop any oxytocin infusion
- Tocolytic therapy (salbutamol 500 µg in 10 ml normal saline IV) may be required
- Hydrostatic method to reduce the inversion (O'Sullivan method) – at least 4 l of warm sterile water connected by IV lines and tubing into the vagina as a douche

- Once uterus is reduced and placenta separated, give ergometrine 500 µg intramuscularly (IM) and then a 40 unit oxytocin infusion
- Prophylactic antibiotics.

Shoulder dystocia

Shoulder dystocia is when the shoulders fail to traverse the pelvis spontaneously after delivery of the head, with the result that the anterior shoulder becomes trapped behind the symphysis pubis, whilst the posterior shoulder may lie within the sacral hollow or above the promontory. The presentation is cephalic, the head is delivered usually slowly and with difficulty, but the neck does not appear and the chin retracts against the perineum. The incidence of shoulder dystocia is approximately 0.5% and has significant risk factors that should enable anticipation and preparation.

- **Risk factors:**
- Fetal macrosomia (estimated weight of >4.5 kg)
- Previous baby >4 kg
- Previous shoulder dystocia
- Excess maternal weight gain or a large-for-dates fetus
- Slow progress in the first and second stage
- Postmaturity.
- **Management:** While this complication cannot be prevented, the results can be improved by recognizing the situations in which it occurs.

    Alert senior medical and midwifery staff when delivery is imminent.
If shoulder dystocia occurs:

- Do not pull hard on the fetal head as this may increase the amount of impaction within the pelvis.
- Position mother in McRoberts position (knee–chest or thighs abducted and hyperflexed on the abdomen supported by an assistant on each side) or on all fours.
- Perform an episiotomy to aid access to fetal shoulders/posterior arm.
- Clear baby's nose and mouth of mucus.
- Apply firm suprapubic pressure and attempt basic method of delivery of the shoulders.

If this fails, attempt delivery of anterior shoulder using the Rubin manoeuvre (Fig. 17.2A):

- Place hand deeply in vagina behind anterior shoulder.
- With next contraction rotate the axis of the shoulders into the more favourable oblique diameter of the pelvis.
- Firm traction is made on the head, deflecting it towards the floor.
- Suprapubic pressure is exerted; this usually succeeds in bringing the anterior shoulder into and through the pelvis.

Extraction of posterior shoulder and arm

If this fails, attempt extraction of posterior shoulder and arm (Fig. 17.2B):

- Place hand deeply into vagina along the curvature of the sacrum and behind the baby's posterior shoulder.
- Identify posterior arm, follow to elbow. Pass finger into the antecubital fossa to encourage flexion of the elbow joint. Grasp forearm and hand and sweep anteriorly across the baby's abdomen and chest to deliver the posterior arm.
- Usually, normal head traction will now deliver the anterior shoulder. If not, rotate the baby 180° so that the anterior shoulder is now in the posterior position. It can then be extracted using the same manoeuvres.

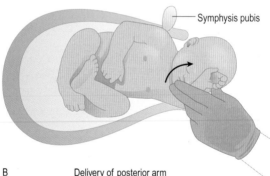

A   Rubin manoeuvre

B   Delivery of posterior arm

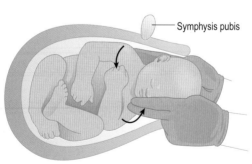

C   Wood's screw manoeuvre

Figure 17.2 Manoeuvres in management of shoulder dystocia.

Woods' screw manoeuvres

If this fails, attempt Woods' screw manoeuvres (Fig. 17.2C):

- Apply suprapubic pressure.
- Place two fingers from each hand on the baby's shoulders.
- Rotate the shoulders anticlockwise through 180° to bring the anterior shoulder to a posterior position and draw it lower in the pelvis. The posterior shoulder should deliver under the pubic arch.
- Rotate the shoulders clockwise through 180° to return the former anterior shoulder to the anterior position. It should then also deliver under the pubic arch.

Other delivery methods

Other delivery methods are extremely rare and require consultant management:

- Zavanelli: an alternative, though controversial, delivery method if dystocia is unresolved by more conventional techniques. The procedure involves replacement of the head under anaesthesia and delivery by caesarean section.
- Symphysiotomy: division of the pubic symphysis.
- Cleidotomy: deliberate fracture of the clavicles to reduce the diameter of the shoulders.

Cord presentation/prolapse

Cord prolapse is the condition in which the cord lies lower than the presenting part with ruptured membranes. It occurs in approximately 1 in 300 deliveries.

This is an obstetric emergency as the fetus is put at risk of losing its blood supply from spasm of the umbilical vessels caused by cooling, drying, altered pH and handling, and mechanical compression of the cord between the presenting part and the bony pelvis.

- Management:
- If the baby is alive, aim to expedite delivery immediately.
- Alert senior medical staff, midwife, paediatrician and anaesthetist.
- Alert theatre staff.
- Stop IV infusion of oxytoxin if in progress.
- Place the woman in the knee–chest, deep Trendelenburg or exaggerated Sims position (with pelvis raised).
- Explain the reason for midwife action to woman and birthing partner.
- With gloved hand use two fingers to replace any loop of cord gently outside the vulva into the vagina to keep it warm and moist. This is not always possible; if the cord cannot be replaced then cover it with warm moist padding.
- Palpate cord for pulsation and ascertain fetal viability.
- Relieve pressure from the cord by pressing up on the presenting part with gloved hand within the vagina until the delivery is imminent.
- If the cervix is greater than 9 cm dilated, the client is multiparous and the presenting part cephalic, the obstetrician may want to expedite delivery by ventouse.
- If the cervix is less than 9 cm dilated an emergency caesarean under general anaesthetic is carried out.
- If the cervix is fully dilated, forceps or breech extraction is the likely outcome.

Repair of episiotomy or vaginal laceration

A spontaneous perineal trauma is classified as:

- First degree: involves fourchette, hymen, labia, skin, vaginal epithelium.
- Second degree: involves pelvic floor, perineal muscle, vaginal muscles.

- Third degree: see below
- Fourth degree: see below.

The aim of repair is to achieve adequate haemostasis and obliteration of dead space so as to avoid potential haematoma or infection. Adequate analgesia is essential and, if regional anaesthesia is not established, then local anaesthesia can be used: lidocaine 1% with a maximum dosage of 20–30 ml. The procedure is as follows (Fig. 17.3):

- Good exposure and lighting are essential.
- Apply local anaesthesia if required.
- Appose all tissue involved in the laceration in a correct anatomical fashion after securing the apex, closing all vaginal epithelial lacerations to the fourchette.
- Use a continuous non-locking suture technique with an absorbable synthetic suture.
- Approximate both the superficial and deep perineal muscles involved in the laceration with either a continuous or interrupted suture.
- Repair the perineal skin using either interrupted or, preferably, a subcuticular suture.
- Perform and document both a vaginal and rectal examination on completion of the repair.
- Perform and document a count of instruments, needles and packs used at the end of the procedure.

Third- and fourth-degree perineal tears

- Anatomical definitions
- A third-degree tear involves partial or complete disruption of the external anal sphincter.
- A fourth-degree tear involves complete disruption of the external and internal sphincters and the anal or rectal mucosa.

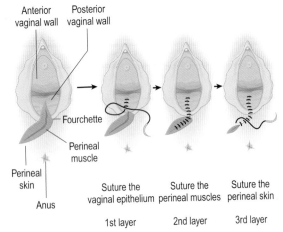

Figure 17.3 Repair of episiotomy or laceration.

Repair

- These tears must be carried out by a senior obstetrician. Very severe injury may require the expertise of an anorectal surgeon.
- Good analgesia is essential, i.e. regional or, rarely, general anaesthesia. Good exposure and lighting are essential to allow meticulous inspection. The repair should be carried out in theatre.
- Any obvious faecal contamination should be cleared away and the area thoroughly drenched with an aqueous antiseptic solution.
- In a fourth-degree tear the rectal mucosa should be repaired with an interrupted absorbable suture, ensuring the knots are not within the rectum or anal canal.
- In a fourth-degree tear the internal anal sphincter is a 'white' muscle attached to the mucosa. This should be repaired in interrupted sutures. There is recent evidence that 3.0 polydioxane (PDS) may be superior for suturing of the sphincters.
- The external anal sphincter ends need to be adequately mobilized and identified to ensure accurate suture placement.
- The external anal sphincter should be repaired with 3.0 polydioxane suture in either an overlapping or end-to-end technique (Fig. 17.4).
- The remainder of the repair is the same as for an episiotomy or second-degree tear, using an absorbable suture.
- A broad-spectrum antibiotic should be commenced intraoperatively and continued for 1 week. Stool softeners can be considered or advice given regarding avoidance of constipation.
- Advice regarding care of the perineum should be given as soon as possible.

Follow-up

- All patients should be reviewed at 6 weeks.
- Symptoms of flatus or faecal incontinence should alert the obstetrician that further investigations and referral may be necessary.
- If the repair has failed, then appropriate referral for a secondary repair may be considered at least 3 months after primary repair.
- At follow-up there should be a discussion regarding future deliveries and consideration should be given to the use of prophylactic episiotomy.

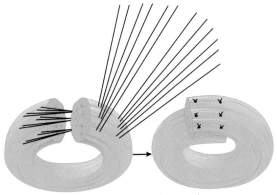

Figure 17.4 Overlapping technique of anal sphincter repair.

Retained placenta

A placenta is 'retained' when it has not been expelled 30 minutes following active management and 60 minutes following physiological management of the third stage. In this event:

- Inform senior medical staff.
- Observe blood loss, pulse and respirations.
- If an epidural is in place and effective, attempts to remove the placenta may take place in the labour ward.
- If there is no epidural, or if it is ineffective, arrange for transfer to obstetric theatre for removal under regional or general anaesthesia.
- Establish IV access and take blood for full blood count and group (consider crossmatch for 4 units).
- Following the procedure continue a Syntocinon infusion (40 units in 500 ml over 4 hours).

Postpartum haemorrhage

PPH is defined as greater than 500 ml of blood loss and is described as primary if it occurs in the first 24 hours, or secondary thereafter up to 6 weeks postpartum. An accurate record of blood loss should be kept in cases of haemorrhage since blood loss is generally underestimated.

Primary postpartum haemorrhage

- **Causes:**
- Retained placenta or retained products
- Uterine atony
- Vaginal lacerations
- Coagulation defect
- Uterine rupture.
- **Risk factors:** PPH can often be anticipated and several risk factors should heighten awareness, so that they are recognized early and preventive measures taken. These risk factors include:
- APH
- Previous history of PPH
- Overenlarged uterus as a result of multiple pregnancy, polyhydramnios or macrosomic fetus
- Placenta praevia
- Prolonged labour
- Grand multiparity
- Uterine fibroids
- Chorioamnionitis
- Bleeding diathesis.
- **Management:** Anticipate the possibility of PPH from recognition of risk factors so that preventive measures can be performed at the earliest opportunity, e.g. ensuring the administration of an oxytocin infusion postpartum in cases of prolonged labour. In the event that haemorrhage occurs (Figs 17.5 and 17.6):
- Alert senior medical and midwifery staff
- Resuscitate and ensure early recognition of cause
- Record maternal observations, pulse, blood pressure, blood loss and fluid balance
- Establish large-bore IV access and take blood for full blood count, coagulation screen and crossmatch for 2–4 units or as necessary.

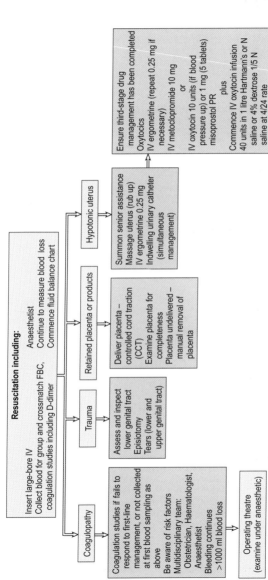

Resuscitation including:

Insert large-bore IV
Collect blood for group and crossmatch FBC,
coagulation studies including D-dimer

Anaesthetist
Continue to measure blood loss
Commence fluid balance chart

Coagulopathy

Coagulation studies if fails to
respond to first-line
management, or not collected
at first blood sampling as
above
Be aware of risk factors
Multidisciplinary team:
Obstetrician, Haematologist,
Anaesthetist
Bleeding continues
>1000 ml blood loss

Operating theatre
(examine under anaesthetic)

Trauma

Assess and inspect
lower genital tract
Episiotomy
Tears (lower and
upper genital tract)

Retained placenta or products

Deliver placenta –
controlled cord traction
(CCT)
Examine placenta for
completeness
Placenta undelivered –
manual removal of
placenta

Hypotonic uterus

Summon senior assistance
Massage uterus (rub up)
IV ergometrine 0.25 mg
Indwelling urinary catheter
(simultaneous
management)

Ensure third-stage drug
management has been completed
Oxytocics
IV ergometrine (repeat 0.25 mg if
necessary)
IV metoclopromide 10 mg
or
IV oxytocin 10 units (if blood
pressure up) or 1 mg (5 tablets)
misoprostol PR
plus
Commence IV oxytocin infusion
40 units in 1 litre Hartmann's or N
saline or 4% dextrose 1/5 N
saline at 4/24 rate

Figure 17.5 Management of primary postpartum haemorrhage. FBC, full blood count.

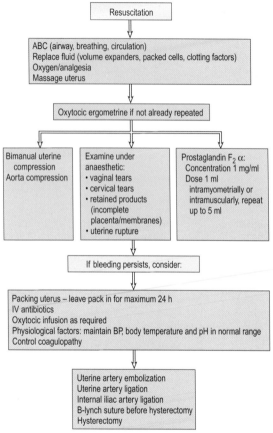

Figure 17.6 Further management of primary postpartum haemorrhage. BP, blood pressure.

- Check to ensure placental delivery was complete: if not, the patient may need an examination under anaesthesia.
- Arrange transfer to theatre for manual removal if the placenta has not been delivered.
- Catheterize the bladder and massage the uterus to encourage contraction.
- Establish what oxytocic drug has already been given for the third stage.
- Administer 200–500 μg of ergometrine stat or, if contraindicated, 10 units of oxytocin IV.
- Commence 40 units oxytocin infusion in 500 ml of Hartmann's over 4 hours if uterus continues to relax.

- Consider vaginal, cervical or uterine laceration if uterus is contracted, but blood loss continues, and prepare for examination under anaesthetic if unable to locate.
- Consider the use of prostaglandin $F_{2\alpha}$ if uterine atony persists, at doses of 250 μg IM or directly into the uterine muscle at 15-minute intervals, to a maximum of 2 grams (8 doses).

Secondary postpartum haemorrhage

- Causes:
- Retained products of conception
- Infection.
- Investigations:
- General examination, including abdominal palpation to assess uterine involution and vaginal examination to confirm that the cervix is closed
- High vaginal swab
- Ultrasound assessment to exclude retained products of conception.
- Management:
- Antibiotics – may need to consider IV cover if there is persistent pyrexia
- Evacuation of retained products of conception (ERPC) should be performed by experienced staff as the postpartum, and possibly infected, uterus is easily perforated
- Consider 24 hours of IV antibiotics if infected and bleeding is not too severe, before ERPC.

Massive obstetric haemorrhage

This is defined as greater than 2000 ml of blood loss and it is essential to be familiar with the unit protocol and in particular that all relevant staff are notified immediately, including senior obstetric, midwifery, anaesthetic and haematological staff, as well as porters and technicians. A catastrophic obstetric haemorrhage, although difficult to separate from a simple APH or PPH, should be suspected when there is unexplained collapse with signs of shock (Fig. 17.6).

Emergency management

- Alert senior medical (obstetric, anaesthetic and haematology) and midwifery staff.
- Lay the patient on her left side, ensuring an adequate airway, and give oxygen via a face mask.
- Check respiration and pulse.
- If postpartum, rub up a contraction of the uterus and give IV ergometrine 250 μg.
- Set up two large-bore IV access lines with colloid and crystalloid while awaiting blood.
- Take blood for crossmatching, full blood count and platelets, clotting screen, urea and electrolytes.
- Delegate duties to other staff, e.g. midwives to take charge of observations and monitoring of pulse, blood pressure, respirations, fluid balance and blood loss using a high-dependency chart; porters to transport specimens to the laboratory and retrieve at least 6 units of blood from the laboratory.
- In cases of placental abruption the estimation of blood loss is frequently severely underestimated and the need for early and adequate blood transfusion, if necessary with O-negative blood, is vital.

- When haemostasis is controlled, 1 unit of fresh frozen plasma should be given for every 10 units of blood. The consultant haematologist must be involved at an early stage if there is a suspected coagulopathy or need for massive blood transfusion. Inappropriate treatment with anticoagulants may worsen the condition.
- Definitive therapy for the catastrophic haemorrhage must accompany attempts at basic resuscitation. For APH this means urgent delivery; for PPH the usual measures include IV ergometrine, oxytocin infusion or intramyometrial prostaglandin injection. IV tranexamic acid can be useful in the control of bleeding from the lower segment.
- If bleeding cannot be controlled by direct uterine compression, oxytocics and control of a coagulopathy, a laparotomy for a B-Lynch suture, internal iliac ligation or a hysterectomy must be considered.
- Patients who have had a massive blood loss and transfusion will almost certainly have a coagulopathy, and will require intensive-care nursing.

Pulmonary embolus

Pulmonary embolus can present in a variety of ways from simple shortness of breath to sudden collapse. Signs include:
- Anxiety, tachycardia and tachypnoea
- Cyanosis, apnoea and unconsciousness
- Chest pain, pleuritic pain or haemoptysis.

Investigations
- Electrocardiogram (ECG)
- Arterial blood gases
- Full blood count and coagulation screen
- Chest X-ray
- Ventilation/perfusion scan
- Doppler examination of both legs to exclude deep-vein thrombosis (DVT)
- D-dimers.

Management
- As in unconscious patient (p. 277)
- Monitor vital signs
- Facial oxygen and pulse oximetry monitoring
- Continuous ECG
- Suggested anticoagulant therapy – IV loading dose of heparin (5000 IU) over 5 minutes followed by an infusion of 1000 IU/ml at 1.6 ml/h.

Thromboprophylaxis in obstetrics

Thromboembolism is a major cause of maternal mortality and caesarean section is a major contributing factor (the risk of thromboembolism is multiplied by 20). The risk of DVT after lower-segment caesarean section (LSCS) is approximately 1–2%. Therefore, all women should be assessed antenatally and again at delivery for risk factors for thromboembolism.

Caesarean section

Risk assessment
- Low risk: Elective LSCS, uncomplicated pregnancy and no other risk factors.

- High risk:
- Emergency LSCS in labour
- Age >35 years
- Obesity – body mass index (BMI) >30 at booking
- Parity 4 or more
- Gross varicose veins
- Current infection
- Pre-eclampsia
- Immobility preoperatively
- Major current illness, e.g. heart or lung disease, inflammatory bowel disease
- Extended surgery, e.g. caesarean hysterectomy
- Patients with a thrombophilia (e.g. antiphospholipid syndrome, activated protein C resistance, protein C or S deficiency).

Management

- Low risk: Intermittent compression stockings perioperatively; early mobilization, hydration, regular pain relief and TED stockings postoperatively.
- High risk: Intermittent compression stockings perioperatively; early mobilization, hydration, regular pain relief, TED stockings and heparin postoperatively.

    Use of heparin in LSCS patients is similar to the guidelines below for gynaecology patients.

Severe pregnancy-induced hypertension

This patient has proteinuria of 2+ or more on dipstick urinalysis and hypertension (diastolic >90 mmHg) and is symptomatic as above, or is thrombocytopenic (platelets <100 × 10^9/l, or has deranged liver function tests (aspartate transaminase >50 IU/l). This includes all women who have an eclamptic fit or who have evidence of haemolysis, elevated liver enzymes, low platelet count (HELLP). The plan should be to stabilize the patient prior to delivery, however the delivery is undertaken.

Antihypertensive therapy

- Patients may already be on oral treatment with methyldopa, but will require additional treatment with hydralazine if the mean arterial pressure is above 125 mmHg.
- Set up a hydralazine or labetalol infusion in a syringe pump, depending on hospital protocol. Hydralazine may result in a tachycardia >120 beats/min or side effects such as headache and dizziness.
- Any antihypertensive infusion should continue until the patient is delivered and after delivery for at least 24 hours, depending on her response. Thereafter, consider oral antihypertensives if necessary.

Anticonvulsant prophylaxis

This should be started in women with severe pre-eclamptic toxaemia who are symptomatic and hyperreflexic with more than two beats of clonus.

    Magnesium sulphate is used in most hospitals for both prophylaxis and the management of pre-eclamptic seizures, and protocols vary. Careful monitoring of patients on magnesium sulphate includes cardiac oxygen saturation monitoring throughout the infusion and testing the patellar reflex hourly. If the patellar reflex is lost or the oxygen saturation is persistently below 95% on air, stop the magnesium infusion and send a serum magnesium level to the lab (2 ml clotted blood). The therapeutic range is 2–4 mmol/l.

    Continue infusion until 24–48 hours after delivery, depending on clinical signs.

Fluid balance

All patients should be catheterized and their urine output measured hourly. If output remains above 100 ml in 4 hours, they should receive 1 l of Hartmann's over 12 hours. This equals 85 ml/h, and should be reduced accordingly if the patient is receiving other fluid (e.g. a MgSO$_4$ infusion).

If output falls below 100 ml in 4 hours, or if the patient is severely unwell, a central venous pressure (CVP) line should be inserted and the CVP recorded hourly.

Eclampsia

Eclampsia occurs in 1:1500 pregnancies and is a major cause of maternal mortality and morbidity. It characteristically will present as hypertension with headaches, visual disturbance and seizures. The resulting cerebral irritability will result in hyperreflexia and clonus and 70% of deaths are due to intracerebral haemorrhage.

The three serious complications of eclampsia are:
1. Cerebrovascular injury
2. Pulmonary oedema
3. Coagulopathy.

Management

As in unconscious patient (p. 277), but the main principles are (Fig. 17.7):
- Secure airway; intubate if necessary
- Anticonvulsant therapy
- Control blood pressure
- Prevent pulmonary oedema by strict management of fluid input and output
- Be aware of impending coagulopathy.

Treatment of eclamptic fit
- MgSO$_4$ 2 grams IV given over 5 minutes

or
- Diazepam or Diazemuls 10–20 mg IV as a bolus followed by MgSO$_4$ 1 g/h IV diluted to 10 ml, monitoring as above.

Treat further fits with another bolus of Diazemuls, but discuss the possibility of transfer to intensive care facilities in case the patient requires ventilation.

GYNAECOLOGICAL EMERGENCIES AND PROCEDURES

Thromboprophylaxis in gynaecological surgery

The risk of DVT is 12% post total abdominal hysterectomy and 35% post-surgery for gynaecological malignancy and so all women who undergo a gynaecological operation should be assessed for their individual risk of thromboembolism.

Risk assessment
- Low risk:
- Minor surgery and no other risk factors.
- Moderate risk:
- Major surgery and laparoscopic surgery and no other risk factors.
- High risk:
- Minor surgery with a personal or family history of DVT, pulmonary embolism or thrombophilia

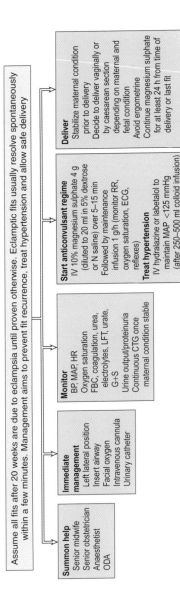

Assume all fits after 20 weeks are due to eclampsia until proven otherwise. Eclamptic fits usually resolve spontaneously within a few minutes. Management aims to prevent fit recurrence, treat hypertension and allow safe delivery

Summon help
Senior midwife
Senior obstetrician
Anaesthetist
ODA

Immediate management
Left lateral position
Insert airway
Facial oxygen
Intravenous cannula
Urinary catheter

Monitor
BP, MAP, HR
Oxygen saturation
FBC, coagulation, urea, electrolytes, LFT, urate, G+S
Urine output/proteinuria
Continuous CTG once maternal condition stable

Start anticonvulsant regime
IV 10% magnesium sulphate 4 g (diluted to 20 ml in 5% dextrose or N saline) over 5–15 min
Followed by maintenance infusion 1 g/h (monitor RR, oxygen saturation, ECG, reflexes)
Treat hypertension
IV hydralazine or labetalol to maintain MAP <125 mmHg (after 250–500 ml colloid infusion)

Deliver
Stabilize maternal condition prior to delivery
Decide to deliver vaginally or by caesarean section depending on maternal and fetal condition
Avoid ergometrine
Continue magnesium sulphate for at least 24 h from time of delivery or last fit

Figure 17.7 Management of eclampsia. ODA, operating department assistant; BP, blood pressure; MAP, mean arterial pressure; HR, heart rate; FBC, full blood count; LFT, liver function tests; G+S, group and save; CTG, cardiotocograph; RR, respiration rate; ECG, electrocardiogram.

- Major surgery with any of the following risk factors:
  - obesity: BMI >30
  - gross varicose veins
  - current infection
  - immobility prior to surgery
  - major current illness, e.g. heart or lung disease, malignancy, inflammatory bowel disease, nephrotic syndrome
  - heart failure or recent myocardial infarction
- Surgery for gynaecological malignancy
- Paralysis or immobilization of the lower limbs
- On hormone replacement therapy or combined oral contraceptive pill preoperatively.

Management

- Low risk:
- Early mobilization, hydration and adequate pain relief.
- Moderate risk:
- Intermittent compression stockings perioperatively; early mobilization, hydration, pain relief and TED stockings postoperatively.
- High risk:
- Intermittent compression stockings perioperatively; early mobilization, hydration, pain relief, TED stockings and heparin postoperatively.
- Use of heparin:
  - low-molecular-weight heparin (LMWH) may be used depending on individual hospital policy
  - for elective surgery, LMWH should be given the evening before the surgery and then given daily in the evening
  - for emergency surgery, LMWH should be commenced postoperatively on the day of the surgery
  - the heparin may be withheld pre- or postoperatively in certain circumstances (e.g. myomectomy)
  - if an epidural is used, there should be 12 hours between the preoperative dose of LMWH and the insertion of the epidural. The epidural catheter should not be removed within 8 hours of a dose of tinzaparin and a further dose should not be given until 2 hours after the catheter is removed.

Other points

Hormone replacement therapy or the combined oral contraceptive pill does not need to be stopped preoperatively before a minor procedure when immediate postoperative mobilization is possible. However, they should be stopped at least 1 week prior to major gynaecological surgery.

Final medicine examination: Questions and answers

QUESTIONS

1. Polyhydramnios is characteristically associated with:
   a. Anencephaly
   b. Intrauterine growth retardation
   c. Placenta accreta
   d. Potter's syndrome
   e. Insulin-dependent diabetes mellitus

2. Hypertensive disease in pregnancy is associated with all of these apart from:
   a. A low serum urate level
   b. A low platelet count
   c. Increased creatinine clearance rate
   d. Increased reflexes
   e. A high haematocrit

3. Down's syndrome
   a. Has a birth prevalence in the region of 4.2 per 1000 in England and Wales
   b. Can be diagnosed using nuchal translucency scanning
   c. Cannot be found in mosaic form
   d. Is associated with anhydramnios
   e. Is associated with a higher rate of miscarriage than in pregnancies with a normal karyotype

4. Regarding urinary tract infection in pregnancy, which of the following statements is not true?
   a. It is associated with preterm labour
   b. It may occur without any symptoms
   c. It is commonly caused by *Escherichia coli*
   d. It may be caused by urethral diverticulum
   e. It is increased in pregnancy due to the progesterone effect on the ureters

5. Regarding rubella in pregnancy:
   a. It is associated with recurrent miscarriages
   b. It is associated with the greatest incidence of congenital malformations when infection occurs during the first trimester
   c. It is indicated by a rise in rubella-specific IgG antibody levels following recent infection
   d. It is associated with neural tube defects in the fetus
   e. All women who lack rubella antibodies should be identified and offered vaccination in pregnancy

6. A 40-year-old woman attends antenatal clinic for booking bloods, including one for hepatitis B. The results show hepatitis B surface antibody positive, greater than 100 surface core antibody negative. Which is the single most likely explanation?
   a. Hepatitis B carrier of high infectivity
   b. Hepatitis B carrier of low infectivity
   c. Laboratory error
   d. Past infection with hepatitis B, not cleared
   e. Previous vaccination for hepatitis B

7. A 22-year-old prostitute presents with persistent perivaginal itching. A speculum examination is performed and shows white plaques. Which is the single most appropriate treatment?
   a. Amphotericin
   b. Clotrimazole
   c. Co-trimoxazole
   d. Doxycycline
   e. Metronidazole

8. A 25-year-old primigravida has been fully dilated for 2 hours, is on Syntocinon and has been pushing for an hour. She is contracting 1 in 3 and the membranes ruptured spontaneously at 4 cm. The fetus is of average size, with 2/5 palpable abdominally. On vaginal examination the presenting part is −2 above the ischial spines, and the position is occipitoposterior with significant caput and moulding. The CTG is normal. Which is the single most appropriate course of action?
   a. Apply Keilland's (rotational) forceps
   b. Apply Silastic vacuum cup
   c. Increase the Syntocinon and review in 2 hours
   d. Continue pushing and review in 2 hours
   e. Perform a caesarean section

9. GnRH analogues
   a. Can be used for long-term treatment of endometriosis
   b. Cause vaginal dryness
   c. Can be administered vaginally
   d. Are administered daily for endometriosis
   e. Act predominantly at the ovarian level

10. Which of the following is not known to cause congenital fetal abnormalities?
    a. Phenytoin
    b. Warfarin
    c. Methyldopa
    d. Alcohol
    e. Aminoglycosides

11. A 38-year-old woman attends for a routine smear at her general practitioner's surgery. Which single sign suggests HIV-related immunosuppression?
    a. Persistent painful vulval ulcers, 2 cm in size
    b. A Gartner's cyst on the right vaginal wall
    c. Recurrent multiple painful ulcers, 1 mm in size
    d. Recurrent offensive, grey milky vaginal discharge
    e. Umbilicated papules on the labia, 4 mm in size

12. Regarding emergency contraception, a 21-year-old woman attends a local pharmacy requesting Levonelle (progesterone-only) emergency contraception as she had unprotected intercourse 2 days ago. She is currently taking amoxicillin for a chest infection. Which is the single most appropriate advice for the pharmacist to give?
    a. She needs a negative pregnancy test before she can be given emergency contraception
    b. She requires a prescription from the doctor to be given emergency contraception
    c. She should be given Levonelle, which may delay her next period, in which case she should have a pregnancy test
    d. She should be given Levonelle, which may induce breakthrough early bleeding, in which case she should have a pregnancy test
    e. The trimethoprim will interact with the Levonelle and make it ineffective, so an intrauterine device would be a better option

13. Concerning sickle-cell disorders in pregnancy:
    a. Sickle-cell disorders are most common in women of Mediterranean origin
    b. The sickle-cell crisis can be precipitated in conditions of lowered oxygen tension
    c. Sickle-cell disorders are not associated with an increased incidence of hypertension during pregnancy
    d. Sickle-cell disease results from a variant on the fetal globin chain
    e. Partner screening is recommended during the second trimester

14. Secondary postpartum haemorrhage:
    a. Is defined as abnormal bleeding that occurs within 24 hours of delivery
    b. Occurs after approximately 5% of normal deliveries
    c. Can usually be diagnosed by ultrasound examination of the uterus
    d. Often requires a B-lynch suture to control the bleeding
    e. May be due to infection

15. Placental abruption:
    a. Is always an indication for delivery
    b. Is usually diagnosed by ultrasound
    c. Has a higher incidence with maternal cocaine use
    d. Can easily be distinguished from arcuate appendicitis
    e. Is always associated with vaginal bleeding

16. A high fetal head in a primigravida at term:
    a. Can be fundal fibroid
    b. Can be caused by minor placenta praevia
    c. May be associated with an arcuate uterus
    d. Is an indication for caesarean section
    e. Has a lower incidence in patients of African origin

17. With regard to breech presentation:
    a. The incidence is 3–4% at term
    b. External cephalic version at 35 weeks' gestation is recommended for all uncomplicated cases
    c. A radiological pelvimetry is recommended for the selection of women suitable for trial of vaginal breech delivery

d. Randomized controlled trials have demonstrated in breech deliveries before 28 weeks' gestation that the perinatal outcome is better with caesarean section than with vaginal delivery

e. Planned elective caesarean section of breech presentation reduces the risk of perinatal mortality by 75% in countries with a high perinatal mortality

18. In an epileptic woman who became pregnant while on valproate treatment:
   a. There is a higher risk of exomphalos
   b. There is a risk of having a child who will develop epilepsy
   c. Breastfeeding is contraindicated if the mother is still on medication during the puerperium
   d. There is a higher risk of miscarriage
   e. Seizures are more likely to occur during or immediately after labour

19. A 28-year-old healthy woman has had miscarriages at 6 and 10 weeks. She is requesting advice regarding her next pregnancy. Which is the single most appropriate management?
   a. Aspirin 75 mg daily
   b. Injectable progestogens
   c. Reassurance
   d. Oestrogen pessary
   e. Oral progestogens

20. With regard to emergency caesarean section, a 25-year-old woman is in spontaneous labour at 38 weeks and is having a trial of previous caesarean section scar (the first caesarean section was an elective one for a breech presentation). Her contractions have worn off and she has been 4 cm dilated for 4 hours. She is in pain despite epidural analgesia. The head is not engaged and blood-stained liquor is draining. CTG shows variable decelerations. Which is the most appropriate next management?
   a. Top-up epidural
   b. Emergency caesarean section
   c. Fetal blood sampling
   d. Observe and reassess in 2 hours
   e. Start Syntocinon

21. With regard to urodynamic investigations:
   a. They involve a pressure catheter in the bladder and the vagina
   b. They are unnecessary in a patient who complains of stress incontinence
   c. Cystometry measures the pressure/volume relationship of the bladder during filling and voiding
   d. If normal, they should show a bladder capacity of 200 ml
   e. They are not indicated with a neuropathic bladder disorder

22. Concerning HIV in the UK:
   a. The prevalence of infection in women has reached a plateau
   b. The majority of new cases of HIV diagnosed in the year 2008 were the results of transmission between homosexuals
   c. The majority of infected heterosexual women are UK-born
   d. Transmission from mother to child can occur in the first trimester
   e. A caesarean section is indicated if a woman is HIV-positive

23. Patients with the following conditions typically present with primary amenorrhoea:
    a. Bicornuate uterus
    b. Anorexia nervosa
    c. Testicular feminization
    d. Polycystic ovarian syndrome
    e. Down's syndrome

24. In a patient with chlamydial infection:
    a. Lymphogranuloma venereum is a recognized clinical presentation
    b. The organism grows well on chocolate agar
    c. Neonatal conjunctivitis appears in the first 48 hours after birth
    d. The diagnosis is made on a high vaginal swab
    e. Erythromycin is the treatment of choice

25. Which of the following is an autosomal-recessive condition?
    a. Duchenne muscular dystrophy
    b. Achondroplasia
    c. Cystic fibrosis
    d. Huntington's disease
    e. Fallot's tetralogy

26. In the management of recurrent miscarriage:
    a. Karyotyping of the partner should be performed
    b. Routine glucose tolerance test is recommended
    c. Steroid therapy is an acceptable form of treatment of antiphospho-lipid syndrome
    d. Cervical cerclage improves pregnancy outcome
    e. Incidence has remained constant at 3%

27. Regarding early pregnancy loss:
    a. Expectant management is associated with more patients having psychological morbidity
    b. Anti-D should always be reserved for women who miscarry after 12 weeks
    c. In surgical uterine evacuation for an incomplete miscarriage, blunt curettage is a preferred technique
    d. Prophylactic antibiotics reduce infection associated with termina-tion of pregnancy
    e. Bed rest is beneficial in patients with threatened miscarriage

28. A 25-year-old nulliparous woman with a BMI of 37 has not had a period for 12 months. She wishes to become pregnant but investiga-tions suggest a diagnosis of polycystic ovarian syndrome. She has no previous medical problems and takes no regular medications. Which is the single most appropriate initial management?
    a. Prescribe clomiphene citrate
    b. Do her partner's semen analysis
    c. Encourage her to lose weight by modifying her diet and increasing exercise
    d. Refer her to an infertility clinic
    e. Check tubal status

29. A 34-year-old woman is planning on having a baby with her partner. She is concerned about the risk of neural tube defects to the fetus as she has a friend with a baby who has spina bifida. She smokes approximately 5 cigarettes a day and has had a pulmonary embolism. Which single intervention is most likely to reduce the incidence of neural tube defect?
   a. Avoid incidental radiation exposure such as high-altitude flights
   b. Change warfarin to low-molecular-weight heparin
   c. Encourage smoking cessation
   d. Prescribe progesterone
   e. Administer prophylactic folic acid

30. *Candida albicans*:
   a. Causes symptomatic vaginitis in most women who have vaginal colonization
   b. Is found more commonly in pregnant rather than non-pregnant women
   c. Is more common in women using the combined oral contraceptive pill
   d. Has a recognized association with cervical dysplasia
   e. Has a recognized association with premature labour

31. The levonorgestrel IUS:
   a. Has been shown to increase the risk of ectopic pregnancy
   b. Has a higher failure rate than laparoscopic sterilization
   c. Has an increased infection rate compared to the copper intrauterine device
   d. Has been shown to reduce CIN significantly
   e. Can be used with transdermal oestrogen replacement therapy without the need for oral progesterones

32. Herpes simplex viral infection of the cervix:
   a. Is not a common cause of dyspareunia
   b. Causes recurrent miscarriages
   c. Can be treated with aciclovir
   d. Causes cervical intraepithelial neoplasia
   e. Can cause pelvic inflammatory disease

33. With regard to bacterial vaginosis:
   a. The vaginal secretions have a pH of less than 4.5
   b. It is associated with overgrowth of lactobacilli
   c. It is associated with an offensive smell due to amines
   d. First-line treatment is amoxicillin
   e. It is associated with prolonged pregnancy

34. In FIGO stage 1 ovarian cancer:
   a. All patients are advised to have postoperative chemotherapy
   b. Peritoneal washings contain malignant cells
   c. Primary surgery should be carried out through a transverse suprapubic incision
   d. The tumour marker CA 125 has no diagnostic value
   e. Conservative surgery preserving fertility is possible

35. A 49-year-old woman has abdominal distension. A CT scan shows an inoperable ovarian carcinoma. Palliative radiotherapy is recommended. Her family requests that she is not told of the diagnosis or prognosis. Which is the single most appropriate action?
   a. Fully inform the patient of the diagnosis and treatment option
   b. Indicate treatment to patient but not the prognosis
   c. Seek advice from the local ethics committee
   d. Seek patient's view of knowledge she wishes to have
   e. Withhold information and diagnosis from patient on grounds of causing patient serious harm

EXTENDED MATCHING QUESTIONS

Contraception

   a. Depot medroxyprogesterone acetate (Depo Provera)
   b. Desogestrol (Cerazette)
   c. Ethinylestradiol and levonorgestrel (Microgynon 30)
   d. Ethinylestradiol and desogestrol (Marvelon)
   e. Ethinylestradiol and norelgestromin (Evra)
   f. Ethinylestradiol and norethisterone (Loestrin-30)
   g. Etonogestrol (Implanon)
   h. Levonorgestrel 1.5mg (Levonelle)
   i. Levonorgestrel (Microval)
   j. Norethisterone (Micronor)

Select the most appropriate answer for the following scenarios:

1. A 38-year-old woman gives a history of severe migraines with focal aura. She is given hormonal contraception and advised to take it continuously each day within the maximum safe period of 12 hours.

2. A 20-year-old woman attends on day 12 of a regular 28-day menstrual cycle 24 hours after unprotected sexual intercourse requesting emergency contraception.

3. A 28-year-old woman attends postnatal clinic requesting contraception. She is not breastfeeding. She decides that a method that she has to use weekly would be best for her.

4. A 24-year-old woman is having problems with acne with her current method of oral contraception. She decides to change to an alternative formulation (third-generation) after discussion about the associated increased risk of venous thromboembolism.

5. A 22-year-old woman attends the clinic asking for contraception. She works shifts and wants a method she doesn't need to take every day. She thinks she will remember to come to clinic regularly at the recommended interval of 12 weeks.

Gynaecology presentation

   a. Aphthous ulceration
   b. Fitz-Hugh–Curtis syndrome
   c. Elevated LH and FSH levels

    d. Elevated LH/FSH ratio
    e. Elevated prolactin levels
    f. Localized provoked vulvodynia
    g. Premature menopause
    h. Rokitansky–Kuster syndrome
    i. Stevens–Johnson syndrome
    j. Turner's syndrome

For each scenario below, select the most likely finding or diagnosis from the list above:

6. A 32-year-old with a history of previous *Chlamydia* infection who now has right upper-quadrant pain.

7. A 25-year-old with irregular menstrual periods and galactorrhoea.

8. A 48-year-old who has not had a menstrual period for 6 months and has night sweats.

9. A 17-year-old who has normal height and sexual development but has not had a period.

10. A 26-year-old who has developed vulval ulceration. Discussion reveals she had mouth ulcers, and these follow the use of mefenamic acid for her periods.

Prenatal diagnosis and screening

    a. Amniocentesis
    b. Chorionic villous sampling
    c. Combined first-trimester screening (nuchal scan, PAPP-A and hCG)
    d. Cordocentesis
    e. Detailed second-trimester testing
    f. Double test (serum AFP and hCG)
    g. Fetal scalp blood sampling
    h. Maternal and paternal karyotyping
    i. Nuchal translucency
    j. Serum AFP

For each scenario below select the most likely/appropriate from the list above:

11. A woman attends antenatal clinic at 8 weeks' gestation. She and her partner both have sickle-cell trait and they wish to know the sickle-cell status of the fetus.

12. A woman presents in her pregnancy at 15 weeks. Her last baby was born with spina bifida and she wants to know whether this baby is also affected. How will she find out?

13. A woman presents at 6 weeks' gestation with a history of four previous first-trimester miscarriages. Her twin sister miscarried a baby with multiple abnormalities. She is concerned. In view of her previous history she would not consider invasive testing under any circumstances. Which test may be useful?

14. A 42-year-old woman is pregnant for the first time. At 10 weeks' gestation she books in at ANC. She would prefer to avoid amniocentesis in
view of the risk of miscarriage and would like you to suggest the most
sensitive early screening test for Down's syndrome.

15. A woman presents at 18 weeks' gestation with a high titre of anti-D
antibodies. On ultrasound there is evidence of fetal anaemia. What can
be done?

ANSWERS

1. a. True
   b. False
   c. False
   d. False
   e. False

2. a. True
   b. False
   c. False
   d. False
   e. False

3. a. False
   b. False
   c. False
   d. False
   e. True

4. a. False
   b. False
   c. False
   d. True
   e. False

5. a. False
   b. True
   c. False
   d. False
   e. False

6. a. False
   b. False
   c. False
   d. False
   e. True

7. a. False
   b. True
   c. False
   d. False
   e. False

8. a. False
   b. False
   c. False
   d. False
   e. True

9. a. False
   b. True
   c. False
   d. False
   e. False

10. a. False
    b. False
    c. True
    d. False
    e. False

11. a. True
    b. False
    c. False
    d. False
    e. False

12. a. False
    b. False
    c. True
    d. False
    e. False

13. a. False
    b. True
    c. False
    d. False
    e. False

14. a. False
    b. False
    c. False
    d. False
    e. True

15. a. False
    b. False
    c. True
    d. False
    e. False

16. a. False
    b. True
    c. False
    d. False
    e. False

17. a. True
    b. False
    c. False
    d. False
    e. False

18. a. False
    b. False
    c. False
    d. False
    e. True

19. a. False
    b. False
    c. True
    d. False
    e. False

20. a. False
    b. True
    c. False
    d. False
    e. False

21. a. False
    b. False
    c. True
    d. False
    e. False

22. a. False
    b. False
    c. False
    d. True
    e. False

23. a. False
    b. False
    c. True
    d. False
    e. False

24. a. True
    b. False
    c. False
    d. False
    e. False

25. a. False
    b. False
    c. True
    d. False
    e. False

26. a. False
    b. False
    c. False
    d. False
    e. False

27. a. True
    b. False
    c. False
    d. False
    e. False

28. a. False
    b. False
    c. True
    d. False
    e. False

29. a. False
    b. False
    c. False
    d. False
    e. True

30. a. False
    b. True
    c. False
    d. False
    e. False

31. a. False
    b. False
    c. False
    d. False
    e. True

32. a. False
    b. False
    c. False
    d. True
    e. False

33. a. False
    b. False
    c. True
    d. False
    e. False

34. a. False
    b. False
    c. False
    d. False
    e. True

35. a. False
    b. False
    c. False
    d. True
    e. False

Contraception

1. b
2. h
3. e
4. d
5. a

Gynaecology presentation

6. b
7. d
8. c
9. h
10. i

Prenatal diagnosis and screening

11. b
12. e
13. h
14. c
15. d

Appendices

NORMAL VALUES

	Non-pregnant range	Pregnant range
Haemoglobin	11.5–16.0 g/dl	10.6–12.8 g/dl
Haematocrit (packed cell volume)	0.37–0.47%	0.31–0.38%
Mean cell volume	76–96 fl	74.4–95.6 fl
White cell count	4.0–11.0 × 10^9/l	4.0–14 × 10^9/l
Platelets	150–400 × 10^9/l	100–400 × 10^9/l
Erythrocyte sedimentation rate (ESR)	(Age in years +10)/2	44–114 mm/h
Serum iron	11–30 μmol/l	Reduced in pregnancy
Plasma ferritin	20–300 μg/l	Reduced in pregnancy
Red cell folic acid	160–640 μg/l	Reduced in pregnancy
Serum B_{12}	>150 ng/ml	Reduced in pregnancy
Urea	2.5–6.7 mmol/l	2.4–4.3 mmol/l
Creatinine	70–150 μmol/l	34–82 μmol/l
Potassium	3.5–5.0 mmol/l	3.5–5.0 mmol/l
Sodium	135–145 mmol/l	135–145 mmol/l
Uric acid	150–390 μmol/l	Number of weeks' gestation × 10
Alanine transaminase (ALT)	5–35 IU/l	5–31 IU/l
Aspartate transaminase (AST)	5–35 IU/l	8–29 IU/l
Bilirubin	3–17 μmol/l	3–14 μmol/l
Albumin	35–50 g/l	22–40 g/l
Total protein	60–80 g/l	55–73 g/l
Alkaline phosphatase	30–300 IU/l	Elevated in pregnancy
Total calcium	2.12–2.65 mmol/l	2.12–2.65 mmol/l
Fasting glucose	4.0–6.0 mmol/l	3.0–6.0 mmol/l
Random glucose	<11.0 mmol/l	<8.7 mmol/l
Glycosylated haemoglobin	6.0–8.5%	6.0–8.5%

(Continued)

	Non-pregnant range	Pregnant range
Thyroid-stimulating hormone (TSH)	0.5–5.7 mU/l	0.5–7.0 mU/l
Free thyroxine	10.0–40 pmol/l	11.0–23 pmol/l
Glomerular filtration rate (GFR)	100–160 ml/min	170 ml/min
24-hour urinary protein	0.03–0.14 g/24 h	<0.3 g/24 h

DEFINITIONS

amniotomy surgical rupture of the membranes to induce or enhance labour

android pelvis a funnel-shaped male-type pelvis with diameters which decrease from above downwards

antepartum haemorrhage bleeding from the birth canal in the period from the 24th week of gestation to the birth of the baby

asynclitism tilting of the fetal head in labour so that the anterior or posterior parietal bone presents

attitude of the fetus relationship of the fetal head and limbs to the fetal trunk, usually flexion

bregma anterior fontanelle

brow the part of the fetal head between the root of the nose and the anterior fontanelle

caput succedaneum oedema from obstructed venous return in the fetal scalp caused by pressure of the head against the rim of the cervix or birth canal

cephalhaematoma collection of blood beneath the periosteum of a skull bone, limited to that bone by periosteal attachments

cervical dystocia difficult labour due to failure of the cervix to dilate, in spite of adequate uterine contractions

chloasma the brown pigmented facial mask of pregnancy

couvelaire uterus the uterus appears purple due to haemorrhage within its musculature; occurs with severe placental abruption

crowning of the head phase in the second stage of labour when a large segment of the fetal scalp is visible at the vaginal orifice, the perineum being distended and the anus dilated

engagement engagement occurs when the widest diameters of the presenting part have passed through the pelvic inlet

erythroblastosis fetalis haemolytic disease of the newborn, usually due to Rhesus antibodies

fontanelle space at the junction of three or more skull bones, covered only by a membrane and skin

fourchette the fold of skin formed by merging of the labia minora and labia majora posteriorly

funnel pelvis (see android pelvis)

hyaline membrane a homogeneous membrane lining the alveoli, alveolar ducts and respiratory bronchioles, and an important cause of death in premature infants

hydrops fetalis gross oedema of fetal subcutaneous tissues together with ascites and pericardial and pleural effusions, usually due to erythroblastosis

kernicterus yellow staining of the baby's brain due to high blood levels of unconjugated bilirubin causing severe neurological damage or death

lie of the fetus relationship of the long axis of fetus to the long axis of the uterus, usually longitudinal but can be transverse or oblique

linea nigra brown or black pigmented line in the middle of the abdominal wall during pregnancy

lochia the discharge from the uterus during the puerperium, initially red, then yellow, then white

lower uterine segment the thin expanded lower portion of the uterus, which forms in the last trimester of pregnancy

moulding alteration in shape and diameter of the fetal head during labour (the fontanelles and sutures permit the force of contractions to compress the head against the bony pelvis and adapt its shape to that of the birth canal)

Naegele's rule to estimate the probable date of confinement add 9 months and 7 days to the first day of the menstrual cycle (correction required if cycle not 28 days)

neonatal death a liveborn infant who dies within 28 days of birth

obstructed labour there is no descent of the presenting part in the presence of good contractions

operculum the plug of mucus that occludes the cervical canal during pregnancy

Pawlik's grip suprapubic palpation with the outstretched hand to identify the presenting part of the fetus, its position, flexion and engagement

pelvic brim or inlet the plane of division between the true and false pelvis. The plane passes from the upper border of the symphysis pubis, along the pubic crest to the iliopectineal eminence, then to the sacroiliac joint, along the wings of the sacrum to the centre of the sacral promontory

pelvic outlet runs from beneath the symphysis pubis along the ischiopubic ramus to the ischial tuberosity along the sacrotuberous ligament to the fifth sacral vertebra

pelvimetry measurement of the size of the pelvis

perinatal mortality stillbirths plus first-week deaths expressed per 1000 total births

placenta accrete absence of decidua basalis, so that the chorionic villi are attached to uterine muscle

placenta circumvallata placenta with a double fold of amnion forming a ring on the fetal surface some distance in from the edge of the placenta

placenta increta chorionic villi are in the uterine muscle

placenta percreta the villi are through the uterine muscle

placenta succenturiata there is one or more accessory lobe of the placenta

position of the fetus the relationship of a defined area on the presenting part (called the denominator) to the quadrants of the maternal pelvis

presenting part that part of the fetus felt on vaginal examination

prolonged pregnancy a pregnancy that lasts longer than term (37–42 completed weeks)

puerperium the period during which the reproductive organs return to their prepregnant condition (usually regarded as an interval of 6 weeks after delivery)

show a discharge of mucus and blood at the onset of labour when the cervix dilates and the operculum (cervical mucus plug) falls out

sinciput that part of the fetal head in front of the anterior fontanelle

Spalding's sign overlapping of the fetal skull bones, seen radiographically after fetal death

station the level of the presenting part within the mother's pelvis (the ischial spines are the reference points on vaginal examination)

symphysiotomy division of the pubic symphysis to enlarge the diameters of the bony pelvis

third-degree tear a perineal laceration passing through the anal sphincter

vasa praevia fetal vessels lying in the membranes in front of the presenting part (there must be an associated velamentous insertion of the cord, succenturiate lobe or bipartite placenta)

velamentous insertion the umbilical cord inserts on to the membranes over which the vessels course to reach the fetal surface of the placenta

vernix caseosa produced by sebaceous glands and prevents waterlogging and maceration of the fetal skin by the amniotic fluid

vertex the area between the anterior and posterior fontanelles and the parietal eminences

Wharton's jelly the mucoid connective tissue supporting the umbilical cord vessels

Index

NB: Page numbers in *italics* refer to figures and tables